Principles of Radiological Physics

£24.95

IC

D1471921

To Diane

Principles of Radiological Physics

Robin J. Wilks BSc PhD

Principal Physicist
Royal Devon and Exeter Hospital
Wonford, Exeter

FOREWORD BY

June P. Smalley FCR TE
Principal,
The Plymouth School of Radiography
Plymouth

SECOND EDITION

CHURCHILL LIVINGSTONE
EDINBURGH LONDON MELBOURNE AND NEW YORK 1987

CHURCHILL LIVINGSTONE
Medical Division of Longman Group UK Limited

Distributed in the United States of America by
Churchill Livingstone Inc., 1560 Broadway, New
York, N.Y. 10036, and by associated companies,
branches and representatives throughout the world.

First edition 1981
Second edition 1987

ISBN 0-443-03780-9

British Library Cataloguing in Publication Data
Wilks, Robin J.
    Principles of radiological physics.—2nd ed.
    1. Radiography   2. Medical physics
    I. Title
    530'.024616   RC78

Library of Congress Cataloging in Publication Data
Wilks, Robin J.
    Principles of radiological physics.
    Includes index.
    1. Radiology, Medical.   2. Medical physics.
I. Title. [DNLM: 1. Physics—programmed instruction.
2. Technology, Radiologic—programmed instruction.
WN 18 W688p]
R895.W54   1987   539.2'024616   86-17526

Produced by Longman Singapore Publishers Pte Ltd
Printed in Singapore.

Foreword

This is the physics book that I have always hoped someone would write. Dr Wilks is a physicist of distinction. He knows radiography students well, having taught them with notable success since 1972. Like many other physicists and radiography teachers, he is only too aware of the problems which arise year after year when teaching physics to student radiographers. In the light of his experience, he has written a brilliantly simple book which introduces the answers almost before the problems can arise. The style is so lucid that there is rarely the need to read and re-read a passage before comprehension takes place. The chapters on mathematics are simple and directly applied, providing both enlightenment and motivation to further learning. I feel this section in particular will be of immense assistance to bridge the gap between 'school mathematics' and radiography physics.

Although particularly relevant to the Diploma (DCR) physics syllabus, this book deals also with the physics of radiography equipment and photography. Because of this, I feel it will have an appeal not only to staff and students in schools of radiography but also to candidates for the Higher (HDCR) examination, and to trainee radiologists. It is my hope that many physicists will read this book, as it sets the radiographer's interpretative level so absolutely right. Above all it is written by one versed in the art of teaching.

1981   J.P.S.

Preface to the Second Edition

There have been significant changes to both the physics syllabus and the examination for the DCR since the first edition of this book was published. Additional material has therefore been included in this edition, in so far as space has permitted, in order to accommodate these changes. The opportunity has also been taken to correct stubborn misprints and other errors, and to rewrite some sections to provide extra clarity.

In particular new sections have been written on the *errors of measurement* and *statistics* (Ch. 6), simple calculations using the *RC time-constant* (Ch. 9), *mains cable resistance* (Ch. 10), primary and secondary *switching* (Ch. 20), *fuses* and *circuit-breakers* (Ch. 21) and, of course, extensive modifications to Chapter 33 on radiation protection following the *Ionising Radiations Regulations 1985*.

I hope that all pupils and teachers who use this book find that these additions and modifications are useful and helpful.

1987   R.J.W.

Note

Whilst every effort has been made to be accurate, the author disclaims any responsibility for any inaccuracies which remain, or for any newer information which supersedes any part of this book, particularly in relation to the impact of legislation on radiation protection procedures and safety levels.

Preface to the First Edition

The writing of this text-book has grown out of a frustration on the part of the author as a result of using currently available physics text-books in the teaching of radiography students. Although many of these books are, in their own way, excellent, none of them seems to be written at the correct level for the average student who usually finds physics something of a struggle to learn and understand. This is a text-book on physics which is intended primarily for the *student*, although it is hoped that others such as teachers, radiologists and even physicists may also find it of use.

My intention has been to assume very little in the way of previous knowledge by the student and I have attempted to work from the 'known' to the 'unknown' in small steps using examples where appropriate. This is particularly so in Parts A and B on *Mathematics and General Physics*, which seem to give more trouble to the students than *Atomic and Radiation Physics*.

There is a Summary at the end of each chapter where the main points are repeated in a condensed fashion. It is hoped that this, together with the exercises included in each chapter, will facilitate revision for those taking examinations, as well as being a useful *précis* of the essential points of each chapter.

For the brighter student, or one who may be mathematically more able, I have included comments under the heading 'Insight' in most of the chapters. It is *not* essential to read these in order to gain an understanding of the topic under consideration, as they are used to introduce other facets of the topic without spoiling the 'thread' of the argument. It is anticipated that particular Insights may help some students and not others, and this is the spirit in which they have been written.

In the sections from *Atomic Physics* to the end of the book, I have used more 'modern' physics than has been customary hitherto. Chapter 23 introduces some concepts of modern physics, and compares this with the classical physics of Chapter 7. 'Mass–Energy Equivalence' and 'Wave–Particle Duality' are outlined, together with a brief description of Heisenberg's *Uncertainty Principle*. Modern physics is also used in the explanation of the production of X-rays (Ch. 28). This is all at an elementary level, and is intended to illuminate rather than to confuse!

The International System of units (SI) has been used throughout (defined in Appendix VII and explained in Ch. 6), although the units of particular relevance to radiography have of course been retained (kV_p, keV, mAs. HU). For example, radiation dosimetry uses the units of gray, sievert, etc., with the value of the earlier units of rad and rem following in brackets. Appendix VI is used to define the units of the Roentgen, rad and rem.

I have not attempted to cover recent developments in the field of equipment for radiography, since space is short and adequate text-books exist already in this specialised subject. However, the general physical *principles* of the design of the X-ray tube (for example) is covered in a general manner (e.g. the factors which lead to adequate heat loss from the anode), rather than a detailed discussion of different types of equipment.

Finally, a general word to all students concerning physics and radiography. Almost every year I am asked by my students: 'What is the point of all this physics? It is obvious that we shall not use much of it when we qualify, so we shall forget it very quickly anyway!' I must confess that I have some sympathy with this point of view, as some of the physics syllabus may seem of somewhat academic interest at first sight, and it *is* possible to operate an X-ray unit with very little knowledge of physics — it happens all over the country every day! However, I usually reply by putting the question the other way round, i.e. 'Suppose that you *were* trained only to operate the X-ray units correctly, and understood very little of their internal workings, or how a radiograph is formed, wouldn't you then complain justifiably of having a very boring occupation indeed?' I hope that this book will show that the role of physics in radiography is to enable you to *understand* what you are doing both to the machine and to the patient each time you take a radiograph. This makes it safer for the patient, more interesting for you, and enables you to quickly recognise any equipment faults and to take any appropriate action. In addition, during your career you will encounter a wide range of professional people with whom you will need to collaborate. This is possible only if you have a 'professional' knowledge of your own subject. *Understanding* is the key to success in physics, as in any other subject, and it is the underlying principles of physics which I have attempted to stress in this book as an aid to understanding.

Maintain your curiosity about the world around you, happy studying and good luck!

1981   R.W.

Contents

Part A
RADIOGRAPHY AND MATHEMATICS

1. Mathematics for radiography

This introductory chapter on the revision of mathematics is directed primarily towards those whose mathematics is a little weak. However, many of the worked examples shown are chosen from topics in radiography and are therefore of interest to all students.

For those studying for examination purposes, the following remarks concerning the requirements of the examiners are included. The examiners frequently complain of cramped, untidy mathematics which is difficult to follow. What they are hoping to see in the answer is a clear statement of the problem and an easy-to-follow development of the mathematics used to obtain a solution. This is more important than actually obtaining the correct numerical answer! In fact, the correct answer recorded on its own with little or no supporting mathematical argument will not achieve good marks. In practice, then, you need to use phrases and sentences to tell the examiner what you are about to do. This works to your advantage and is a good habit to cultivate, as it helps you to think more clearly about what you are doing, and is a positive boon when checking your own working! A study of the worked examples will clarify these points.

1.1 ALGEBRAIC SYMBOLS

The letters of the English and Greek alphabet (see Table F at the end of this book) are often used to represent the magnitude of an unknown quantity. For example, an electrical potential difference may be represented by V volts, an angle by θ (i.e. 'theta') degrees or radians and an energy by E joules. Such a practice enables the symbols to be used in place of the actual numerical values of the quantities, and is of great practical use in the solving of equations (1.4).

1.1.1 Suffixes

Suffixes are used to denote a specific value of a particular quantity. If we use the symbol I to denote the intensity of radiation from a particular source, then I will depend upon the distance from the source at which the intensity is measured (Ch. 4). We may call a particular distance x, say, and denote the intensity of this distance by I_x — meaning 'the intensity at x'. For another distance y, the corresponding value of intensity is I_y.

Similarly, if a quantity N changes with time, t, the value of N at any given time may be denoted by N_t.

Suffixes are used, then, to avoid ambiguity and are used as such in many chapters of this book.

1.2. FRACTIONS AND PERCENTAGES

1.2.1 Percentages

If a quantity increases in value by 50 per cent (%), then it is meant by this that it has become greater by one-half of its previous value. Thus, if the electric current passing through an X-ray tube was 200 mA (6.4.2) then an increase of 50% would bring this to 300 mA. Alternatively, it may be said that the new value is 150% of the original value.

In general terms, if a is the original value of a quantity and b is its new value, then:

(i)   the *percentage change* $= 100 \times \dfrac{b-a}{a}$

(ii) $\dfrac{100b}{a}$ is the 'percentage of b compared to a'

(iii) y% of a is just $\dfrac{y}{100} \times a$.

Examples
a.   Original value $= 60$; new value $= 80$
The percentage change is then $100 \times \frac{20}{60} = 33\frac{1}{3}$% and the new value is $100 \times \frac{80}{60} = 133\frac{1}{3}$% of the original.
b.   A quantity has reduced by 25%. What is the new value if it was 600 originally?
25% of 600 is just $\frac{25}{100} \times 600 = 150$, so that the new value is $600 - 150 = 450$.

A percentage is a special case of a fraction, where one number is divided by another. The following sections describe how fractions may be added together and multiplied.

1.2.2 Addition of fractions

Suppose we have the fraction a/b, where a and b represent general numbers. Now the addition or subtraction of a/b to another fraction c/d rests on the fact that we can take any fraction and multiply top and bottom by the same factor (k, say) *without* altering its value.

ie. $\dfrac{a}{b} = \dfrac{ka}{kb}$ (because the ks cancel)

It is the appropriate selection of k for each fraction which makes for the easy addition of fractions. For example, suppose we have:

$$\frac{2}{3} + \frac{5}{6}$$

If we multiply $\frac{2}{3}$ by 2 (top and bottom), we shall have a fraction expressed in sixths, just like the second fraction.

i.e. $\frac{2}{3} + \frac{5}{6} = \frac{2 \cdot 2}{2 \cdot 3} + \frac{5}{6} = \frac{4}{6} + \frac{5}{6} = \frac{9}{6} = 1\frac{1}{2}$

Notice that we multiplied only the first fraction — we need not do the same thing to the second. This method is often very quick, particularly when only two or three simple fractions are involved, and is in fact entirely equivalent to the more general method of using the Lowest Common Denominator (LCD), as illustrated in the following example:

$$\frac{2}{3} + \frac{3}{4} - \frac{5}{6} = \frac{4 \cdot 2 + 3 \cdot 3 - 2 \cdot 5}{12} = \frac{8 + 9 - 10}{12}$$
$$= \frac{7}{12}$$

(*Note:* The symbol '.' is often used — as in this example — to denote multiplication).

Here, the LCD of the denominators 3, 4 and 6 is 12 and is therefore used as the overall denominator on the right-hand side. The individual denominators are then divided into 12, the result being multiplied by the respective numerator and summed (observing the correct signs,) as shown in the example.

Exercise 1.1 (answers at the end of the book)

a. $\frac{11}{12} - \frac{5}{6}$

b. $\frac{7}{9} + \frac{2}{3}$

c. what is 20% of 50?

d. $\frac{2}{3} - \frac{1}{4} + \frac{3}{5}$

e. $\frac{7}{11} + \frac{2}{9} - \frac{2}{3}$

f. what is the percentage change if a quantity increases from 80 to 90?

1.3 MULTIPLYING AND DIVIDING

1.3.1 Positive and negative numbers

It is obvious that $1 \times 8 = 8$, but what are -1×8, -1×-8 and 8×-1?

To avoid having to work out such problems from first principles every time, a simple rule has been developed which we may call Rule 1:

RULE 1

  When multiply or dividing two numbers together
    Two (+)s make a (+).
    Two (−)s make a (+).
    A (+) and a (−) make a (−).

i.e. only when the signs are dissimilar is the result negative.

Examples

  a. $-3 \times 4 = -12$ b. $14 \div -7 = -2$ c. $\dfrac{-40}{-4} = 10$

  d. $-2 \times -4 \times -3 = 8 \times -3 = -24$

Exercise 1.2

  a. $28 \div 7$ b. $\dfrac{-36}{6}$ c. $\dfrac{144}{-4}$ d. -13×-3

  e. $-7 \times \dfrac{-8}{-2}$

1.3.2 Fractions

The *multiplication* of two or more fractions is just a matter of simplification by cancellation (where possible) and then multiplying all the nominators together to form the new nominator, and all the denominators together to form the new denominator.

Examples

  a. $\frac{2}{3} \times \frac{7}{5} = \frac{14}{15}$ (no cancellation possible)

  b. $\dfrac{2}{3} \times \dfrac{9}{4} = \dfrac{\overset{1}{\cancel{2}}}{\cancel{3}} \times \dfrac{\overset{3}{\cancel{9}}}{\underset{2}{\cancel{4}}} = \dfrac{3}{2}$

  The *division* of two fractions is straightforward provided that the following rule is obeyed:

RULE 2

  When dividing by one or more fractions, turn those in the denominator upside–down and multiply.

Let us say, by way of illustration, that we wish to divide 4 by $\frac{1}{2}$

  i.e. $\dfrac{4}{\frac{1}{2}}$

Applying Rule 2, we turn $\frac{1}{2}$ upside-down and multiply:

$$\frac{4}{\frac{1}{2}} = 4 \times \frac{2}{1} = 8$$

Is this the answer we would expect intuitively? Well, the problem may be expressed as 'how many halves are there in 4?', and then it is obvious that the answer is 8. Some more examples to clarify the method:

a. $\quad 7 \div \frac{14}{9} = 7 \times \frac{9}{14} = \frac{9}{2}$

b. $\quad \dfrac{\frac{3}{8}}{\frac{7}{11}} = \frac{3}{8} \times \frac{11}{7} = \frac{33}{56}$

c. $\quad \dfrac{\frac{4}{9}}{\frac{-8}{27}} = \frac{4}{9} \times \frac{-27}{8} = -\frac{3}{2}$

d. $\quad \dfrac{\frac{2}{3}}{\frac{4}{7} \times \frac{3}{5}} = \frac{2}{3} \times \frac{7}{4} \times \frac{5}{3} = \frac{35}{18}$

Exercise 1.3

a. $\quad \dfrac{\frac{-4}{11}}{\frac{7}{22}}$

b. $\quad \dfrac{\frac{2}{9}}{\frac{7}{3} \times \frac{-2}{11}}$

c. $\quad \dfrac{\frac{1}{3} \times \frac{2}{9}}{\frac{9}{1} \times \frac{1}{2}}$

1.3.3 Brackets

A bracket links two or more quantities together such that the bracket and its contents may be treated mathematically as a single quantity. If we wish to *remove* the brackets, then care over the plus and minus signs must be taken (Rule 1).

Examples

a. $2 \times (a - b) = 2 \times a - 2 \times b = 2a - 2b$

Thus, each term in the bracket is multiplied by the term outside the bracket, with due regard for the sign convention.

b. $-4(c - 2d) = -4c + 8d$

Note that the multiplication sign, present in example a, has been omitted, as is usually the case.

c. $-3\left(\dfrac{-2a}{3} + b - \dfrac{1c}{7}\right) = 2a - 3b + \dfrac{3c}{7}$

Multiplying two or more brackets together can become quite involved. However, it is rare for problems in radiography to require even the multiplication of two brackets, but the method is outlined below for the sake of completeness.

Assume we wish to calculate:

$(a + b)(c + d)$
i.e. $(a + b)$ multiplied by $(c + d)$

To perform this calculation, we take the first term of the first bracket, a, and multiply it by $(c + d)$. Then we add the result to the multiplication of the second term, b, by $(c + d)$:

i.e. $(a + b)(c + d) = a(c + d) + b(c + d)$
$= ac + ad + bc + bd$

Again, we must be careful of the sign convention (Rule 1), as the following two worked examples show:

Examples

a. $(7 + c)(d - 8) = 7(d - 8) + c(d - 8)$
$= 7d - 56 + cd - 8c$

b. $(4 - a)(3 - b + 2c) = 4(3 - b + 2c) - a(3 - b + 2c)$
$= 12 - 4b + 8c - 3a + ab - 2ac$

Exercise 1.4

a. $7a - 4(a - 2)$ b. $-6(-x + y - 3)$
c. $2(3a - 4) - 3(-a + 6)$

1.4 SOLVING EQUATIONS

The types of equations encountered in problems associated with radiography are those in which a single 'unknown' (whose numerical value we wish to calculate) is 'mixed-up' with several other numbers which may occur on both sides of the equation. (The solution of several equations involving several unknowns, i.e. simultaneous equations, is not normally required, and so will not be discussed here.) Our task, then, in the equations encountered, is to 'unscramble' the unknown so as to leave it on one side of the equation and all the numbers on the other side — the equation is then said to be 'solved'. This process is straightforward, provided that the following simple rule is obeyed:

Rule 3
   Always perform the same operation to *both* sides of an equation.

This rule is intuitively obvious if it is imagined that the equals sign of the equation is the pivot of a pair of scales which is in exact balance. Whatever weight we now add to or subtract from one scale-pan must be added to or subtracted from the other or the scales will no longer be in balance. Similarly, if we double (say) the weight on one side we must do the same to the other — thus, provided we multiply by the same factor, balance is preserved and one side is equal to the other side. For example, consider the simple equation:

$$x - 2 = 3$$

If we add 2 to the left-hand side (LHS) of this equation the -2 will be cancelled, leaving x only. However, in accordance with Rule 3 above, we must add 2 to the right-hand side (RHS) in order to preserve equality.

i.e. $x - 2 + 2 = 3 + 2$ thus $x = 5$

Putting $x = 5$ in the original equation, we have $5 - 2 = 3$, which is correct.
   As another example, consider: $15 - y = 7$. Subtracting 15 from both sides so as to eliminate it from the LHS,

$$15 - y - 15 = 7 - 15$$
i.e. $- y = -8$

Multiplying both sides by -1 in order to make both terms positive (Rule 1), we have:

$$-1 . - y = -1 . -8 \quad i.e. \quad y = 8$$

Substituting our solution into the original equation to serve as a check, as in the previous example, we have:

$15 - 8 = 7$, thus verifying our answer.

It is apparent from these examples that a convenient way of picturing this type of mathematical operation is that of 'transferring a quantity from one side to the other and *changing its sign*'. Obviously, this only applies to the elimination of variables by addition or subtraction, *not* multiplication, which will be discussed in the next example.

Example

$$2 = 7 - \frac{5x}{2}$$

proceeding as before, $\dfrac{5x}{2} = 7 - 2 = 5$

i.e. $\dfrac{5x}{2} = 5$

We cannot now add or subtract anything to leave x on its own — we have to multiply by 2/5:

i.e. $\dfrac{2}{5} \cdot \dfrac{5x}{2} = \dfrac{2}{5} \cdot 5$

i.e. $x = 2$

This last step is known as *cross-multiplication* and may be pictured in the following manner:

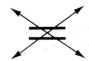

(Cross-multiplication)

The double-ended arrows indicate that movement may be in either direction. Note that there is no change of sign.

One *incorrect* use of cross-multiplication occurs so frequently that it is worth a special mention here. Suppose we have the equation:

$$\dfrac{7x}{2} = \dfrac{3}{8} + \dfrac{x}{3}$$

if we cross-multiply in the following manner:

$\dfrac{7x}{2} \diagdown \dfrac{3}{8} + \dfrac{x}{3}$ (Incorrect)

we obtain

$$x = \dfrac{2 \cdot 3}{7 \cdot 8} + \dfrac{x}{3} \quad \text{(Incorrect)}$$

The fault lies, of course, in the fact that Rule 3 has been disobeyed, i.e. the term $x/3$ remains unaltered although we were intending, by our cross-multiplication, to multiply both sides by $\frac{2}{7}$. Hence, if we wished to cross-multiply at this stage, we should have obtained:

$$x = \dfrac{2 \cdot 3}{7 \cdot 8} + \dfrac{2 \cdot x}{7 \cdot 3} \quad \text{(Correct)}$$

which may be further simplified to solve for x.

Exercise 1.5

a. $\frac{2}{3}x = 4$

b. $\frac{7}{9}y - 1 = 13$

c. $q + \frac{3}{10} = \frac{5}{12}q$

d. $3\frac{3}{5}I - 12\frac{4}{5} = 1\frac{2}{5}I - \frac{7}{10}$

1.5 POWERS (INDICES)

An *index* is written at the top right of a quantity (the *base*) and refers to the number of times the quantity is multiplied by *itself*. For example, 5^3 means $5 \times 5 \times 5$ (i.e. 125). It is a convenient mathematical 'shorthand' to write powers of a number in this way. In this example, the index is a positive integer (i.e. 3), but this need not be the case for it may be positive, negative, fractional or decimal, as described below.

1.5.1 Combining indices

Let us assume that we have two numbers, 2^3 and 2^2, which we wish to combine by addition, multiplication and division in order to elicit general rules for the handling of indices.

Addition
Using the definition of an index as described above.

$$2^3 + 2^2 = 2 \cdot 2 \cdot 2 + 2 \cdot 2 = 8 + 4 = 12$$

Thus, when adding such numbers, each term is calculated separately prior to addition (or subtraction).

Multiplication
Again, from first principles, we have:

$$2^3 \cdot 2^2 = \underbrace{2 \cdot 2 \cdot 2}_{= 2^3} \cdot \underbrace{2 \cdot 2}_{= 2^2} = 2^5 = 2^{(3+2)}$$

Hence, when multiplying two or more such numbers together, the rule is to *add* the indices.

Division

$$\frac{2^3}{2^2} = \frac{2 \cdot 2 \cdot 2}{2 \cdot 2} = 2 = 2^{(3-2)}$$

Thus, when dividing such numbers, the rule is to *subtract* the indices.

1.5.2 Negative indices

Suppose that we wish to divide 4^2 by 4^4. From first principles (1.5), we have

$$\frac{4^2}{4^4} = \frac{4 \cdot 4}{4 \cdot 4 \cdot 4 \cdot 4} = \frac{1}{4^2} \qquad \text{Equation 1.1}$$

Also, by the rule on division as described above, we may subtract indices:

$$\frac{4^2}{4^4} = 4^{2-4} = 4^{-2}$$

Equation 1.2

Since equations (1.1) and (1.2) are equal,

$$4^{-2} = \frac{1}{4^2}$$

In general, therefore,

$$x^{-n} = \frac{1}{x^n}$$

Equation 1.3

i.e. to change a negative index to a positive index, just take the reciprocal, as shown in Equation 1.3.

Examples

a. $10^{-2} = \frac{1}{10^2} = \frac{1}{100}$

b. $\dfrac{1}{\dfrac{1}{10^{-6}}} = \dfrac{1}{\dfrac{1}{10^6}} = 1 \times \dfrac{10^6}{1} = 10^6$

c. $\dfrac{420 \times 10^2}{2 \times 10^4} = 210 \times 10^{-2} = \dfrac{210}{10^2} = \dfrac{210}{100} = 2 \cdot 1$

1.5.3 Fractional indices

What is meant by, say, $x^{1/2}$?

Now, $x^{1/2} \cdot x^{1/2} = x^{1/2 + 1/2} = x^1 = x$

Also, $\sqrt{x} \cdot \sqrt{x} = x$ from the definition of a square root.

Thus, from inspection of these two equations,

$$x^{1/2} = \sqrt{x}$$

i.e. $x^{1/2}$ is just the square root of x.

Similarly, $y^{1/3}$ is the cube root of y, $q^{5/8}$ is the eighth root of q raised to the fifth power, etc.

Examples

a. $9^{1/2} = \sqrt{9} = \pm 3$

b. $9^{3/2} = (9^{1/2})^3 = (\pm 3)^3 = \pm 27$

c. $64^{1/3} = \sqrt[3]{64} = 4$

1.5.4 The zero index – x^0

A general number x raised to a power m is x^m. If we divide x^m by itself, the answer will obviously be one. But $x^m \div x^m$ is x^{m-m} by the rules discussed above. Thus $1 = x^{m-m} = x^0$. Since we took any general number, this result is also general (except for 0^0, which is indeterminate).

Thus any number raised to the power zero is *unity*.

1.5.5 Indices to different bases

A problem on the Inverse Square Law (see Ch. 4) frequently involves a calculation of the form:

$$\frac{a \cdot b^2}{c^2}.$$

Here a, b and c represent numbers whose values are known, having been specified by the problem. We wish to determine the best way of obtaining the final result, since b and c are frequently large numbers, whose squares are therefore even larger. This means that the probability of making an arithmetical error can be quite high if a laborious method of simplification is undertaken. However, a great simplification is possible if we remember that:

$$\frac{b^2}{c^2} = \left(\frac{b}{c}\right)^2 \qquad\qquad\qquad \text{Equation 1.4}$$

Example

If $b = 90$ cm and $c = 60$ cm, then $\dfrac{b^2}{c^2}$ the 'hard' way is:

$$\frac{b^2}{c^2} = \frac{90^2}{60^2} = \frac{8100}{3600} = \frac{81}{36}$$

which may be cancelled to give 2.25 — this exercise being left to the reader. The 'easy' way is to use Equation 1.4:

i.e. $\dfrac{b^2}{c^2} = \left(\dfrac{b}{c}\right)^2 = \left(\dfrac{90}{60}\right)^2 = \left(\dfrac{3}{2}\right)^2 = 1\cdot5^2 = 2\cdot25$

Note that the answers are the same, as we would expect, but that the second method involves cancelling of smaller numbers so that there is less likelihood of an arithmetical error.

1.6 POWERS OF 10

When 10 is used as a base for indices, all the findings of the previous section apply. In addition, however, powers of 10 are very useful when measuring very large or very small quantities of a given unit, as shown in Table 1.1.

Table 1.1 Names for powers of 10

Prefix	Symbol	Power of 10	Example
mega	M	10^6	$1\ MW = 10^6\ watt$
kilo	k	10^3	$1\ kV = 10^3\ volt$
milli	m	10^{-3}	$1\ mA = 10^{-3}\ ampere$
micro	μ	10^{-6}	$1\ \mu F = 10^{-6}\ farad$
nano	n	10^{-9}	$1\ nm = 10^{-9}\ metre$
pico	p	10^{-12}	$1\ pF = 10^{-12}\ farad$

Other names not shown in the table exist (see Table A at end of book), but these are all that we shall need. It is advisable for the student to memorise these terms as they are in very common usage in radiography. The following exercise is included for this purpose:

Exercise 1.6

   a.   An X-ray tube has a current of 0·05 amperes passing through it. How many milliamperes (mA) does this correspond to?

   b.   If the X-ray tube has a peak potential difference of 125 000 volts across it, what is the value in kilovolts (kV_p)?

   c.   Express a capacitance of 0.000065 farads in microfarads (μF).

   d.   A photon of light has a wavelength of 550 nanometres (nm). What is this in metres?

1.7 PROPORTIONALITY

1.7.1 Direct proportion

If a car is travelling at constant speed such that the petrol consumption is a steady 40 mpg, then:

   0·5 gallons have been used after 20 miles
   1·0 gallons have been used after 40 miles
   1·5 gallons have been used after 60 miles, etc.

Thus, the amount of petrol consumed is in *direct proportion* to the number of miles travelled, and we may write:

   gallons $\propto$ mileage

where the sign '$\propto$' means 'is proportional to'. Alternatively, we may write:

   gallons $= \frac{1}{40} \times$ mileage

In general, therefore, if two quantities y and x are directly proportional to each other, then:

$$y \propto x \quad \text{or} \quad y = kx$$

where k is called the 'constant of proportionality'. Some examples of direct proportionality which are discussed in later chapters include:

    a.   The electric current (I) — through a metallic conductor is proportional to the potential difference (V) across it (i.e. $I \propto V$, Ohm's Law — Ch. 10).

    b.   Intensity of an X-ray beam $\propto$ tube current (mA).

    c.   Intensity of an X-ray beam $\propto$ kilovoltage squared (i.e. Intensity $\propto$ kV^2 — Ch. 28).

1.7.2 Inverse proportion

Suppose that we have many rectangles of equal area, k, but of differing heights (h) and widths (w). However, in each case the area is the same, so that:

$$h \times w = \text{constant } (k)$$
$$\text{or, } h = \frac{k}{w}$$

Then, since k is constant, we may write:

$$h \propto \frac{1}{w}$$

In this case, therefore, h and w are in *inverse* proportion, since w is halved if h is doubled, and vice versa. This is opposite to *direct* proportion, of course, where doubling (say) one quantity also doubles the other.

    Examples of inverse proportion discussed in subsequent chapters include:

    a.   The capacity (C) of a parallel-plate capacitor is inversely proportional to the separation (d) between its plates, i.e. $C \propto 1/d$ (Ch. 9).

    b.   The intensity (I) from a point source of electromagnetic radiation is inversely proportional to the square of the distance (x) from the course, i.e. $I \propto 1/x^2$ (Ch. 4).

    c.   The electrical resistant (R) of a given length of wire varies inversely as the area of cross-section (A), i.e. $R \propto 1/A$ (Ch. 10).

1.8 GRAPHS

1.8.1 Drawing and interpretation

A good understanding of the construction and interpretation of graphs is invaluable for radiography, the lack of which is a frequent complaint made by the examiners. Therefore, the following simple, but effective, rules are offered for guidance in the drawing of good graphs:

a.   Each graph should take at least a third of a page — give yourself plenty of room!

b.   Each graph should have a clear, appropriate title.

c.   The axes should be of approximately equal length and must be drawn with a ruler — freehand is not good enough!

d.   Both axes must be labelled clearly, and with the units (eg. cm, secs, etc.) where appropriate.

e.   The *independent* variable is normally drawn on the X axis, and the *dependent* variable on the Y axis. To express this in different words, the variable which is being measured is plotted on the Y axis, while the variable which *causes* the changes in Y is plotted on the X axis. An example of an independent variable is time, while the corresponding dependent variable might be the radioactivity of a sample.

The following examples have been chosen to illustrate both the drawing and interpretation of graphs.

Example 1 — Direct proportion

As described in the last section, two quantities, x and y, are directly proportional to each other if $y = kx$, where k is a constant. Figure 1.1 shows $y = kx$ in graphical form.

The following points should be noted:

a.   The graph passes through the origin, since $y = 0$ if $x = 0$.

b.   The slope of the straight line obtained is a measure of how 'steep' it is, and is defined as the 'change in y divided by the corresponding change in x'. Since the graph passes through the origin, changes in both x and y may be measured from there, so that the slope $= y/x = k$. Thus the slope increases as k increases.

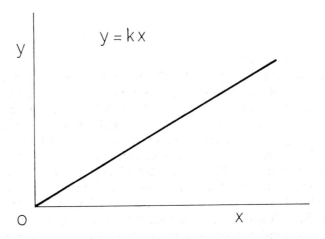

Fig 1.1 Graph of $y = kx$, illustrating direct proportion.

c. The general equation of a straight line would be of the form $y = mx + c$, where m is the slope, and c is the intersection of the line with the y axis (i.e. the value of y when $x = 0$).

Example 2 — Inverse proportion

Figure 1.2 shows a graph of the inverse relationship between the electrical capacity, C, of a parallel-plate condenser and the distance of separation of its plates, d, where $C = \dfrac{1 \cdot 0}{d}$ for a particular condenser.

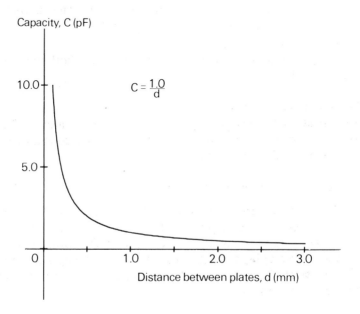

Fig. 1.2 Graph of $C = 1 \cdot 0/d$, illustrating inverse proportion.

Example 3 — Rating Charts

Rating charts are supplied by the manufacturers of X-ray tubes, and contain a lot of information in graphical form which is an essential guide to the radiographer for the selection of 'safe' exposure factors, i.e. the combination of focal-spot size, kV_p, mA, and exposure time which will not cause damage to the X-ray tube. An example of a rating chart is given by Figure 1.3, where a family of curves represent the maximum permissible exposure factors for different settings of kV_p. The use of rating charts is discussed in detail in Chapter 22, and we only need to make the point here that points below a particular curve for one kV_p setting are 'safe', while points above it lead to tube damage by overheating the anode.

Note the non-linear (logarithmic) scale on the X axis. Logarithmic scales are discussed further in section 5.4.

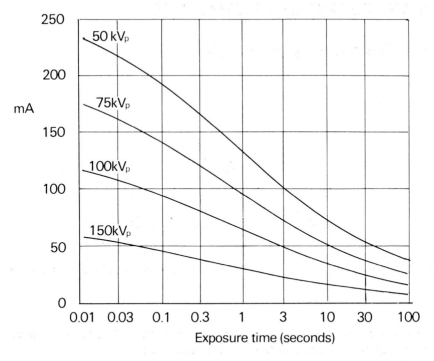

Fig. 1.3 Rating chart for an X-ray tube. Note the non-linear (logarithmic) scale on the X-axis.

1.8.2 Interpolation and extrapolation

It is often the case that a graph is drawn using a relatively small number of points, and that these points are joined together with a curve or straight line passing through them. The smooth curve or line makes it possible to 'read off' values from the graph, even when such values lie between the original points used to construct the graph. This procedure is known as *interpolation* and is one of the advantages obtained from the graphical method.

If it is desired to determine the value of one of the plotted variables when it lies outside the range of the points used to plot the graph, the curve may be extended, or *extrapolated*, to reach this region. However, such an extrapolation can lead to large inaccuracies, since several different curves may seem equally suitable and there may be no way of knowing which one is correct!

Exercise 1.7
   a.   Draw a graph of $y = 0.2x$, choosing values of x from 1 to 10 in steps of 1. Hence read from the graph the value of y when x is (i) 1.5, (ii) 9.5, (iii) 12, (iv) 0.5. Verify your answers by substitution into the original equation.
   b.   Repeat the same procedure for the equation $y = 0.2x^2$. (Note the increased uncertainty in obtaining the extrapolated value of y when $x = 12$.)

1.9 THE GEOMETRY OF TRIANGLES

1.9.1 The right-angled triangle

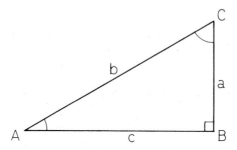

Fig. 1.4 A right-angled triangle. See text for definition of sine, cosine and tangent of an angle.

Consider the right-angled triangle shown in figure 1.4. The trigonometric functions of sine, cosine and tangent are defined as:

$$\sin A = \frac{\text{opposite}}{\text{hypotenuse}} = \frac{a}{b}$$

$$\cos A = \frac{\text{adjacent}}{\text{hypotenuse}} = \frac{c}{b}$$

$$\tan A = \frac{\text{opposite}}{\text{adjacent}} = \frac{a}{c}$$

Note that:

$$\frac{\sin A}{\cos A} = \frac{\dfrac{a}{b}}{\dfrac{c}{b}} = \frac{a}{b} \cdot \frac{b}{c} \qquad \text{(by Rule 2)}$$

i.e $\dfrac{\sin A}{\cos A} = \dfrac{a}{c} = \tan A$

Exercise 1.8
    a. Write down expressions for sin C, cos C, tan C from Figure 1.4.
    b. What is the value of $\sin^2 A + \cos^2 A$?

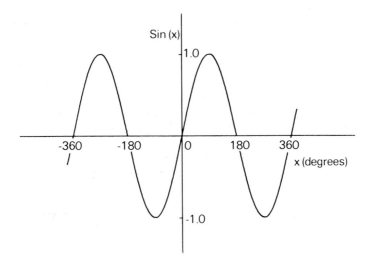

Fig. 1.5 A sine-wave. The curve repeats itself every 360°.

The sine function occurs frequently throughout this book, e.g. in the geometry of triangles and in alternating current theory (Ch. 15). Its graphical form is shown in Figure 1.5.

This graph is known as a 'sine-wave', and always lies between plus one and minus one. Also, the shape of the curve is *cyclical*, repeating itself every 360°.

1.9.2 Similarity of triangles

The two triangles shown in Figure 1.6 are said to be 'similar' because one is just a bigger version of the other, while retaining the same *shape*. Thus, the corresponding angles of the two triangles are equal, but the lengths of the

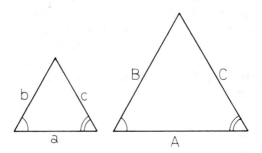

Fig. 1.6 Two similar triangles.

corresponding sides need not necessarily be so. However, if one side has a length which is double (say) that of the corresponding side of the other triangle, then *all* the sides will be doubled compared to the other triangle. Generally, then, we may write:

$$\frac{A}{a} = \frac{B}{b} = \frac{C}{c}$$

Equation 1.5

In many practical examples in radiography, however, the similar triangles look more like those shown in figure 1.7.

These two types of similar triangles are discussed further in section (3.2) to (3.4). In each case, the ratios of the corresponding sides are equal, in agreement with equation 1.5.

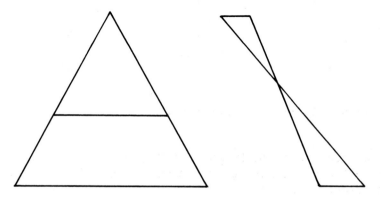

Fig. 1.7 Further example of similar triangles.

1.10 CALCULATIONS IN THE EXAMINATION

The examining body of the College of Radiographers does not now permit students to take their own scientific tables into their examinations, as all necessary tables and information are provided. However, slide-rules and pocket calculators belonging to students may be used in the examinations. Neverthless, the great majority of numerical calculations set in the examinations are chosen so that they are able to be solved by 'hand' fairly easily, so that a long tedious calculation is normally the result of a numerical slip or poor method and should therefore be viewed with suspicion. As mentioned in the introductory remarks of this chapter, the examiners are attempting to test understanding of principles rather than great numerical dexterity, although a little of the latter helps.

1.10.1 Pocket calculators

The recent advent of Large-Scale Integration (LSI) silicon 'chips' has enabled manufacturers to offer quite powerful pocket calculators at very reasonable prices, the cheaper varieties of which are well within almost everybody's budget. It is recommended that a pocket calculator be purchased rather than a slide-rule, as it is easier to use, quicker and more accurate.

For convenience, the calculator should be able to take *square roots* of numbers at the press of a key. This facility is in addition to the usual calculator functions of addition, subtraction, multiplication and division, of course. The ability to raise a number to a power (e.g., squaring) is useful if it may also be accomplished with one key-stroke, but it is not essential as it may be performed by successive multiplications of the number. The ability to perform trigonometric functions is also useful, but not essential for the examinations. However, many quite inexpensive calculators contain these and many other functions which may conceivably be of some use in daily life, so unless personal finances are very low it may be worthwhile paying a little more for a lot more calculating power; the choice is the individual's. The obvious course of action is to try a friend's calculator, or one in a shop, with some typical problems (e.g., on the Inverse Square Law — Exercise 4.1) to see if it is suitable.

One cautionary note — make sure that the battery is charged prior to the examination.

1.10.2 Slide-rules

Although quick and reasonably accurate in skilled hands, the slide-rule has been almost completely superseded by the pocket calculator. It is therefore assumed here that those students who possess a slide-rule and intend to use it already know how to, and that those who do not own one are about to purchase a calculator — hence no attempt is made in this book to explain either the theory or practice of its use.

1.10.3 Logarithms

For those who prefer to use logarithms, the following section is offered.

If $y = b^x$, then x is the 'logarithm of y to the base b', and is written $x = \log_b y$. In practice, b usually has a value of either 10 or 'e', which is a number which is particularly useful in mathematics, and is approximately equal to 2·7183. This is the same 'e' as used in the exponential law (e.g. $N_t = N_0 e^{-\lambda t}$ — Ch. 5), but we shall consider the base 10 only here. This is also used in the definition of the optical density of the radiograph (Ch. 31).

If we have two numbers, a and b, then $a = 10^x$ and $b = 10^y$, where x and y are the logarithms of a and b to the base 10, and may be found from suitable tables. Supposing that we wish to multiply a and b together, then $ab = 10^x . 10^y = 10^{x+y}$ (see 1.5.1) so that the logarithm of ab is just $x + y$, the addition of the two individual logarithms. The antilogarithm of $x + y$ may then be obtained from tables to find the final answer (i.e. the value of ab). Similarly, $\dfrac{a}{b} = 10^{x-y}$, so that the individual logarithms are subtracted when numbers are divided. An example of this is shown below. Since it is easier and quicker to add and subtract than to multiply and divide, the use of logarithm and antilogarithm tables simplifies the handling of long, or 'awkward' numbers.

These rules for adding logarithms when multiplying numbers and subtracting logarithms when dividing numbers seem always to be well understood by all students. However, many find logarithms difficult because of the effort of having to memorise the apparently arbitrary rules for determining what number to place before the decimal point of the logarithms, and the care that needs to be taken with $\bar{1}$, $\bar{2}$, etc. These difficulties mar what is otherwise a simple and convenient method for multiplying and dividing 'awkward' numbers, and it is better to ignore them totally! From example, suppose that we wish to divide 1243 by 34·21.

Now, $\log_{10} 1243 = 0944$; $\log_{10} 34·21 = 5341$ (from tables), completely ignoring all the rules regarding the decimal point, etc. Since we are dividing, we must subtract the logarithms:

i.e. $0944 - 5431 = 5603$, ignoring numbers further to the left.

From tables, antilog$_{10}$ 5603 = 3634, and our only remaining problem is to determine the position of the decimal point.

If we had obeyed all the rules of taking logs and antilogs, the position of the decimal point would have been specified, but we may determine this by performing the calculation with *approximate* numbers:

i.e.   1243 is approximately 1200
and 34.21 is approximately 34

so that the result is approximately $\dfrac{1200}{34} = \dfrac{600}{17}$

$$= \dfrac{600}{20} \text{ (approx.)}$$

$$= 30$$

Thus we know that the answer is about 30 (rather than 3 or 300) so the accurate answer is 36·24.

A little practice of this method will establish that sensible approximations always give a result which is sufficiently accurate to fix the decimal point quite quickly. In any case, it is important to check the results of any calculations are reasonable and that no arithmetical error is present. This simplified method therefore provides a 'built-in' check of the answers as well as removing what is for many a potential source of difficulty.

However, it must be stated that, as is the case for slide-rules, the pocket calculator has superseded the general use of logarithms.

SUMMARY

1.   When multiplying or dividing, two $+$s (or two $-$s) make a $+$; one $+$ and one $-$ make a $-$.

2. When dividing by a fraction, turn it upside-down and multiply.
3. $x^a . x^b = x^{a+b}$; $x^a/x^b = x^{a-b}$; $x^{-a} = 1/x^a$; $x^{1/2} = \sqrt{x}$; $x^0 = 1$

4. $\dfrac{b^m}{c^m} = \left(\dfrac{b}{c}\right)^m$ (useful for inverse square law calculations — when $m = 2$).

5. Direct proportion: $y \propto x$ or $y = kx$
   Inverse proportion: $y \propto 1/x$ or $y = c/x$
   where k and c are 'constants of proportionality'.

6. $\sin \theta = \dfrac{\text{opposite}}{\text{hypotenuse}}$; $\cos \theta = \dfrac{\text{adjacent}}{\text{hypotenuse}}$; $\tan \theta = \dfrac{\text{opposite}}{\text{adjacent}}$

7. Sine (and cosine) functions are cyclical, repeating themselves every 360°.
8. When drawing graphs, take at least a third of a page, draw the axes with a ruler, label both axes and use a title.
9. Similar triangles (i.e. having corresponding angles equal) have the ratios of their corresponding sides equal.
10. Use a pocket calculator.

2. Principles of radiography

The radiographic applications of the mathematics introduced in Chapter 1 are discussed more fully in Chapter 3. However, a brief outline of the basic principles of radiography will first be given in this chapter in order to put the mathematics into practical perspective.

Radiography is a *diagnostic* investigation, where a visual image (on film or fluorescent screen) is produced of the structures within a patient's body. Normally, of course, we cannot see inside each other's bodies because light rays, to which our eyes are sensitive, are absorbed and reflected very close to the surface of the bodily tissues. Hence, light does not penetrate sufficiently far inside the body to be useful for our purpose. However, other parts of the electromagnetic spectrum, of which light rays are but a small part (Ch. 24), *are* capable of significant penetration through bodily tissues, the most useful being X-rays, which are photons or quanta (Ch. 23) of higher energy than light. For example, photons of 'blue' light have energies of about 3 eV while X-rays for radiographic imaging are about 50 keV per photon (see 6.4.3 for the definition of 'eV').

Unfortunately, it is not possible to focus X-rays with lenses and mirrors, unlike light rays, so only 'shadow-like' images may be obtained, rather like an optical 'pin-hole' camera. In radiography, however, the image is produced by the *transmission* of a beam of X-rays, and there is only one source of 'illumination' — the X-ray tube. Referring to Figure 2.1, the source of X-rays, S, is a small area on the anode of the X-ray tube.

The X-rays are emitted in all directions from S, but are absorbed either by the anode or by thin lead foil wrapped inside the casing of the X-ray tube housing (Ch. 21), except for the radiation emitted in the direction of the patient. The X-rays travel at the speed of light (24.1) in straight lines, and it is this latter property which enables them to produce a 'shadow' of the patient onto the photographic film. First, however, they must pass through beam limiters, called diaphragms, which are adjusted so as to 'illuminate' just that part of the body under investigation. The X-rays pass through the patient, some being totally absorbed, some being deflected ('scattered') and some being unaffected. It is the latter category of X-rays which is used to form an image of the film, i.e. the *transmitted* X-rays. Now the lower the energy of the X-ray beam, the more are absorbed within the patient, so that fewer X-rays reach the film. There thus comes a point when X-rays of a sufficiently low energy give only a radiation dose to the patient and contribute nothing to the film blackening. Such low-energy X-rays are undesirable and are therefore 'filtered' out by a thin layer of aluminium placed between the glass envelope of the X-ray tube and the diaphragm assembly (Ch. 29). Of the 'useful' X-rays left, then, those that pass through bone are more absorbed than those that pass through soft tissue (muscle and fat). If B in figure 2.1 represents a bone, then the number of X-rays reaching C (along SABC) will therefore be fewer than those reaching E (along SDE). A photographic film placed just behind the patient will therefore produce an image (when developed and 'fixed') which is blacker at point E than C, so that the contrast between levels of blackness (corresponding to the transmission of the X-rays) constitutes the radiographic image. However, such an image will be poor in practice owing to the contribution of the scattered X-rays to the image (as shown by FG). These events cause a 'halo' of blackness on the photographic film around small objects, so that they blur and smear detail. The larger the X-ray beam the worse this effect becomes, which is why the smallest practicable size of beam is used, as mentioned above.

The function of the grid (explained in Ch. 31) is to absorb the majority of such scattered X-rays, thus restoring picture quality so that fine detail may be revealed. The 'screen' is a fluorescent material (Ch. 27) which greatly reduces the exposure times required to produce the radiograph, thus reducing the radiation dose which the patient receives during an exposure. However, this is at the cost of a small increase of overall unsharpness (3.4).

Finally, then, the transmitted X-rays form an 'X-ray image' of the patient's internal structure onto the photographic film. After photographic processing,

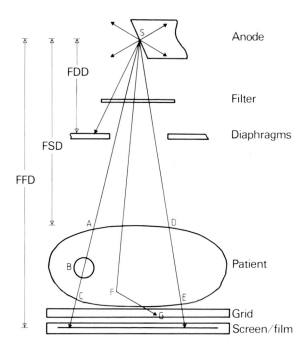

Fig. 2.1 The formation of a radiograph.

the resultant image may then be used for diagnosis by the Radiologist. Obviously, the better the quality of the photographic image, the easier is his task, and it is therefore the radiographer's prime function to be able to select all the necessary parameters (kV_p, mAs, FFD, focal spot size, screen/film combination) in order to obtain the necessary high-quality images.

The next Chapter shows some geometric aspects of image formation in more detail, while Chapters 30 and 31 discuss the physical processes which affect the quality of the radiograph obtained.

3. Geometrical radiography

Many of the concepts and calculations encountered in radiography are based on the geometry of triangles (1.9) — hence the title of this chapter. Some commonly used terms and abbreviations will first be defined:

    Field size — the size and shape of the cross-section of an X-ray beam at a specified distance from the *focus,* or source of radiation

    FFD — Focus-to-Film Distance
    FDD — Focus-to-Diaphragm Distance
    FSD — Focus-to-Skin Distance

The influence of these quantities on the geometrical formation of the X-ray image is described in the following sections.

3.1 EFFECTIVE (APPARENT) FOCAL SPOT SIZE

As described in Chapter 21, an electron beam within an X-ray tube flows from cathode to anode and produces X-rays when suddenly slowed down within the tungsten anode 'target'. The shape of the area bombarded by the electrons is actually a thin rectangle (referred to as a 'line' focus), but is made to appear much more like a small square when 'viewed' from the position of the X-ray film. This is accomplished by imposing an angle on the anode, as shown in Figure 3.1. If the anode is viewed from position A, then the 'true' or 'real' size

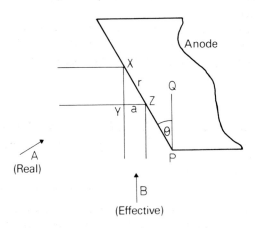

Fig. 3.1 Real and effective focal spot sizes.

of the focal spot is perceived, i.e. the length XZ or r. However, when viewed from B, the line focus appears to be only as long as YZ, owing to the effect of the anode angle θ. The distance YZ is known as the 'effective' or 'apparent' focal spot size. The apparent reduction in focal spot size may be understood by viewing a piece of paper (say) at 90° to its surface, and then rotating the paper until an 'edge' view is obtained. During the rotation of the paper, its apparent width becomes steadily smaller, although its actual width remains unchanged.

Considering the triangle XYZ in Figure 3.1 the angle YXZ is the same as ZPQ $(=\theta)$, since PQ and XY are parallel.

Also, $\sin \theta = \dfrac{a}{r}$ (see 1.9.1)

where a is the size of the effective focus.
Cross-multiplying, we have therefore:

$a = r \sin \theta$ Equation 3.1

This means that the effective (or apparent) focal spot size is obtained simply by multiplying the real size by the sine of the anode angle.

Example
Supposing that the real focal spot size is 2 mm, and the anode angle is 17° (a typical value), then the effective size is:

$2 \sin 17° = 2 \times 0.2924 = 0.5848 = 0.6$ mm (approx)

Thus the effective size is about one third of the real focal spot size, resulting in radiographic images of smaller 'unsharpness' as described in 3.4.

3.2 FIELD SIZE AND FFD

Figure 3.2 shows the divergence (in two dimensions) of an X-ray beam with the increasing distance from the source F.

It is obvious from the figure that the field size, S, is proportional to the distance from the source. If we wish to relate field size to diaphragm setting, d, then we may make use of the similarity of triangles FJB and FGD:

$$\frac{S/2}{FFD} = \frac{d/2}{FDD}$$

(dropping the suffix notation as S and FFD are general values).

---

i.e $S = d \cdot \dfrac{FFD}{FDD}$ Equation 3.2

If, however, we wish to relate the field size at one FFD to the field size of another FFD *without* moving the diaphragms, then we consider the similar triangles FGD and FHP:

$$\frac{S_1/2}{FFD_1} = \frac{S_2/2}{FFD_2}$$

i.e $\dfrac{S_1}{FDD_1} = \dfrac{S_2}{FFD_2}$ Equation 3.3

This is the more common example of the two, and equation 3.3 is both easy to derive and to remember.

Example

An X-ray beam has a field size of 20 cm × 20 cm at an FFD of 50 cm. At what FFD will the field size be 30 cm× 30 cm?

We may draw a diagram similar to Figure 3.2 (but with no necessity to include the diaphragms), and relate the similar triangles as described above, where $S_1 = 20$ cm; $FFD_1 = 50$ cm; $S_2 = 30$ cm, and FFD_2 is unknown.

$$\therefore \quad \frac{20}{50} = \frac{30}{FFD_2} \quad \text{(from Equation 3.3)}$$

Cross-multiplying:

$$FFD_2 = \frac{30 \times 50}{20} = 75 \text{ cm}$$

i.e. the field size will be 30 cm × 30 cm at a distance of 75 cm.

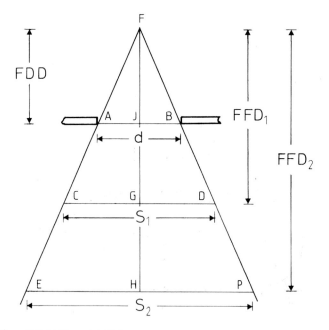

Fig. 3.2 Variation of Field Size with FFD.

(Useful check: The field size has increased by 50% (i.e. from 20 cm to 30 cm), so the FFD would also increase by 50% (as they are directly proportional to each other). Thus, 50% of FFD$_1$ is 25 cm, so that FFD$_2$ = 50+25=75, agreeing with our answer.)

3.3 FILM MAGNIFICATION

In Figure 3.3, XY represents a structure within the patient volume (e.g. a bone or foreign body) which is at a distance t from the photographic film. X-rays emanating from F travel in straight lines, so that point X is 'imaged' onto the film at point X' and Y at Y', so that X' Y' is the photographic image of XY produced by the X-rays. Obviously, X' Y' is greater than XY, so that the image is said to have been *magnified.*

Triangles FX'Y' and FXY are similar since corresponding angles of both are equal. The ratios of their corresponding sides are therefore equal (1.9.2)

$$\therefore \quad \frac{X'Y'}{XY} = \frac{F'Y'}{FY} \qquad\qquad \text{Equation 3.4}$$

Also, triangles FYZ, FY'M are similar, giving:

$$\frac{FY'}{FY} = \frac{FM}{FZ} = \frac{FFD}{FFD - t} \qquad\qquad \text{Equation 3.5}$$

since FM = FFD and FZ = FFD $- t$

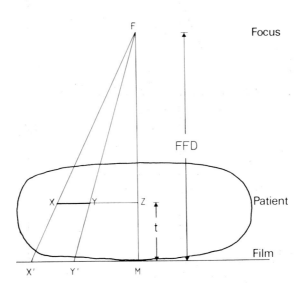

Focus

FFD

Patient

Film

Fig. 3.3 Film magnification: the image of *XY* is *X'Y'* such that *X'Y'* is larger than *XY*.

Equations 3.4 and 3.5 both contain the term $\dfrac{FY'}{FY}$ in isolation on one side of the equations — hence the other quantities must also be equal. Therefore:

$$\frac{X'Y'}{XY} = \frac{FFD}{FFD - t}$$

Now, the *magnification factor*, m, is just defined by the ratio of the image size to the object size, i.e. $\dfrac{X'Y'}{XY}$

$$\therefore \quad m = \frac{FFD}{FFD - t} \qquad\qquad \text{Equation 3.6}$$

Note that the magnification factor does not depend upon the position of the object XY relative to the centre of the beam, but only upon its distance from the film and the FFD.

The most important practical consequence of the above expression for radiography is the fact that the magnification factor, m, varies as t is changed. For example, if $t = 0$ (i.e. the object being radiographed is touching the film), then Equation 3.6 simplifies to $m = \dfrac{FFD}{FFD} = 1$, so that the magnification is unity, as may be verified by drawing the appropriate figure. Also, as t increases, $FFD - t$ decreases, making m larger (from Equation 3.6). Therefore, objects in the patient further away from the film give different film magnifications from objects close to the film, so that all radiographs give a *distorted* image compared to the true shape of the object being radiographed. This effect is slight in most cases, however, and may be reduced by increasing the FFD if required.

3.4 GEOMETRIC UNSHARPNESS (PENUMBRA)

Figure 3.4 represents the effect of the finite size of the focal spot on the 'blurring' of the structures within the patient on the radiograph. To enable simple calculation, the focal spot size is taken to be the effective size (3.1) AB, of length a, and P is a very small object or structure within the patient.

Lines APD, BPC are the X-rays from the extreme edges of the source which pass through P and produce a blurred image of P over the length CD on the photographic film. By analogy to the casting of optical shadows (e.g. from the Sun), this length is referred to as the *geometric penumbra* or *geometric unsharpness* (U). The magnitude of U may be calculated by using the properties of the similar triangles (1.9.2) PCD and PBA:

$$\text{i.e.} \quad \frac{PD}{PA} = \frac{U}{a} \qquad\qquad \text{Equation 3.7}$$

Also, triangles PDE, PFA are similar, so that:

$$\frac{PD}{PA} = \frac{PE}{AF} = \frac{t}{FFD - t} \qquad \text{Equation 3.8}$$

Combining equations 3.7 and 3.8, and solving for U:

$$U = \frac{at}{FFD - t} \qquad \text{Equation 3.9}$$

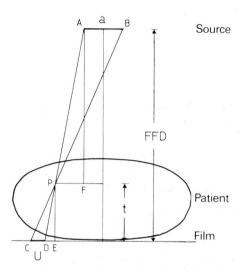

Fig. 3.4 Penumbra or Geometric Unsharpness, U, caused by finite size of effective focal spot, a.

Notice that, as for magnification (3.3), the geometrical unsharpness does not depend upon the position of the object relative to the central ray (or axis) of the X-ray beam. Thus, if P had been placed at F in Figure 3.4 the value of U would have been the same. It is desirable to have as small a geometric unsharpness as possible in order to produce radiographs of good photographic definition. From Equation 3.9 this may be accomplished by:

a. Reducing a (i.e. using as small an effective focus as possible).
b. Increasing the FFD (i.e. moving the patient and film further from the X-ray tube).
c. Reducing t. In practical terms, this means that for a radiograph of a right lateral skull, for example, it is the *right* side of the patient's skull which is placed closest to the film in order to achieve the best possible image of structures on the right side of the skull.

Exercise 3.1

Sketch figures similar to Figure 3.4 and alter a, t and FFD in turn to verify the above conclusions.

The *total* unsharpness U_t, is composed of three unsharpness factors; film/screen, patient movement and geometrical. In some cases, a smaller total unsharpness may be obtained when using a short exposure time and a relatively large focal spot rather than a long exposure and a small focal spot, owing to the effect of patient movement during the exposure. A small focal spot may require a longer exposure time if the rating of the X-ray tube is not to be exceeded (Ch. 22). Mathematically, the total unsharpness U_t, may be related approximately to the constituent sources of unsharpness by the equation:

$$U_t{}^3 = U_1{}^3 + U_2{}^3 + U_3{}^3$$

Equation 3.10

An alternative, more rigorous, method of expressing imaging performances of the separate causes of unsharpness is the Modulation Transfer Function (MTF) as described in Appendix III.

3.4.1 Penumbra from diaphragms

Figure 3.5 demonstrates the action of a movable diaphragm in defining the size of the X-ray beam. Two such diaphragms at right-angles to each other are required in order to completely define the beam. Alternatively, detachable 'cones' of different sizes may be used, but the calculation of the penumbra is exactly the same.

The penumbra, p, is the 'shadow' of the edge of the diaphragm or cone formed by the finite size, a, of the X-ray source. The calculation follows exactly the same progression as in the calculation in the previous section, and is therefore left as an exercise in similar triangles for the student. By substitution of the appropriate values into equation 3.9 we may obtain:

$$p = a \, \frac{\text{FFD} - \text{FDD}}{\text{FFD}}$$

Equation 3.11

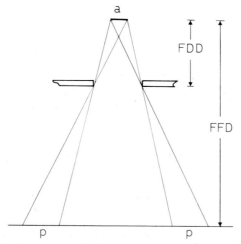

Fig. 3.5 Penumbra, p, due to the diaphragms.

The calculation of the penumbra from beams of X- or gamma-radiation is important in teletherapy treatment (34.2), where it is necessary to know the radiation dose to the whole of the treatment volume within the patient. It is of limited practical use in radiography.

3.5 FOREIGN-OBJECT LOCALISATION

If a foreign object is to be removed from a patient by surgical procedures, the surgeon must know where the object is located relative to the patient's anatomy. This information cannot be determined fully from a single radiograph, since no estimate of the depth of the body can be made. Two radiographs at right-angles to each other may be used to locate the object's position more precisely, therefore. Alternatively, layer tomography (3.6) is capable of establishing the depth of the object. It is also possible that 'computerised tomography' (CT) will play a useful role in this problem, particularly where very accurate localisation relative to adjacent anatomical structures is required. (CT is described in Appendix IV.) However, only one of the more conventional two-radiograph methods is described here. All such methods are very similar in principle, and rely on the properties of similar triangles.

The foreign object is first located by 'screening' with movable X-ray tube and image intensifier combination, where an 'under-couch' tube is the usual configuration. When the object has been located in the *centre* of the image on the television monitor, the screening is terminated and a mark placed on the patient's skin on the beam axis — point A in Figure 3.6. A film cassette is then positioned at a known distance, a, above the patient and a radiograph taken using one half of the usual value of mAs to avoid overexposure on the second radiograph.

Next, the X-ray tube is moved a known distance, s, horizontally to position F_2 while the film remains stationary. Another radiograph is then taken on the

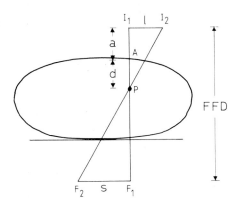

Fig. 3.6 Localisation of a foreign object, P. Two exposures are made (at F_1 and F_2) without moving the film. Separation of images, I_1 and I_2, enables calculation of object's depth, d.

same film. If the object is located at position P at a distance d below the skin, the image of P due to an exposure at F_2 is at I_2 on the film, where $I_1 I_2 = l$, and is measured on the radiograph.

The triangles $PF_1 F_2$ and $PI_1 I_2$ are similar (1.9.2), so that:

$$\frac{PF_1}{PI_1} = \frac{F_1 F_2}{I_1 I_2}$$

$$\therefore \quad \frac{FFD - (a + d)}{a + d} = \frac{s}{l}$$

Cross-multiplying and simplifying (1.3.3):

$$lFFD - la - ld = sa + sd$$
$$\therefore \quad lFFD - la - sa = d(s + l)$$
$$\therefore \quad d = \frac{lFFD - a(s + l)}{s + l}$$
$$\therefore \quad d = \left(\frac{l}{s + l}\right) . FFD - a$$

In particular, if the film cassette is placed in contact with the patient's skin, then $a = 0$, and above expression simplifies to:

$$d = \left(\frac{l}{s + l}\right) . FFD \qquad\qquad \text{Equation 3.12}$$

This expression for d, the depth of the foreign object, is in terms of quantities which are known or measurable, so that d may be calculated.

Example

If $FFD = 50\,cm$, $s = 10\,cm$ and l is measured to be $2.0\,cm$ on the radiograph, then d may be calculated by substitution into Equation 3.12:

$$\text{i.e.} \quad d = \frac{2}{12} . 50 = 8\tfrac{1}{3}$$

i.e. $d = 8.3\,cm$ (approximately)

3.6 TOMOGRAPHY

'Tomography' is the term given to the techniques used to obtain sharp images of thin sections within the patient. There are two types of tomography: layer and axial. The former produces radiographs which are similar in appearance to 'conventional' radiographs, except that structures which do not lie within the chosen layer (the 'slice') appear blurred. In Computerised Tomography (CT) a cross-section of the body is imaged as explained in Appendix IV. Tomography of both types constitutes a very broad and somewhat specialised subject which is impossible to cover fully here. However, the simplest system of layer tomography (linear tomography) will be discussed in order to establish the general principles.

The linear system of tomography, as illustrated in Figure 3.7, involves movement of both the X-ray tube and the film, but in opposite directions. This is usually accomplished by a bar joining the two and rotating about a fulcrum. If the fulcrum is positioned at level P in the figure, then structures at level P are imaged sharply on the film at all points of its motion (i.e. the image falls on the same part of the film) while structures above and below P are 'smeared' out and contribute little to the detail of the image obtained. Thus, with the focus at F_1, P is imaged at I_1, and when the focus has reached F_2 the film has moved to I_2, so that I_1 and I_2 are the same point as far as the film is concerned. A point Q directly below P is imaged at a different point of the film for each value of the angel θ (except $\theta = 0$), and so is blurred on the resulting radiograph.

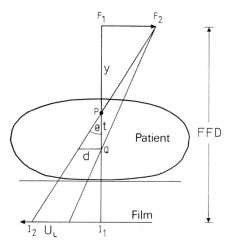

Fig. 3.7 Linear tomography. The X-ray tube and film move about P as a fulcrum. Objects in the plane containing P are always imaged onto the same points on the film — they are 'in-focus', while objects above and below are increasingly 'out-of-focus'.

3.6.1 Thickness of 'slice'

The thickness of 'slice', i.e. the useful thickness of the tomographed layer, is defined in terms of the geometrical unsharpness (3.4) of the two surfaces of the layer. This calculation is performed using the assumption that there is a point source of X-radiation.

Referring to Figure 3.7, if the X-ray tube and film have rotated through an angle θ, then a point Q at a distance t from the plane of best sharpness has a geometrical unsharpness, U_L, as shown marked. This represents the distance between where Q would be perfectly imaged, i.e. at I_2, to where it actually is imaged.

Now, $\tan \theta = d/t$ (see 1.9.1).

i.e. $t = d/\tan \theta$ Equation 3.13

Also, as shown for the case of magnification (3.3):

$$\frac{U_L}{d} = \frac{FFD}{y + t}$$

$$= \frac{FFD}{y} \text{ approx. (since } t \text{ is much smaller than } y \text{ in practice)}$$

$\therefore \; d = \dfrac{U_L y}{FFD}$ Equation 3.14

Substituting 3.14 into 3.13:

$$t = \frac{U_L y}{FFD} \cdot \frac{1}{\tan \theta}$$

The total slice thickness is $2t$, as the same arguments apply to points above P. Therefore, the slice thickness, T, is just given by:

$T = \dfrac{2\,U_L y}{FFD \,.\, \tan \theta}$ Equation 3.15

Thus, for a given value of the unsharpness, U_L, the thickness of the tomographic layer T may be reduced by:
   a.   reducing y
   b.   increasing FFD
   c.   increasing $\tan \theta$, i.e. increasing θ,

Example
   If $U_L = 2$ mm; FFD $= 50$ cm: $y = 20$ cm: $\theta = 45°$

   then $T = \dfrac{2 \times 0.2 \times 20}{50 \times 1} = \dfrac{8}{50} = 0.16$ cm

   $\therefore \; T = 1.6$ mm

Other types of tomography (e.g. 'multilayer' and 'hypocycloid') are adequately explained in many textbooks specialising in X-ray equipment and so will not be dealt with here, as they add little further to the basic principles of tomography as outlined above.

Exercise 3.2
   a.   What are the 'anode angle', 'line focus', 'real' and 'effective (apparent)' focal spot sizes?

b.   The real focal spot size is 3 mm on an anode of angle 15°. What is the effective size? (sin 15° = 0.26)

c.   If the effective size on the same anode had been 0.52 mm, what would the real size have been?

d.   The size of an X-ray beam is 10 cm × 12 cm at a distance of 40 cm from the focus. What is the size of the beam at a distance of 50 cm? Also, at what distance is the beam size 8 cm × 9.6 cm?

e.   Why is the image on a radiograph larger than the true size of the object? What magnification would you expect if an object was 10 cm from the film and the FFD was 60 cm? If the size of the object as measured on the radiograph was 12 cm, what was the true size of the object?

f.   What is meant by geometric unsharpness (penumbra)? If the effective focal spot size is 0.5 mm and an object is 8 cm from the film, what would be the size of the penumbra if the FFD was:
(i) 48 cm
(ii) 72 cm?
Why is the penumbra smaller in the second case?

g.   What method or methods are used in your hospital to locate foreign objects within patients? Illustrate your answer with appropriate diagram(s) and verify any formula used, by means of the properties of similar triangles, or otherwise.

h.   What is meant by 'tomography'? Explain the action of linear tomography and state the factors which influence the effective thickness of the tomographic layer.

SUMMARY

1.   Effective spot size, $a = r \sin \theta$.

2.   Field size, $s \propto \text{FFD}$, so $\dfrac{s_1}{\text{FFD}_1} = \dfrac{s_2}{\text{FFD}_2}$

3.   Film magnification depends upon FFD and position of structure within the patient, leading to distorted image.

4.   Very small structures (or edges of larger structures) are slightly blurred on the radiograph owing to the finite size of the focal spot. This is known as 'Geometric Unsharpness' or 'penumbra', of magnitude given by Equation 3.9.

5.   The blurred image of the edge of the diaphragms is also known as 'penumbra'.

6.   The location of foreign objects is performed by taking a double exposure on one film with the X-ray tube in two known positions. The application of similar triangles is then used to calculate the depth of the body.

7.   Tomography is accomplished by simultaneous motion of X-ray tube and film(s). This achieves sharp images of thin layers and blurred images of structures either side of this layer. The 'slice' thickness is adjusted by the selection of the total angle of movement of the X-ray tube.

4. The Inverse Square Law

The Inverse Square Law is important both in practical radiography and radiation protection. It is a consequence of two factors: that electromagnetic radiation travels in straight lines and that space is three-dimensional.

4.1 INTENSITY OF RADIATION

To understand the Inverse Square Law we have also to understand what is meant by the term 'Intensity'.

As shown in Chapter 23, electromagnetic waves are composed of 'quanta', each of which has an energy of hv, where h is Planck's constant and v is the frequency of vibration of the quantum. If we draw a square of unit area at right-angles to the path of a uniform beam of electromagnetic radiation (X-rays, say), then the *total* energy per second from all the quanta passing through the square is defined as the *Intensity* of the beam, so that:

Definition
> The *Intensity of a beam of electromagnetic radiation* at a given point is the total energy per second flowing past the point when normalised to a unit area.

For example, if 0·01 joules of energy pass through an area of 1 square centimetre every second, then the Intensity is $0·01 \times 100 \times 100 = 100$ joules per second per square metre (or W m^{-2} — see 6.3.6 on SI units).

4.2 A POINT SOURCE OF RADIATION

Referring to Figure 4.1, P is a point source of electromagnetic radiation (e.g X-rays, light) which is emitting its radiation *isotropically* (i.e. equally in all directions).

Consider a square of side one unit at a distance x units away from P (where x is much greater than 1) such that an Intensity I_x of radiation passes through this square, where the Intensity may be measured in any convenient units.

If we now extend the marginal rays containing this square out to a distance $2x$ (the rays travelling in straight lines), then we shall be able to draw a square of side 2 units in this position, by the properties of similar triangles (1.9.2).

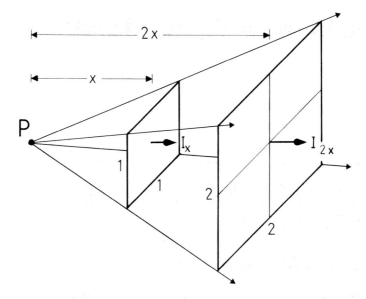

Fig. 4.1 Explanation of the Inverse Square Law — the area through which the radiation passes is proportional to the square of the distance, so that the intensity is inversely proportional to the square of the distance (e.g. $I_{2x} = I_x/4$).

Now, assuming that none of the rays has been absorbed or deflected ('scattered'), then the same number of rays per second which passed through the small square will now pass through the large square.

However, remembering that 'Intensity' means the energy/second per *unit* area, it is clear that, since the area is four times larger, the Intensity must be four times smaller, i.e. $I_{2x} = I_x/4$.

Similarly, it may be argued that, at $3x$, the Intensity has been reduced by a factor of $3 \times 3 = 9$, at $4x$ by a factor of 16 and so on. Thus, as Table 4.1 shows, the Intensity falls as the 'inverse square' of the distance.

Table 4.1 The relationships between distance from a point source of radiation and the intensity passing through and area as shown in Figure 4.1. The intensity is seen to be proportional to the inverse square of the distance — the Inverse Square Law.

Distance	Area	Intensity	$1/(Distance)^2$
x	1	I_x	$1/x^2$
$2x$	4	$I_x/4$	$1/4x^2$
$3x$	9	$I_x/9$	$1/9x^2$
...	...	...	...
$10x$	100	$I_x/100$	$1/100x^2$
...	...	...	...

4.3 STATEMENT OF INVERSE SQUARE LAW

The preceding arguments lead to the following statement of the Inverse Square Law:

The Inverse Square Law
The Intensity of the radiation emitted from a small isotropic source is proportional to the inverse square of the distance from that source, provided that there is negligible absorption or scattering of the radiation by the medium through which it passes.

Note that this statement of the Inverse Square Law also gives the conditions under which the law may be directly applied:

   a.   small source — in practice, this means small when compared to the distance from the source
   b.   isotropic source — in order that the intensity of radiation is independent of the *direction* from the source
   c.   no absorption or scattering of radiation — so that the radiation passing through a given area is not affected by the medium through which the radiation passes.

Of course, if any of these conditions is not met, then the Inverse Square Law must be applied with caution, perhaps with a statement of the direction from which the intensity is measured, or the application of appropriate correction factors (e.g. absorption due to air).

An additional constraint is that there should be no reflection or scattering back of the beam from other structures further in the path of the beam.

4.4 INVERSE SQUARE LAW AND THE X-RAY BEAM

Strictly speaking, none of the conditions outlined above for the validity of the Inverse Square Law is true for an X-ray beam, because:

   a.   the X-rays are not emitted from a true point source
   b.   they are not emitted equally in all directions (the anode 'heel effect' — see 21.1.3) — the intensity varies across the beam for equal distances from the source
   c.   absorption and scattering of the X-rays occurs in the air through which the beam passes.

However, these effects are small and may be ignored for X-ray beams generated at about 50 kV_p or over, so that the Inverse Square Law may be applied to such beams.

Insight

Situations where the Inverse Square Law would not apply include the light radiation emitted by a searchlight or laser. This is because the light is essentially parallel, so that the intensity is constant and does not depend on distance from the source. These are examples of non-isotropic sources of radiation.

4.5 MATHEMATICAL EXPRESSION FOR THE INVERSE SQUARE LAW

If I_x is the Intensity of the radiation at a distance x, then the mathematical statement of the Inverse Square Law is:

$$I_x \propto \frac{1}{x^2}$$

Equation 4.1

The proportional sign may be replaced by an equals sign if a 'constant of proportionality' is introduced (1.7):

i.e. $I_x = \dfrac{k}{x^2}$

Equation 4.2

Here, k represents the 'source strength' in terms of the total energy emitted per second by that source.

A problem frequently encountered in radiography is that of calculating the Intensity of radiation at one distance from the source, from a knowledge of the Intensity at another distance. If the new distance is called y, and the Intensity at y is I_y, then we may apply the Inverse Square Law at this new distance, in exactly the same way as in Equation 4.2.

i.e. $I_y = \dfrac{k}{x^2}$

Equation 4.3

Notice that the ks are the same, since it is assumed that the source strength is unaltered.

Rearranging equations 4.2 and 4.3 by cross-multiplication (1.4) we have:

$$k = I_x \cdot x^2 \quad \text{and} \quad k = I_y \cdot y^2$$

$\therefore \; I_x \cdot x^2 = I_y \cdot y^2$

Equation 4.4

This is a very useful formula and is easy to remember, since the equation is symmetrical on both sides.

Insight

A quicker, and at the same time, more rigorous proof of the Inverse Square Law is given by considering a small isotropic source at the centre of two concentric spheres of radii x and y. The total energy per second passing through the surface of the sphere B is the same as that passing through the surface of sphere A (in the absence of absorption or scatter). Let this be E units.

The Intensity of radiation at the surface of sphere A is (by definition) the energy passing through unit area per second (4.1).

i.e. $\quad I_x = \dfrac{E}{4\pi x^2}\quad$ or $\quad I_x \cdot x^2 = \dfrac{E}{4\pi}$

(remembering that the surface area of a sphere is $4\pi r^2$).

Similarly, for the sphere B.

$\quad I_y = \dfrac{E}{4\pi y^2}\quad$ or $\quad I_y \cdot y^2 = \dfrac{E}{4\pi}$

Thus,

$I_x \cdot x^2 = I_y \cdot y^2\quad$ as before.

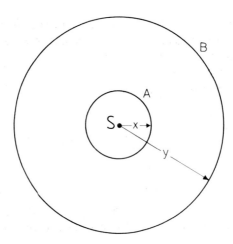

4.5.1 Units and calculations

The unit of Intensity used to derive Equation 4.4 was expressed in watts per square metre (4.1). In the measurement of the amount of light energy (i.e. 'photometry'), for example, the luminous intensity of a visible source of radiation is expressed in candelas (see Chapter 6), and the flow of energy per unit area per unit time (i.e. the Intensity) is the 'luminous flux per unit area' and is expressed in 'lux'. However, the most convenient way of measuring the 'quantity' of X or γ radiation is by the collection of the charged ions formed by the ionisation for air (32.3.1). The various types of interaction of X-rays with matter are discussed more fully in Chapter 30, and we may merely note here that there is no simple relationship between the Intensity of an X-ray beam and the rate of production of ions in the air *unless* the energy distribution (the 'spectrum') of the beam is unaltered. In practice, this means that the rate of production of ions in the air through which the X-rays pass is proportional to the Intensity provided that the potential difference (kV_p — see 6.4.1) across the tube is unaltered. (Altering the kV_p affects the number and energy of the X-rays emitted by the X-ray tube, and the amount of ionisation in the air also depends on the energy of the beam.)

The SI unit used to measure the ionisation of air is the *Exposure*, which has units of coulombs per kilogram of air (C kg^{-1}). The Exposure rate is thus $Ckg^{-1}s^{-1}$. Alternatively, we may use the unit of *absorbed dose*, the gray (Gy), as a measure of the Intensity of the X-ray beam subject to the same proviso that the kV_p is unaltered. The gray is expressed in joules per kilogram (J kg^{-1}), and is described more fully in (32.1.2).

However, it is not necessary at this stage to understand in detail the units of Exposure and absorbed dose in order to solve simple problems using the Inverse Square Law; the values of either unit are simply substituted directly for I_x or I_y in Equation 4.4, as shown in the following two examples.

Examples

a.   The absorbed dose rate in air at a distance of 60 cm from the focal spot of an X-ray tube is 0.5 mGy s^{-1}. What is the absorbed dose rate at 75 cm?
Using the Equation 4.4 $I_x \cdot x^2 = I_y \cdot y^2$
where $I_x = 0.5$; $x = 60$; $y = 75$; $I_y = ?$
We have by substitution:

$$0.5 \times 60^2 = I_y \times 75^2$$

$$\therefore \quad I_y = 0.5 \times \frac{60^2}{75^2} = 0.5 \times \left(\frac{60}{75}\right)^2 \quad (see\ 1.5.5)$$

$$\therefore \quad I_y = 0.5 \left(\frac{4}{5}\right)^2 = 0.5 \times \frac{16}{25} = 0.32.$$

Thus the absorbed dose rate at 75 cm is 0.32 mGy s^{-1}.

b.   In the above example, at what distance would the absorbed dose rate be 2.0 mGy s^{-1}?
We may substitute into the same equation as before, to give:

$$0.5 \times 60^2 = 2.0 \times y^2$$

$$\therefore \quad y^2 = \frac{0.5 \times 60^2}{2.0} = \frac{60^2}{4} = \left(\frac{60}{2}\right)^2.$$

Taking the square root of both sides removes both of the squares, so that:

$$y = \frac{60}{2} = 30\ cm$$

so that the absorbed dose rate is 2.0 mGy s^{-1} at 30 cm. (*Note:* A doubling of the distance must reduce the Intensity by a factor of four, by the Inverse Square Law, so that the above calculation is seen to be correct.)

Exercise 4.1

a.   The Exposure rate in an X-ray beam is 81×10^{-6} C kg^{-1} s^{-1} (18·8 R/min) at a distance of 80 cm from the focus. If the field size is 10 cm $\times$ 10 cm at this distance, at what distance is the field size 15 cm $\times$ 15 cm (see 3.2), and what is the Exposure rate at this distance?

b.   For the previous example, at what distance will the Exposure rate be 16×10^{-6} C kg^{-1} s^{-1} (3·7 R/min)?

c.   The absorbed dose rate in air from a small source of radioactivity is 520 mGy/hr (52 rad/hr) at a given distance. What is the absorbed dose rate at ten times this distance?

4.6 mAs AND THE INVERSE SQUARE LAW
[*See* (6.4.2) for the definition of mAs.]

There is another, more common, use of the Inverse Square Law in radiography which may be paraphrased as follows:

We know that a given setting of mAs gives a good picture at this FFD, but what mAs would be needed at a different value of FFD?

Here it is assumed that the kV$_p$ control is unaltered for both exposures (but see 4.7). For the purposes of this section, all we need to know is that the mAs is directly related to the total number of X-rays emitted by the source. In these calculations it is assumed that the absorption of the X-rays by the patient is the same at both distances.

It is important to form a mental picture of the essential difference between the straightforward measurement of the Inverse Square Law, where the source strength remains the same, and using the Inverse Square Law to determine what the new mAs should be to give equivalent X-ray films at the two distances.

The Intensity (I_x) at a given distance x is composed of two factors:

a.   The distance from the source — as in the Inverse Square Law.

i.e. $I_x \propto \dfrac{1}{x^2}$

b.   the total energy emitted per second from the source — this is proportional to mA,

i.e. $I_x \propto$ (mA)$_x$ (*see* 6.5.2)

Therefore, combining (a) and (b) above, we have:

$I_x \propto \dfrac{(\text{mA})_x}{x^2}$, where (mA)$_x$ is the mA setting for distance x.

The total energy per unit area reaching the X-ray film is known as the 'photographic exposure', and determines the optical density, or blackening, of the film. The exposure, E_x, is given simply by the multiplication of the Intensity, I_x, by the time, t, for which the X-rays are emitted, so that

$E_x = I_x . t$, into which expression we may substitute the value of I_x obtained above   to produce:

$$E_x \propto \frac{(mA)_x}{x^2} . t$$

Now, $mA \times t$ is the mAs, by definition of mAs (6.4.2)

$$\therefore \quad E_x = \frac{c(mAs)_x}{x^2} \qquad\qquad \text{Equation 4.5}$$

where c is the constant of proportionality which relates all the units together. Similarly, for distance y,

$$E_y = \frac{c(mAs)_y}{y^2} \qquad\qquad \text{Equation 4.6}$$

As mentioned above, it is the exposure at the film which determines the degree of film blackening. Hence, if we wish to produce two pictures which look 'the same' at two different distances (apart from magnification, of course) we must have equal exposures at the two distances,

i.e. $E_x = E_y$.

Thus, combining Equations 4.5 and 4.6 we have

$$\frac{c(mAs)_x}{x^2} = \frac{c(mAs)_y}{y^2}$$

Cancelling the constant c from both sides,

$$\frac{(mAs)_x}{x^2} = \frac{(mAs)_y}{y^2}$$	Equation 4.7

for equivalent radiographs at distances x and y.

Notice that this equation is symmetrical, as is equation 4.4, but now the x^2 and y^2 terms are used as denominators.

It is not necessary to remember in detail the steps which led to Equation 4.7 in order to carry out the calculations, but an appreciation of the reason for the difference between Equation 4.4 and 4.7 is necessary for intelligent use of the Inverse Square Law. Also, it is not *essential* to use Equation 4.7 as the numerical examples may be solved by the application of Equation 4.4 and 'common-sense', as shown in the example below. However, the remembrance and practise of both formulae is recommended for examination purposes, as it is not always easy to think at one's best in such circumstances.

Example

1. At a focus-to-film distance (FFD) of 50 cm the required exposure is 6 mAs. What would the exposure need to be if the FFD was increased to 100 cm?

Method 1 — Use of Equation 4.7:

The Inverse Square Law implies the following relationship if radiographs are to be comparable at two distances x and y:

$$\frac{(mAs)_x}{x^2} = \frac{(mAs)_y}{y^2}$$

where $(mAs)_x$ is the mAs value associated with the radiograph taken at distance x, and $(mAs)_y$ is the corresponding value at y.

Now, $x = 50$ cm; $(mAs)_x = 6$; $y = 100$ cm.

$$\therefore \quad \frac{6}{50^2} = \frac{(mAs)_y}{100^2} \quad \text{by substitution}$$

Cross-multiplying:

$$(mAs)_y = 6 \times \frac{100^2}{50^2} = 6 \times \left(\frac{100}{50}\right)^2$$

$$\therefore \quad (mAs)_y = 6 \times \left(\frac{2}{1}\right)^2 = 6 \times 4 = 24$$

i.e.   *24 mAs* is the required exposure at an FFD of 100 cm.

Method 2 — Use of Equation 4.4:

The mathematical statement of the Inverse Square Law applied to two different distances x and y is

$$I_x \cdot x^2 = I_y \cdot y^2$$

where I_x is the Intensity of the X-ray beam at x and I_y is that at y.

We know that $x = 50$ cm and $y = 100$ cm, but we do not know I_x or I_y.

Now, $\dfrac{I_y}{I_x} = \dfrac{x^2}{y^2}$, by cross-multiplication

i.e. $\dfrac{I_y}{I_x} = \dfrac{50^2}{100^2} = \left(\dfrac{50}{100}\right)^2 = \left(\dfrac{1}{2}\right)^2 = \dfrac{1}{4}$

This means that, *everything else being equal*, the X-ray Intensity at 100 cm would be *four times less than at 50 cm*. Thus, for the same exposure time, the film would be severely underexposed; therefore the radiographer may increase *either* the exposure time *or* the mA by a factor of four to obtain the same photographic effect. This is equivalent to increasing the mAs value by a factor of four, i.e. the mAs associated with a distance of 100 cm is just $4 \times 6 = 24$ *mAs*, giving the same result as Method 1.

Which of methods 1 or 2 is used is a matter of personal preference. Method 1 has the advantage of being shorter and quicker without the need to keep checking whether the multiplying factor is round the right way.

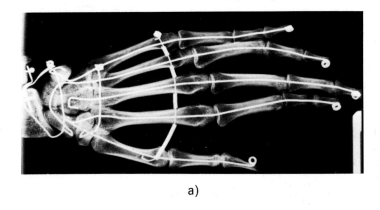

a)

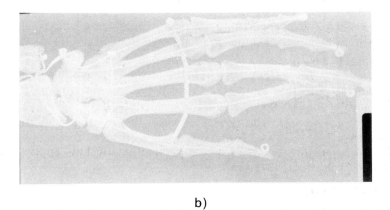

b)

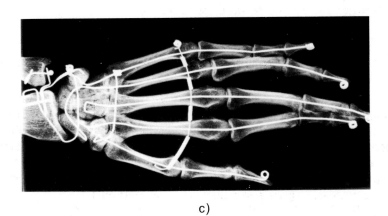

c)

Plate I mAs and the Inverse Square Law. (a) 50 cm FFD; 6 mAs, (b) 100 cm FFD; 6 mAs, (c) 100 cm FFD; 24 mAs 50 kV_p for each image.

Plate I illustrates the practical application of the last example, where all the values are as in the problem. Plate I(a) shows the original radiograph taken on a 'phantom' hand at an FFD of 50 cm and an exposure of 6 mAs. When the FFD is increased to 100 cm , Plate I(b) shows the underexposed film for 6 mAs. Using the calculated factor of four, however, results in a visually identical radiograph for an exposure of 24 mAs, in agreement with our solution.

4.7 GRIDS, SCREENS AND kV_p

The previous sections have assumed no changes in kV_p, grid or screen/film combination between two exposures of the same subject. If this is not the case, then some method of calculating the effect of such changes must be developed. Before this is discussed, however, two definitions are needed:

a. The grid factor g, is the factor by which the photographic exposure must be increased to achieve the same photographic density obtained when not using any grid (31.1.2).

b. The relative screen/film speed S, is the factor by which one screen/film combination is 'faster' than another, i.e. the ratio of exposures to give the same photographic effect (27.5.1).

We must now investigate the quantities which determine the photographic density in order to relate them to the preceding sections of this chapter.

Firstly, the Intensity of the X-ray beam I is related to the following variable quantities:

a. $I \propto kV_p^2$ (see 28.2.2)

b. $I \propto mA$

c. $I \propto \dfrac{1}{d^2}$ } as discussed in Sections 4.5 and 4.6.

Combining all these factors, we have

$$I \propto \frac{mA \cdot kV_p^2}{d^2} = \frac{c \cdot mA \cdot kV_p^2}{d^2}$$

where c is a constant of proportionality (1.7).

The film exposure, E, is just the intensity multiplied by the exposure time t (see 4.6) so that the film exposure obtained when using no grid or screen is given by:

$$E = I \cdot t = \frac{c \cdot mA \cdot t \cdot kV_p^2}{d^2} = \frac{c \cdot mAs \cdot k_p^2}{d^2}$$

The effect of using a grid is to reduce the photographic exposure by the grid factor, g, while a screen has a two-fold effect:

a. The screen has a greater absorption of the X-rays than the film, and this absorption increases with increasing values of kV_p over the useful 'diagnostic' range of kV_p settings. It is usual to approximate this effect by changing the kV_p^2 term in the above equation to kV_p^4, which also includes the effect of increased penetration of the beam through the patient's tissues as the kV_p is increased.

b.   The light emitted by the screen produces a greater photographic effect than the X-rays alone (the 'Intensification Factor' — see 27.5.1). When comparing the effects of two screens on the radiographs, it is only the *relative* speeds which need to be considered, however.

Thus, the photographic exposure obtained when using both a grid (of grid factor g) and screen (of relative speed S) is given by:

$$E = \frac{c \cdot mAs \cdot kV_p^4 \cdot S}{d^2 \cdot g} \qquad \qquad \text{Equation 4.8}$$

If two radiographs are to have the same photographic density (31.2) i.e. to look the 'same', then the film exposures must also be the same. This is true no matter what combination of grids, screens, mAs, kV_p or FFD are used. Hence, if the value of E in the above equation is kept constant (i.e. is the same for the two radiographs), then both radiographs will look the same.

---

i.e. $$\frac{mAs_1 \cdot kV_{p1}^4 \cdot S_1}{d_1^2 \cdot g_1} = \frac{mAs_2 \cdot kV_{p2}^4 \cdot S_2}{d_2^2 \cdot g_2} \qquad \qquad \text{Equation 4.9}$$

---

where the suffixes 1 and 2 refer to the value of each quantity for the first and second radiographs respectively.

If we take the example of Section 4.5, where the mAs and FFD may be varied but everything else remains constant, then Equation 4.9 reduces to:

$$\frac{mAs_1}{d_1^2} = \frac{mAs_2}{d_2^2}$$

This is the same formula as 4.7.

Now, Formula 4.9 is not particularly easy to remember, so we may resort to the use of a mnemonic to help us! Such a mnemonic may be:

'MASKS over GRID2'   Equation 4.10

---

where $MAS \equiv mAs$; $K \equiv kV_p^4$; $S =$ relative screen factor; $GRID \equiv$ grid factor; $D2 \equiv d^2$ (i.e. Inverse Square Law).

Thus, the only extra feat of memory is that of K being raised to the fourth power if a screen is used, and the second power if no screen is used.

Example

The first exposure has a combination of factors as follows: mA = 500; time = 0·04 sec; kV_p = 60;   screen   speed = 2;   grid   factor = 3; FFD = 90 cm. The required combination for the second exposure is: mA = 200; kV_p = 120;   screen   speed = 3;   grid   factor = 4;   FFD = 180 cm.

What exposure time is required to achieve the same photographic effect?

Using the mnemonic of 4·10:

$$\frac{500 \times 0{\cdot}04 \times 60^4 \times 2}{3 \times 90^2} = \frac{200 \times t \times 120^4 \times 3}{4 \times 180^2}$$

Cross-multiplying (*without* multiplying out the indices),

$$t = \frac{500 \times 0{\cdot}04 \times 2 \times 60^4 \times 180^2 \times 4}{3 \times 90^2 \times 200 \times 120^4 \times 3}$$

$$= \frac{500 \times 0{\cdot}04 \times 2 \times 4}{3 \times 200 \times 3} \times \left(\frac{180}{90}\right)^2 \times \left(\frac{60}{120}\right)^4$$

$$= \frac{16}{180} \cdot 2^2 \cdot \frac{1}{2^4} = \frac{16}{180 \times 4} = \frac{2}{90} \text{ sec}$$

$$\therefore \quad t = 0{\cdot}02 \text{ sec (approximately)}$$

Note the collection of terms containing the same indices, enabling easy simplification (1.5.5).

Exercise 4.1
   a.   At an FFD of 60 cm the required exposure is 15 mAs. What would the exposure need to be at an FFD of 72 cm?
   b.   Why is the mAs required to produce a given photographic density
        (i)   increased if a grid is used
        (ii) decreased if a screen is used
        (iii) increased at a larger FFD
        (iv) decreased if a higher kV_p is used?
   c.   What is meant by the 'grid factor' and the 'relative screen factor'?
   d.   An exposure was made using the following values: $90kV_p$, 120 mAs, 75 cm FFD, grid factor = 4. What value of mAs would be needed if the values are changed to $60\ kV_p$, 100 cm FFD, grid factor = 3, assuming that the screen used in the second exposure is twice as 'fast' as that used in the first exposure?
   e.   What would have been the mAs value for the second exposure in the previous question if no screens were used in either exposure?

SUMMARY

1.   The Inverse Square Law is a consequence of space being three-dimensional and electromagnetic radiation travelling in straight lines.
2.   Statement of Law: 'The Intensity of radiation emitted from a small isotropic source is proportional to the inverse square of the distance from that source, provided that there is no absorption or scatter of the radiation by the medium through which it passes.'

3.   Mathematical statement of the Law is $I_x \propto \dfrac{1}{x^2}$

4.   Intensities at two distances x and y:

$$I_x \cdot x^2 = I_y \cdot y^2$$

5.   The mAs settings for equivalent radiographs at two distances x and y:

$$\frac{(mAs)_x}{x^2} = \frac{(mAs)_y}{y^2}$$

6.   If mAs, kV_p, screens and grids may be changed between exposures, then for equal film densities:

$$\frac{mAs \cdot kv_p^{\,4} \cdot S}{d^2 \cdot g} \quad \text{is constant}$$

(Mnemonic: 'MASKS over GRID2'.)

5. The Exponential Law

5.1 DESCRIPTION OF THE EXPONENTIAL LAW

This Law is fundamental to the understanding of radioactive decay and X-ray attenuation in matter. Many students find this one of the more difficult aspects of radiographic physics — hence its treatment within this separate chapter.

Perhaps the best example of the Exponential Law to which we are accustomed in our everday life concerns money. If £100 has been invested in a Building Society, at an annual interest rate of 5%, then there will be a total of £100 plus 5% of 100 = £105 after one year. During the second year, the 5% interest will apply to the £105, so that there will be £105 plus 5% of £105 = £110·25 after two years. If we draw a graph of the money in the Building Society against time, and draw a smooth line through the points, we shall have a curve as shown in Figure 5.1. Notice that the rise in the amount of money is initially quite small, but becomes greater and greater. This is an example of a curve of exponential *growth*, as we shall see later.

For a second example we shall suppose that the tax system is such that each

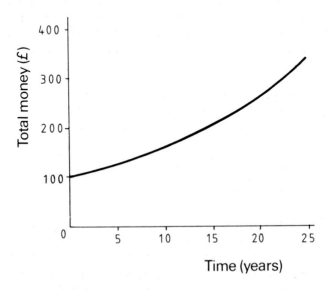

Fig. 5.1 Growth of £100 at 5% interest per annum. Note that the rate of growth becomes greater with time. This is an example of *exponential growth*.

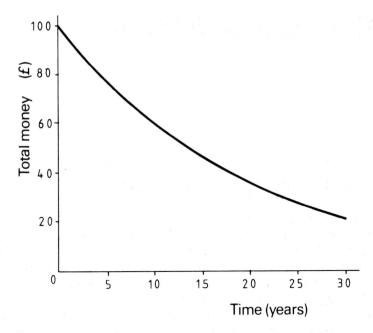

Fig. 5.2 'Decay' of £100 at 5% tax per annum. The rate of decay decreases with time, and the curve never reaches zero. This is an example of *exponential decay*.

year 5% of the money is taken in tax fees. Thus, considering £100 as the initial sum, after the first year there will be £95 left, after the second year £91·75 and so on. Again, constructing a graph, we shall see a curve as shown in Figure 5.2. In this case, the fall in the amount of money left is greater initially and then tends to level off. Also, notice that there is *always something* left, i.e. the curve never reaches zero. This type of curve is an example of exponential *decay*.

The common factor in these two examples is the 5% *change* in a given time. This is the characteristic of all exponential change, and may be expressed as:

Definition
   A quantity y is said to vary *exponentially* with x if equal changes of x produce equal *fractional* (or percentage) changes in y

---

Insight
   For those students familiar with the Calculus, the mathematical equivalent of the above statement is
$$\frac{dy}{y} = k\,dx, \quad \text{or} \quad \frac{dy}{dx} = ky$$

Integrating, we have $y = y_0 \cdot e^{kx}$
Here the independent variable x forms part of the exponent of the number e, hence the term 'exponential' law.

The two major examples of the exponential Law in radiography are radioactive decay and X-ray attenuation by matter. Both of these are described in the following sections.

5.2 RADIOACTIVE DECAY

Radionuclides are said to 'decay' when they change from one nuclear configuration to another. This decay may take several forms, including the ejection of alpha particles, electrons (positive and negative) and gamma rays from the nucleus. These, and other, modes of decay are discussed more fully in Chapter 26. However, the particular mode of decay is not important to our purpose in this section, as the exponential law is valid for all, and may be stated as:

Definition

The law of radioactive decay states that the rate of decay of a particular radionuclide (i.e. the number of nuclei decaying per second) is proportional to the number of such nuclei left.

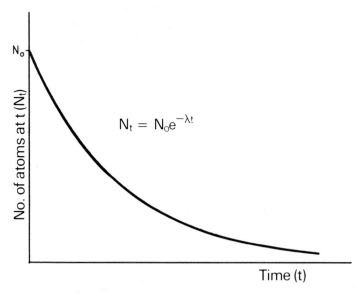

$$N_t = N_o e^{-\lambda t}$$

Fig. 5.3 Exponential decay of the number of atoms of a particular radionuclide. Note the similarity to Fig. 5.2.

At first sight this does not appear to be very similar to the above definition of an exponential change, but it is, in fact, exactly analogous to the example of 5% tax per annum. Here the 'rate of decay' is analogous to 'the *loss of money* per year', which from the law of radioactive decay stated above is seen to change quickly initially, but to slow down as less and less of the original nuclei (or analogously the original money) is left. Figure 5.3 shows a graph of the decay of a radionuclide. This is exactly the same type of curve as Figure 5.2. Note the relatively high early decay rate and the way the curve never reaches zero.

5.2.1 Activity

In practice it would be extremely difficult to measure a curve as shown in the above figure, as we would have to be able to measure the number of nuclei of a particular sort which is present at any given time. However, what we can measure more easily is the *effects* of the nuclear disintegrations by 'counting' the gamma rays (for example) with a suitable detector (e.g. scintillation counter — Appendix II). In this way we may make an estimate of the total number of disintegrations per second occurring within the radioactive sample at any given time. This quantity is known as the 'activity' of the radioactive sample and is measured in becquerels (where 1 becquerel (Bq) ≡ 1 disintegration per second), or previously in curies (where 1 curie (Ci) ≡ 3.7×10^{10} disintegrations per second). The actual units are not important to an understanding of the decay curve, however, and we may now plot 'activity' against 'time' and obtain exactly the same shape of curve, i.e. activity decays exponentially with time, as shown in Figure 5.4.

As shown in Figure 5.4 are the decay curves for a quickly decaying radionuclide and a slowly decaying radionuclide.

A quantity called the 'half-life' is used in describing the rate of decay of a particular radionuclide, as described in the next section.

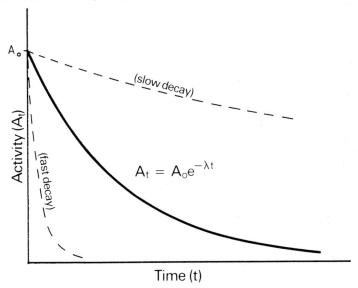

$$A_t = A_o e^{-\lambda t}$$

Time (t)

Fig. 5.4 Exponential decay of the *activity* of a radionuclide.

5.2.2 Half-life and decay constant

An illustration of the half-life of a particular radionuclide is shown in Figure 5.5. Here, the original activity at $t = 0$, is A_0. When the disintegration rate has decayed to one half of this (i.e. $A_0/2$) a certain time has passed $t_{1/2}$. It is this time which is called the 'half-life' and may be defined as:

Definition
    The *half-life* of a radionuclide is the time required for the activity of a radioactive sample to decay to one half of its original value.

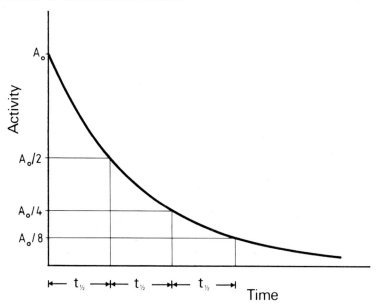

Fig. 5.5 Half-life ($t_{1/2}$) and radioactive decay. Each $t_{1/2}$ reduces the activity by one-half.

If now another half-life $t_{1/2}$, passes then the activity is reduced by a further factor of two, i.e. $A_0/4$, and so on for further half-lives. Notice that, as in our monetary example (5.1), the curve never reaches zero activity, so that no radioactive source is ever completely 'dead'.

In addition, Figure 5.4 shows the mathematical formula for the exponential law:

$$A_t = A_0 e^{-\lambda t} \qquad\qquad \text{Equation 5.1}$$

Here, λ is the 'decay constant' and is related to the half-life by the relationship:

$$\lambda = \frac{0{\cdot}693}{t_{1/2}} \qquad\qquad \text{Equation 5.2}$$

The decay constant is thus measured in units of time^{-1}, since it is inversely related to the half-life. For example,

$$\lambda = 0{\cdot}115 \text{ h}^{-1} \quad \text{for } ^{99}\text{Tc}^m.$$

Thus Equation 5.1 may also be written

$$A_t = A_0 e^{-(0{\cdot}693t/t_{1/2})} \qquad\qquad \text{Equation 5.3}$$

Another important point is that it does not matter from which time the half-life begins to be measured. Figure 5.6 shows the decay of a radionuclide over a time of one half-life starting at any arbitrary time, T. Thus, over an interval of $t_{1/2}$ the activity has been reduced by a factor of two, independent of the starting time, T.

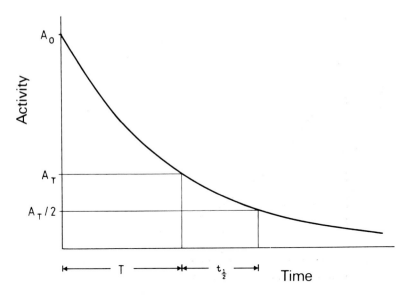

Fig. 5.6 The half-life, $t_{1/2}$, is measured from an arbitrary time, T, in the above figure. It is found that the value of $t_{1/2}$ so obtained does not depend upon the value of T, so that half-life may be measured from any starting time.

Insight

1.   The 'law of radioactive decay' is, as defined in Equation 5.2, the 'rate of decay $\propto$ number of nuclei left'.

i.e. $-\dfrac{dN}{dt} \propto N = \lambda N$

Thus, the decay constant, λ, is just introduced as a constant of proportionality (1.7).

Integrating, $N = N_0 e^{-\lambda t}$.

2. $-\dfrac{dN}{dt} = \lambda N$ and $N = N_0 e^{-\lambda t}$

$\therefore$ $-\dfrac{dN}{dt} = \lambda N_0 e^{-\lambda t}$ by substitution.

Now $-\dfrac{dN}{dt} = A$, the activity; and λN_0 is the activity at $t = 0$, i.e. A_0

$\therefore$ $A = A_0 e^{-\lambda t}$, as shown in Figure 5.5.

3.   After time $t_{1/2}$, A has been reduced to $A^0/2$ (by definition)

$\therefore$ $\dfrac{A_0}{2} = A_0 e^{-\lambda t_{1/2}}$

$\therefore$ $2 = e^{\lambda t_{1/2}}$

$\therefore$ $\log_e 2 = \lambda t_{1/2}$

$\therefore$ $\lambda = \dfrac{0 \cdot 693}{t_{1/2}}$, as stated in Equation 5.2.

Example

A radioisotope of Iodine, ^{131}I, has a half-life of eight days. Its activity was measured to be 14·4 MBq at 9.00 on 3rd February. What will be its activity at 9.00 on 27th February?

Questions of this type invariably involve calculating the number of half-lives through which the radionuclide has decayed. In this case, the time of decay is 24 days, and since the half-life is eight days, this is equivalent to three half-lives.

Now 1 half-life reduces the activity by a factor of 2
2 half-lives reduce the activity by a factor of $2 \times 2 = 4$
3 half-lives reduce the activity by a factor of $4 \times 2 = 8$.

i.e. each successive half-life reduces the activity by a factor of 2.

$$\therefore \quad \text{the activity after 3 half-lives} = \frac{14\cdot4}{8} = 1\cdot8 \text{ MBq}$$

This example gives a clue as to the general method of solution of such problems, for assuming n half-lives of decay, then the decayed activity, A_n, is

$$A_n = \frac{A_0}{2^n} \qquad\qquad \text{Equation 5.4}$$

where A_0 is the original activity.

Similarly, if we wish to know the activity n half-lives *before* the known activity A_0, the factor 2^n will be the other way up, i.e.

$$A_n = 2^n A_0 \qquad\qquad \text{Equation 5.5}$$

Exercise 5.1

a. Use Equation 5.4 to verify the result of the previous worked example.

b. The radionuclide ^{99}Tc^m has a half-life of six hours. If a sample of ^{99}Tc^m has an activity of 128 MBq at 9.00 hours, what is its activity at 15.00 hours on the following day? What is this in microcuries (from Table B at the end of the book)?

c. Define half-life and decay constant. What is the relationship between them? If one radionuclide has a decay constant of 0·5 sec^{-1} and another has a decay constant of 0·05 sec^{-1}, which decays faster, assuming that they both start with the same activity?

d. Explain the law of radioactive decay, using a graph as illustration.

5.3 ATTENUATION OF ELECTROMAGNETIC RADIATION BY MATTER

The attenuation of X-rays by matter constitutes the other major example of the exponential law in radiography.

The types of interactions which electromagnetic radiation undergoes when passing through matter are explained more fully in Chapter 30. For our purposes here, however, we need to know only that electromagnetic radiation (which includes light, X-rays and gamma rays — see Ch. 24) either passes straight through matter, or is absorbed or deflected ('scattered') by the matter itself (e.g. a car's headlights shining through fog.) For example, if a slab of material only allows 10% of the incident radiation through (i.e. 10% is 'transmitted'), then the 'attenuation' is 90%. The exponential law describes in quantitive terms the relationship between the attenuation of the radiation and the thickness of the absorber. The subtle difference between *absorption* and *attenuation* is explained in Chapter 30.

Consider that there is a narrow parallel beam of X-rays (say) which is incident upon a slab of absorbing material of thickness x, as shown in Figure 5.7. Supposing that there is a 10% attenuation, then 90% of the original beam is transmitted. Now, if we put a further identical absorber in the path of the beam, then it is found by experiment that this also transmits 90% of the radiation incident upon it, so that the total amount which is transmitted through the two absorbers is $0.9 \times 90 = 81\%$. A third identical absorber will transmit 90% of this amount, i.e. 72.9%, and so on for further absorbers.

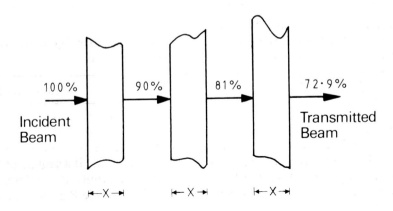

Fig 5.7 Exponential attenuation of electromagnetic radiation in matter. Equal thickness (x) of absorber transmit equal fractions of intensity of radiation incident upon them (9/10 in the figure).

Thus, we may say that 'equal changes of x produce the same fractional (or percentage) change of the transmitted X-ray intensity'. This from 5.1 above, is just the definition of an exponential change, so that the attenuation of electromagnetic radiation is said to vary exponentially with absorber thickness. (This is not necessarily true of other 'radiations' e.g. an electron beam, where there exists a definite range beyond which the electrons cannot travel).

A graph of the transmitted intensity, I_x, through an absorber of thickness x is shown in Figure 5.8. The incident radiation is the value of I_x when there is no absorber at all, i.e. $x = 0$, and is therefore denoted as I_0 and corresponds to the

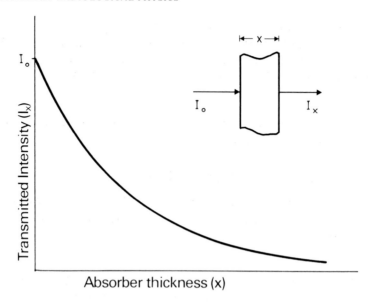

Fig 5.8 Exponential attenuation of electromagnetic radiation. Note the similarity to Fig. 5.3.

point where the curve touches the 'ordinate' or 'y-axis'. The mathematical relationship between all these quantities is:

$$I_x = I_0 e^{-\mu x}$$ Equation 5.6

Here μ is the 'total linear attenuation coefficient', so called because it takes *all* processes of attenuation into account ('total') and refers to the variation of transmittance with 'linear' distance x. As the figure shows, I_x never becomes zero — an accustomed result of exponential decay.

Definition
The *total linear attenuation coefficient* is the fractional change of intensity of a parallel beam of electromagnetic radiation per unit thickness of absorber.

Insight
Equation 5.6 give $I_x = I_0 e^{-\mu x}$.
Differentiating with respect to x,

$$\frac{dI}{dx} = \mu I_0 e^{-\mu x} = -\mu I$$

i.e. $\mu = -\dfrac{dI}{I} \bigg/ dx$

verifying the definition of μ above

Note the similarity between Figures 5.4 and 5.8 and Equations 5.1 and 5.6,
- i.e. there is an exact parallel between radioactive decay and the attenuation of

electromagnetic radiation as examples of the exponential law. Is there a corresponding parallel term to 'half-life', then, as described in 5.2.2? The answer to this rhetorical question is, as one might expect, in the affirmative! The equivalent term is 'Half Value Thickness', abbreviated to HVT.

Exercise 5.2
Before reading further, try to describe what is meant by HVT, by analogy to radioactive half-life (see 5.2.2).

5.3.1 Half-Value Thickness (HVT)

Refering to Figure 5.9, we see that successive thickness of HVTs reduce the Intensity by successive factors of two. We are therefore in a position to define HVT more precisely.

Definition
   The Half-Value Thickness (HVT) is that thickness of substance which will transmit exactly one half of the intensity of the radiation incident upon it.

The HVT therefore depends upon the substance itself and the penetrating power of the beam of electromagnetic radiation incident upon it. In general, the penetrating power increases as the energy of the beam increases.
   To complete the analogy with radioactive decay, Equation 5.2 is paralleled by:

$$\mu = \frac{0\cdot693}{HVT}$$

Equation 5.7

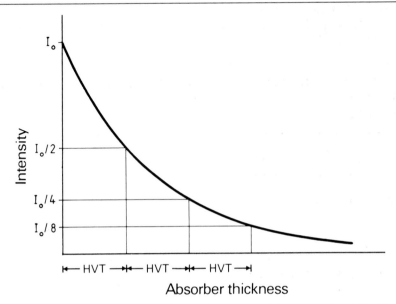

Fig. 5.9 Half-Value-Thickness (H.V.T) and electromagnetic radiation. Each H.V.T. of absorber reduces the intensity by one-half.

Example

The HVT of lead to a particular beam of X-rays is 2 mm. What thickness of lead must be placed in the X-ray beam such that only 0·1% of it is transmitted?

Most questions of this sort hinge on the calculation of the number of HVTs required to achieve a given transmission. (Note the similarity to the calculation of the number of half-lives in examples on radioactive decay.)

There are several ways of tackling this and similar problems. The following method is recommended as being easy to follow, easy to check and providing less opportunity for making arithmetical slips.

100% of the X-ray beam is incident upon the lead, and 0·1% is transmitted. This gives a factor of

$$\frac{100}{0·1} = 1000$$

between these two figures.

Now each HVT gives a factor of two between incident and transmitted intensities, and we may therefore construct the following simple table:

Number of HVTs	Intensity Reduction Factor
1	2
2	4 (i.e. 2 × 2)
3	8 (i.e. 4 × 2, etc.)
4	16
5	32
6	64
7	128
8	256
9	521
10	1024

A table of this sort is easy to check, since only whole numbers are used. The factor of 1024 is reached after 10 HVTs — this is very close to our required factor of 1000.

Thus 20 mm of lead must be used (i.e. 10 HVTs) to reduce the transmitted intensity to 0·1% of the incident intensity.

Again as in the case of the examples of radioactive half-life (5.2.2) we may generalise by writing the following formula:

$$I_n = \frac{I_0}{2^n} \qquad \qquad \text{Equation 5.7}$$

where I_0 is the incident intensity of radiation and I_n the transmitted intensity after passing through n HVTs.

5.3.2 Tenth-Value Thickness

It should be clear at this stage that other values of absorber thickness than the

HVT will also produce equal fractional changes in transmission, so that it is possible to define a 'Fifth-Value Thickness' or a 'Hundredth-Value Thickness', etc. Although the HVT is a very common method of measuring the attenuation of electromagnetic radiation through matter, the 'Tenth-Value Thickness' is also of use when considering large amounts of attenuation. An example of this would be when designing the walls of a radiotherapy treatment room when a very high intensity of radiation from the treatment machine must not be allowed to penetrate the wall in any significant quantities. One Tenth-Value Thickness would reduce the intensity by a factor of 10 (by a similar definition to HVT), two would reduce the intensity by 100, and so on.

A similar argument applies to radioactive decay, of course, where a 'Tenth-Life' would be the time taken for the activity to decay by a factor of 10.

5.4 LOGARITHMIC GRAPH PAPER AND THE EXPONENTIAL LAW

The use of logarithmic graph paper greatly simplifies the plotting of both radioactive decay and X-ray attenuation, as it transforms the curved lines on all the previous figures into straight lines. The scale on the ordinate of logarithmic graph paper is non-linear as may be seen from Figure 5.10.

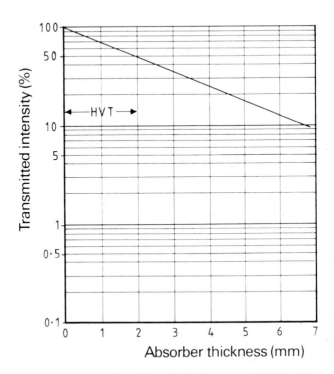

Fig. 5.10 An example of a logarithmic scale applied to the exponential law. The exponential *curve* of previous figures has become a *straight* line. The H.V.T. is 2 mm, as read from the graph. Half-lives may also be determined in this manner.

The characteristic feature of a logarithmic scale is that equal spacings on the paper (e.g. the distance between 0·1 and 1·0) give rise to the same fractional or percentage change in *values* on the scale. From inspection of the logarithmic scale of Figure 5.10 it may be seen that the physical distance between 100 and 10 is the same as between 10 and 1, which is the same as between 1 and 0·1 and so on. Thus, the logarithmic scale *never reaches zero*, and anything plotted on it has its high values 'squashed' together and its low values 'expanded', which is exactly what is wanted to make Figure 5.9, for example, 'straighten out'.

In principle only two points need to be known in order to draw the whole graph. In practice, more than two points may be obtained in order to provide a more accurate straight line, since each experimental point is subject to errors of measurement (6.5). The 'best' straight line may then be drawn through the same points plotted on the logarithmic graph paper.

Thus, in measuring HVT, for example, the transmitted intensities through a series of thin absorbers is measured and the best straight line may be drawn as shown in the graph. The thickness corresponding to 50% transmission (i.e. the HVT) is then read off the graph as shown.

The graphical logarithmic scale saves us the trouble of *calculating* the logarithms — we can just plot the values of I_x directly and thus obtain a straight line very simply.

Insight

Let us suppose that we wish to plot

$$I_x = I_0 e^{-\mu x}$$

on logarithmic paper. Rearranging this equation we have

$$\frac{I_x}{I_0} = e^{-\mu x}$$

or $\log_e \dfrac{I_x}{I_0} = -\mu x$ (from the definition of a logarithm 1.10.2)

∴ $\log_e I_x - \log_e I_0 = -\mu x$
∴ $\log_e I_x = \log_e I_0 - \mu x$

Thus, if we plot $\log_e I_x$ against x we shall have a straight line ('$y = mx + c$')

Exercise 5.3

a.   What is an exponential change? Illustrate your answer by considering the attenuation of a parallel beam of electromagnetic radiation passing through matter.

b.   What is meant by the Half-Value Thickness (HVT) of a material? Why does the HVT of a material vary with the energy of the incident radiation?

c.   What is meant by the 'total linear attenuation coefficient' of a material? However is this related to HVT? If a radiographic screening session resulted in a radiation Exposure of $1·28 \times 10^{-5}$ Coulombs/kg to a lead apron, what was the Exposure at the other side of the lead apron, assuming that the apron is equivalent to 2 mm of lead and the HVT of lead was 0·5 mm to that radiation?

    d.   How many HVTs are required to reduce the incident radiation by

   (i)   a factor of at least 100

  (ii)   a factor of at least 1000

 (iii)   a factor of at least 8000?

SUMMARY

1.   Exponential change: A quantity of y is said to vary exponentially with another quantity x if equal changes of x produce equal fractional (or percentage) changes in y.

2.   Law of radioactive decay: The rate of decay $\propto$ number of atoms left of the radionuclide.

3.   Half-life: The time interval required for the activity of a radioactive sample to decay to one half of its original value.

4.   Half-Life may be measured from any starting time.

5.   Radioactivity never decays exactly to zero.

6.   Half-Value Thickness (HVT): The thickness of a substance required to reduce the transmitted intensity to one half of the incident intensity.

7.   The transmitted intensity is never reduced to zero.

8.   Logarithmic graph paper makes exponential curves straight and graphical measurement of half-life and HVT easier.

Part B
GENERAL PHYSICS

6. Experimental measurement – units, errors and statistics

6.1 THE SCIENTIFIC METHOD

Science may be described as a systematic and rational study of reality. It has three fundamental 'tools' which it uses in its attempt to understand the external world: experimental measurements, logic and theory. The theoretical aspects of science lead to the formulation of concepts and laws (such as Ohm's Law — 10.5) which explain certain phenomena and may be used in an attempt to predict other phenomena. However, the essential point is that it is the experimental evidence which is crucial, so that if experiment and theory do not agree, it is the theory which must be scrapped or modified.

For example, 'phlogiston' was once thought to be a substance essential for the explanation of combustion. However, the experimental evidence clearly showed that a body became *heavier* after burning (if all the gases were collected) and not lighter, as would have been the case if the body had 'lost its phlogiston'. The concept of phlogiston was replaced by that of the combination of the atoms of the body to oxygen atoms and the liberation of energy in the combustion process.

Similarly, 'Newtonian Physics' (see next chapter) was very successful in predicting the behaviour of a body undergoing acceleration (e.g. the orbits of planets around the sun), but was shown by Einstein to be an approximation to the truth (albeit a close one) when the velocities of the bodies were insignificant compared to the velocity of light. However, Newtonian physics has not been abandoned, unlike phlogiston, since it is sufficiently accurate for situations occurring in everyday life.

Problems arise when making experimental measurements as to what quantities to measure and how to measure them. In particular, the *units* in which the quantities are to be expressed must be precisely defined in order to achieve reproducible measurements in practice. Also there are obvious advantages if one set of units is universally adopted as a basis for all measurements.

Each of the 'base' units discussed in the next section relies on an appropriate *standard* to which each measurement is compared (directly or indirectly.) Thus, there are units of standard length, standard mass, a standard time interval, and so on. A measurement of 0.5 metre is equivalent to a distance of one half of that of the 'standard metre', for example. Without such standards no really accurate measurements can be made, which in turn retards the development of adequate theories, or models, of the world.

6.2 SI BASE UNITS

The International System of Units (SI), if universally adopted, will gradually replace the present plethora of systems of units used throughout the world by one which is based on seven standards only. These standards are termed 'base' units, and represent the fundamental questions which may be asked concerning a body:

   (i)   how big is it, and where is it? (length — metre)
  (ii)   how massive is it? (mass — kilogram)
 (iii)   how bright is it? (luminous intensity — candela)
 (iv)   how much electric charge (or flow of charge) does it possess? (electric current — ampere)
  (v)   how many elementary particles does it contain? (amount of substance — mole)
 (vi)   how hot is it? (temperature — kelvin)
(vii)   how do all the above quantities vary with time? (time — second).

Table 6.1 SI base units

Quantity	Name	Symbol
Mass	kilogram	kg
Length	metre	m
Time	second	s
Electric current	ampere	A
Temperature	kelvin	K
Luminous intensity	candela	cd
Amount of substance	mole	mol

The appropriate SI base unit is shown in parentheses after each question, and summarised in Table 6.1. The very precise modern definitions of these units are somewhat specialised and do not concern us further, although Appendix VII may be consulted for those who wish to see them.

The base units of mass, length and time are also termed 'fundamental' units, since one or more of them is always involved in the measurement of any quantity. The measurement of electric current, for example, is based on the standard of 1 ampere which involves the measurement of force between two wires separated by a given distance (13.3.1).

These seven SI base units may be combined into 'derived' units, as described below.

6.3 DERIVED SI UNITS

Many derived units, formed by combinations of the seven units described above, are sufficiently important to be given their own names. Some of these are shown in Table 6.2 and discussed in the following sections. Further derived units are considered as they present themselves in subsequent chapters.

Table 6.2 Derived units and their definition

Quantity	Definition	SI Unit	Scalar/vector
Speed	Distance travelled in unit time	metre/second ($m\ s^{-1}$)	scalar
Velocity	Distance travelled in unit time in a given direction	metre/second ($m\ s^{-1}$)	vector
Acceleration	Change of velocity in unit time	(m/second)/second ($m\ s^{-2}$)	vector
Force	Unit force on unit mass produces unit acceleration	newton (N) ($kg\ ms^{-2}$)	vector
Pressure	Force per unit area	pascal ($N\ m^{-2}$)	vector
Weight	Gravitational force on a body	newton	vector
Work	Force times distance moved by force	joule (J)	scalar
Energy	Kinetic energy: work required to bring body to rest Potential energy: work able to be performed by virtue of position or state of system	joule	scalar
Power	Rate of doing work	watt (W) (Js^{-1})	scalar
Momentum	Mass times velocity of a body	($kg\ m\ s^{-1}$)	vector

6.3.1 Speed and velocity

The speedometer in a car is calibrated in terms of miles per hour (mph) or kilometres per hour (kph), either of which serves to show that 'speed' means the distance travelled in unit time.

In SI units, therefore, speed (S) is related to distance travelled (d) in time (t) by the expression

$$S = \frac{d}{t}$$

where d is in metres, t in seconds and S therefore is metres/second, or $m\ s^{-1}$. The speedometer in the car gives no information as to the *direction* in which the car is moving. In fact, it is possible to imagine a constant speed with continuously changing direction (circling a roundabout, for example). *Velocity* is measured in the same units as speed, i.e. $m\ s^{-1}$, but the instantaneous direction in which the body is moving must be stated. Any such statement of direction makes the quantity being measured a 'vector' quantity rather than a 'scalar' quantity — e.g. the speed of a particular body may be '400 m s⁻¹' whereas the velocity of the same body might be '400 m s⁻¹ in a north-easterly direction'.

6.3.2 Acceleration

Acceleration implies a changing velocity, and is defined as the 'change in velocity per unit time'. For example, the acceleration due to gravity is approximately 9·8 metres per second per second (9·8 m s⁻²). This means that the velocity changes by 9·8 m s⁻¹ after each second. Thus, if a body is dropped, the velocity is 9·8 m s⁻¹ downwards after the first second, 19·6 m s⁻¹ after the next second and so on.

Notice that acceleration is also a vector quantity, as the acceleration has direction.

6.3.3 Force

Newton's Second Law of Motion (see 7.4) shows that the net force on a body is proportional to the mass of the body multiplied by the acceleration produced on the body. The units of force are therefore kg m s⁻² in SI units. However, the special name of a 'newton' is given to this quantity, which may be defined as:

Definition
> A net force of 1 *newton* on a body of mass 1 kg causes it to have an acceleration of 1 m s⁻²

Force is a vector quantity, as it has direction. Obviously, the force and the acceleration act in the same direction.

6.3.4 Pressure

Pressure is defined as the 'force exerted per unit area', and has the special unit of the 'pascal', where 1 pascal is 1 newton per square metre (Nm^{-2}). Pressure is therefore a vector quantity, since it has direction. The difference between force and pressure may be readily appreciated if one's foot is trodden upon by someone wearing a narrow-heeled shoe. The force exerted by the same person wearing a flat heel would have been the same, but all the force is concentrated upon a small area of one's foot, and hence is very painful!

6.3.5 Weight and mass

The mass of a body may be somewhat ambiguously described as the 'amount of matter' contained by the body. However, it is better to visualise mass as giving a body 'inertia', i.e. resistance to a change of motion when a force is applied to it. As already described above, mass is a 'fundamental' unit which is measured in terms of the standard kilogram.

The weight of a body is the downward force on the body due to the gravitational attraction of the earth. Hence, the weight of a body is expressed in newtons (not kg). The relationship between the weight, w, and the mass, m, is given by

$$w = mg$$

where g is acceleration due to gravity

A body therefore has weight *only* in the presence of a gravitational field, while it always possesses mass. Hence, a body has no weight in deep space, but it has mass since it still requires a force to change it from its path (i.e. it has inertia).

6.3.6 Work and energy

Both work and energy are measured in the same units. If a force F is applied to a body and the point of application of that force moves a distance d, then the amount of work performed, W, is defined as

$$W = F \times d$$
Equation 6.1

Thus work is just the 'force times the distance moved by the force', and is measured in *joule* where:

Definition
   1 *joule of work* is performed when a force of 1 newton moves through a distance of 1 metre.

Energy is measured in terms of work, and may be defined as 'the capacity of a body to do work'. Two *types* of energy must be distinguished, however: kinetic and potential energy.

a. Kinetic energy
Kinetic energy is the energy a body possesses by virtue of its motion, which may either be translational (i.e. movement of the whole body along a path) or rotational, or both. In both cases the amount of kinetic energy possessed by the body is just the work which would have to be done on the body to bring it completely to rest. As we shall see (7.4), a body of mass m moving at velocity v has a kinetic energy of $\frac{1}{2}mv^2$.

b. Potential energy
Potential energy is the energy possessed by a body by virtue of its condition or state. The body (or system) may be completely stationary, and only awaiting the conditions to occur which will enable it to give up its 'stored' energy. Examples of potential energy include explosives, electrical batteries and gravitational energy. In each case the amount of potential energy in the system is measured by the work the system performs while it brings its potential energy to zero. Thus, if a body of mass m is at height h above some arbitrary level, then the amount of work required to put it there in the first place is given by 'force $\times$ distance' $= mgh$ (see above). The potential energy of the body is therefore mgh, and if dropped, mgh joule of work would be performed by the body.
   Work and energy are scalar quantities, since they do not have direction.

6.3.7 Power

A particular car may reach a speed of 60 mph (or kph) in under six seconds. If another car of equal mass does the same in 20 seconds, then we would say that the first car was more *powerful*. The kinetic energy of both cars at 60 mph, given by $\frac{1}{2}mv^2$, is the same, but the first car reached that energy more quickly. Hence, *power* expresses the *rate* of energy expenditure, and since energy and work are basically the same thing, we may say that:

Definition

Power is the rate of doing work.

Thus, power is measured in joule per second ($J\ s^{-1}$). However, power is such a well-used quantity that it has its own unit, the *watt*, where

1 watt = 1 joule/second

or

$$\text{watts} = \frac{\text{joules}}{\text{seconds}} \qquad \text{Equation 6.2}$$

Example

a. If 4 kJ of work are performed over a time of 1 minute, what is the power?

From equation 6.2, the power in watt, W, is just

$$W = \frac{4000}{60} = 66\cdot7 \text{ watts}$$

b. 10 kW of power is generated for 2 minutes. What is the total energy? Again from 6.2, total energy is

$$J = 10 \times 10^3 \times 2 \times 60$$
$$\therefore \quad J = 1\cdot2 \times 10^6 \text{ joule} = 1\cdot2 \text{ MJ.}$$

6.3.8 Momentum

In everyday speech, 'momentum' expresses the ability of a moving body to 'keep going', which depends both on the mass and the velocity of the body. In scientific use, where all terms are to have an exact meaning, the momentum is defined as the mass of a body multiplied by its velocity. Since momentum has a direction, it is a vector quantity. Momentum is discussed further in the next chapter (7.3).

6.4 UNITS USED IN RADIOGRAPHY

Many derived units are used in radiography, as in other subjects, e.g. joule, watt, coulomb, etc. However, other units outside the strict adherence to the SI system are especially useful to radiography and are unlikely to be discontinued owing to their practical convenience. These are shown in Table 6.3 and described below.

Table 6.3 Special units for radiography

Unit	Definition
kV_p	Maximum kilovoltage applied across X-ray tube in forward direction
mA	Average electric current passing through X-ray tube in milliampere
mAs	mA × time of exposure in seconds (1 mAs = 1 millicoulomb of charge)
keV	Energy imparted to electron passing through potential difference of 1 kV
HU	kV_p × mAs — a measure of heat energy deposited on anode by one exposure

6.4.1 (kV$_p$)

The potential difference (Ch. 9) existing between the cathode and anode of an X-ray tube is measured in kilovolts, where $1 \text{ kV} = 10^3 \text{ V}$ (see 1.6). However, in many X-ray units this potential difference is not constant but varies as a result of the frequency of the electrical supply. Hence, it is conventional practice to quote the *peak* (i.e. maximum) value of the potential difference which exists across the X-ray tube. Thus, a unit operating at, say, 50 kV$_p$ has a maximum, or peak, potential difference of 50 kV. Obviously, the suffix 'p' stands for 'peak'.

In addition, the kV$_p$ setting determines the maximum energy of the X-ray photons emitted (see Ch. 28), so that a 50 kV$_p$ potential difference yields a maximum photon energy of 50 keV (see 6.4.3). The *average* energy of the X-ray photons is $\frac{1}{3}$ to $\frac{1}{2}$ of this value.

As we shall see later (Ch. 28 and 29), the kV$_p$ alters both the *intensity* and *quality* of the beam.

6.4.2 mA and mAs

Production of X-rays occurs when a fast moving beam of electrons from the cathode of an X-ray tube strikes the anode (Ch. 21). The intensity of the X-ray beam is proportional to (1.7) the rate at which the electrons strike the anode, which is intuitively what we would expect. Now, the number of electrons flowing per second is just a measure of the electrical *current* (Ch. 10) flowing through the X-ray tube. The SI unit of current is the ampere (A), and is such that there is a flow of approximately 6.0×10^{18} electrons/sec for 1 A. This is too large a unit for practical radiography, so that milliamperes (mA) are used to measure current flow through an X-ray tube, where $1 \text{ mA} = 10^{-3} \text{ A}$ (1.6).

It is theoretically possible, of course, to keep 200 mA (say) flowing through the tube indefinitely (although damage would result in so doing). Thus, any radiographic film used in taking a radiograph would become blacker until totally useless for diagnostic purposes. Hence, a time limit is required to produce a diagnostically acceptable image on the film. This time limit is called the 'exposure time', and depends on many factors, such as kV$_p$, film type, grid ratio, focus to film distance (FFD), etc. However, if all these other factors are kept constant then it is the *total* number of X-rays reaching the film that determines the photographic exposure. Now, from the foregoing arguments, the total number of electrons striking the anode determines the total number of X-rays emitted by the anode. This number of electrons may flow either over a short or a long exposure time, but the photographic exposure will be the same, since the same number of X-rays will have reached the film.

The unit used to describe the total electron flow through an X-ray tube is the milliampere-second (mAs), and is obtained by *multiplying* (NOT dividing) the mA by the exposure time in seconds (s).

For example, if 60 mAs is required to produce an acceptable photographic image (all other factors being specified), then this may be delivered in any of the following ways:

a. 10 mA for 6 seconds

b.   20 mA for 3 seconds
c.   30 mA for 2 seconds
d.   300 mA for 0·2 seconds, etc.

In each case, the mA value times the exposure time is constant at 60 mAs.

As we shall see (Ch. 10), the mAs is equivalent to the *millicoulomb* (10^{-3} C), which is a unit of electrical charge and therefore proportional to the *total* number of electrons striking the anode during an exposure. However, the mAs is used in preference to the millicoulomb as it makes it obvious that it is both tube mA and exposure time that are able to be adjusted on the X-ray unit.

6.4.3 keV

The electron-volt (eV) is a unit of energy of great convenience in physics, radiography and radiotherapy. The kiloelectron-volt (keV) is just 10^3 eV.

If an electron is accelerated from rest across a potential difference of 1 volt, then the kinetic energy it attains is defined as 1 eV.

In general, the energy, E, is given by:

$E = eV$ joule   Equation 6.3

Where e is the electrical charge on the electron ($1·6 \times 10^{-19}$ coulomb) and V is the potential difference in volts (Ch. 9 and 10). Thus,

1 eV $= 1·6 \times 10^{-19}$ joule

If, therefore, an X-ray tube is subject to a potential difference of 75 kV$_p$, then we know that the energy of the electrons striking the anode must be 75 keV. This is because the X-ray tube is basically a device for accelerating electrons, which travel across a potential difference of the kV$_p$ of the tube. Thus, some X-rays will also be emitted at an energy of 75 keV, corresponding to the whole of the energy of some of the electrons being converted directly to X-ray photon energy (Ch. 28).

6.4.4 Heat Units (HU)

When the energetic electrons strike the anode of the X-ray tube, they are quickly brought to rest within the tungsten (Ch. 28). Thus, they deposit all their energy onto a small area of the 'target'. Some of this energy is converted into X-rays, but most (95–99%) is converted into heat, i.e. the atoms in the tungsten target are given a higher kinetic energy by the decelerating electrons (Ch. 8). It is important to know how much heat a particular exposure, or series of exposures, will deposit on the target area, for too much heat may easily damage the anode and make the X-ray tube useless. A convenient unit for such a purpose is the Heat Unit (HU) which gives a useful measure of the heat energy imparted to the anode. In Chapter 10 it is shown that the total energy dissipated by a current I driven by a potential difference V is given by

$E = VIt$ joule

Where V is in volts, I in amperes and t in seconds.

This equation is correct only if V and I remain constant for the time t, which is not necessarily the case for an X-ray tube. Strictly, then, the 'effective' or 'RMS' values of V and I should be used (15.2.3) to obtain an absolute measure of the energy imparted to the anode, but this is not essential, as long as each X-ray tube is *calibrated* in terms of convenient measures of V and I. Such units are, of course, kV_p and mA.

However, mA $\times$ t = mAs (6.4.2), so that we obtain finally:

Heat units = kV_p $\times$ mAs   Equation 6.4

To reiterate, provided that the manufacturer quotes the maximum permissible heat loading in terms of Heat Units, then an accurately quantitive measure of heat energy in joule is not required. The permissible value of HUs is dependent on the type of rectification, focal spot size, anode rotation speed, anode cooling characteristics and frequency and time of exposure(s) as described in Chapter 22.

6.5 EXPERIMENTAL ERRORS

6.5.1 How exact is accurate?

As outlined above, Physics attempts to be an exact science based on accurate measurements of defined quantities such as mass, length, temperature and time. However, no instrument is able to give a truly exact value of the quantity being measured, since errors of measurement or of observation will always be present. Used in this sense, an error of measurement is not the same thing as a mistake but just an uncertainty as to the correct value of a measured quantity.

For example, suppose that we are using a moving-coil meter (17.5) to measure an electrical current. Among many possible sources of error, the following may be present:

a. an observational error due to the thickness of the pointer on the scale
b. an observational error due to incorrect interpolation between scale markings
c. an observational error due to poor technique (e.g. not looking at right-angle to the scale)
d. a measurement error due to an incorrect 'zero', i.e. the pointer is not on the scale zero mark when no current flows
e. a measurement error due to the scale being incorrectly calibrated
f. a measurement error due to the act of measuring the current changing the current being measured (17.2).

Finding and reducing the effects of possible sources of error in a measurement is essential if an accurate, even if not exact, reading is to be taken.

How accurate do we need to be? Well, this depends upon why a particular measurement is being performed. If we make an error of 2 mm in an FSD

(Ch. 2) setting of 50 cm, then the effect will be negligible on a conventional radiograph. However, a fault in an X-ray tube which produced the same error of 2 mm in an effective focal spot size of 1 mm (3.1) will have the observable effect of increasing the unsharpness (3.4) quite markedly. The fractional (or percentage) error is important, therefore, and is discussed in more detail in Section 6.5.3.

Basically, the errors of measurement are sufficiently small if they do not affect the conclusions drawn from a result of a measurement or affect a procedure being undertaken (e.g. radiograph or radiotherapy treatment). In radiography or radiotherapy practice, errors of 1 mm when setting a distance or 1 degree when setting an angle are usually considered to be sufficiently accurate.

6.5.2 Random and systematic errors

Random errors are those errors which, on repeated measurements of the same quantity, are variable in size and have no discernible pattern or sequence. This may be due to the quantity itself varying in a random manner (e.g. number of radioactive disintegrations per second — Appendix V) or due to slight differences in the measurement technique of the observer on each occasion. Alternatively, the ambient conditions of temperature, pressure or humidity etc. may affect the instrument being used in an apparently random manner.

Systematic errors may arise either from the observer or from the instrument itself, and may be a constant or vary in some regular (i.e. non-random manner). For example, the measurement of a length using a ruler with the zero incorrectly positioned will give rise to results which are systematically in error by a constant amount, e.g. 10·3 cm and 4·6 cm when the correct values are 10.0 cm and 4.3 cm respectively, when the zero is displaced by 3 mm.

Many sources of error are wholly random or systematic, but most errors encountered in practical situations are the result of both types. The reader may like to inspect the list of meter errors in the previous section and decide where the random and systematic errors might lie!

The existence of random and systematic errors leads to the concept of *accuracy* versus *precision*. Precision is a measure of the repeatability of a series of measurements, while accuracy is a measure of the correspondence between the result obtained and its exact value. The precision of a series of readings may be quite high in that they all might lie close to each other, but the accuracy may be poor if there is a significant systematic error involved. A faulty scale on a meter or a ruler, for example, will give the 'wrong' answers even though the readings taken from the scale may be highly repeatable. Precision leads to accuracy, therefore, if the systematic errors have been eliminated or corrected. It is the usual practice in physics to record a result with the estimated error in the form:

true value = measured value ± estimated error

If we have the statement that FSD = 50·0 ± 0·2 cm, then it is implied that the true value of the FSD lies somewhere between the values 49·8 cm and 50·2 cm.

Mathematically, if the error is e, the measured value is m and the true value is t, then $e = m - t$, since the error is just the difference between the measured and true values. Rearranging this, we have:

$$m = t + e$$ Equation 6.5

where the error e may be positive or negative.

The magnitude of e may be reduced by careful measurement technique and where possible, the recording of a large number of readings so that a mean value (6.6.1) may be taken.

6.5.3 Fractional and percentage errors

In practice, it is often useful to express an error in relation to the magnitude of the quantity being measured. If it is possible to measure to within 1 mm when using a particular ruler, then this error will become progressively less important as lengths of 1 cm, 10 cm, 1 m, 1 km are taken. Expressing the error of 1 mm as a fraction of the measured value, we obtain 0·1, 0·01, 0·001, 0·000001 or 10%, 1%, 0·1%, 0·0001% respectively. This concept of a fractional or percentage error is important because it helps us to predict what accuracy we need for our individual measurements in order to achieve a given percentage error in the final result. If we wish to measure the area of a rectangle to within 1%, for example, then it may be shown (6.5.4) that it is necessary to measure the sides to an accuracy of 0·5%. Hence, a 10% error would be much too high while a 0·001% error would be unnecessarily restrictive for our purpose. A knowledge of the accuracies required also has an effect on the experimental apparatus used, for a 0·5% error in a 1 mm length is 0·005 mm — well beyond the capabilities of a ruler, so that a travelling microscope would be more suitable — while a 0·5% error in a length of 10 cm is 0·5 mm, enabling an accurate ruler to be used.

If we give the fractional error in a quantity the symbol f, then f is just the size of the error (i.e. measured value, m, minus true value, t) divided by the true value, t, of the quantity, so that $f = (m - t)/t$. Rearranging this equation, we have

$$m = t(1 + f)$$ Equation 6.6

6.5.4 Combining errors

This section illustrates how to combine errors in some simple examples to obtain an error in the final result.

Error in a product
To take the previous example of measuring the sides of a rectangle, then the measured area A is just the product of the measured lengths of the sides. Now, if the exact lengths are a and b, and the fractional errors are taken as f_a and f_b,

then from Equation 6.6 the measured lengths are just $a(1 + f_a)$, $b(1 + f_b)$ respectively. Hence:

$$A = a(1 + f_a) \cdot b(1 + f_b) = ab(1 + f_a) \cdot (1 + f_b)$$
$$= ab(1 + f_a + f_b + f_a \cdot f_b)$$

Now, the product $f_a \cdot f_b$ is very small compared with f_a and f_b (e.g. if f_a and $f_b = 0 \cdot 01$, then $f_a \cdot f_b = 0 \cdot 0001$) and may be neglected, so that we obtain:

$$A = ab(1 + f_a + f_b)$$

We now relate this to f_A, which is the fractional error in the exact area, ab, due to the errors involved in measuring the sides a and b. Equation 6.6 gives us: $A = ab(1 + f_A)$, so by comparison with the above formula we have finally that $f_A = f_a + f_b$. Hence, the fractional error in the area, f_A, is just the sum of the fractional errors f_a, f_b produced when measuring the two sides.

Generally, if we have a product involving several terms then, in words:

> The fractional (or percentage) error in a product is the sum of the individual fractional (or percentage) errors of each term in the product.

As another example, if the mA is in error by $+5\%$ and the exposure time is in error by -2%, then the percentage error in the mAs (6.4.2) is $+3\%$. Frequently, however, the sign of the errors in unknown, so they are both taken as either positive or negative to obtain an error band about the measured value. This constitutes the 'worst case' size of the error.

Error in a quotient
If we divide one measured value of an exact quantity, a, by another measured value of an exact quantity, b, then the result obained, R, is given by:

$$R = \frac{a(1 + f_a)}{b(1 + f_b)}$$

where f_a and f_b are the fractional errors in a and b.

$$\therefore \quad R = \frac{a}{b} \cdot (1 + f_a)(1 - f_b) \qquad \text{(approximately)}$$

Expanding the two brackets (1.3.3), and ignoring $f_A \cdot f_B$ as described above, we have:

$$R = \frac{a}{b} \cdot (1 + f_a - f_b)$$

So that the fractional error in R is $f_a - f_b$. Hence, the fractional error in a quotient is obtained by subtracting the fractional error of the denominator from that of the nominator. If the signs of the errors are unknown, however, then the worst case is obtained by *adding* the fractional errors.

Error in a sum
If S is obtained by summing measured quantities a and b (whose exact values

are $a0$ and $b0$, and whose errors are e_a, e_b), then:

$$S = (a0 + e_a) + (b0 + e_b) = a0 + b0 + e_a + e_b.$$

Hence, as may be expected, the error in a sum is just the sum of the individual errors. As in the two previous sections, if the signs of the errors are unknown, then the worst case error is still obtained by adding the magnitudes of the errors, i.e. assuming both are either positive or both negative. The fractional error in S, f_S is given by the formula:

$$f_S = \frac{a0 \cdot f_a + b0 \cdot f_b}{a0 + b0}$$

so that the fractional error in a sum depends upon the relative magnitudes of the individual terms and their fractional errors.

Insight

Calculus may be used to obtain an expression for an error by differentiating and treating dx and dy as errors in x and y, as shown in the following examples:

Expression	Error	
$y = a + b$	$dy = da + db$	(see paragraph above)
$y = a \cdot b$	$dy = a \cdot db + b \cdot da$	
	$\therefore\ dy/y = db/b + da/a$	(fractional error in $a \cdot b$)
$y = a/b$	$dy = (b \cdot da - a \cdot db)/b \cdot b$	
	$\therefore\ dy/y = da/a - db/b$	(fractional error in a/b)
$y = x^2$	$dy = 2x\, dx$	
	$\therefore\ dy/y = 2\, dx/x$	
$y = k/x^2$	$dy = -2k\, dx/x^3$	
	$\therefore\ dy/y = -2\, dx/x$	

The last example shows that the relative error in the measurement of radiation from a source when using the Inverse Square Law decreases as the distance from the source increases, i.e. dx/x decreases as x increases.

6.5.5 Examples of errors in practical radiography

Whenever a measurement is made or a procedure is undertaken, inexact quantities will be involved. These are present in even the best and most careful of techniques and do not necessarily invalidate the results of the measurements or procedures performed. It is important to be aware of the magnitude of the errors, however, in order to be confident of the validity of the procedure. This is particularly important in radiotherapy, where the radiation dose delivered to the patient over a course of treatment must be as accurate and as reproducible as can be realistically achievable. For example, an inherent 'chain of errors' exists in the calibration procedure of a therapy machine which involves errors in the following:

— errors of measurement from an ionisation chamber (32.3.1) placed in the beam

— errors in correcting the above reading for temperature and pressure (32.2.2)

— errors in correcting for various calibration factors (32.3.1)

— errors in the positioning of the chamber

— errors in the reproducibility of the therapy machine's output doserate

— 'switch-on' and 'switch-off' errors, i.e. the output doserate does not immediately assume its steady value on switch-on, nor immediately drop to zero on switch-off

— errors in relating the measured doserate to the '100%' value of an isodose distribution (34.2.1) since, in many cases, it is not practicable to measure the 100% value, but some known percentage depth-dose at, say, 5 cm in water.

If all these errors act in the same direction, for example all tending to make the doserate larger than it really is, then an overall error of 5% or greater is possible. Hence, great attention to detail is required in order to reduce the percentage error to 1% or less.

Further examples of areas where significant errors may occur are shown in Table 6.4.

Table 6.4

Measurement/ procedure	Method	Potential sources of error	Comment
FSD/SSD setting	Applicator Pointer Optical Indicator	Incorrect length Reading error Incorrect alignment	Systematic Random and systematic Systematic
Field Size adjustment	Motorised Collimators	Calibration error; mechanical backlash	
Focal spot size measurement	Pinhole in lead sheet	Size of pinhole; 'off-focal' radiation; distances in error	
Film magnification	Object of known size on skin, and film taken	Estimation of patient's thickness; movement; estimate of image size on film; angle of object to central ray	(see 3.3)
Quality/Filtration of X-ray beam	Ardran-Crookes penetrameter/Multiple detector system controlled by microprocessor	Optical density estimate; rectification system; regulation with mA	Multiple detectors may also be used to measure kVp
Output Doserate measurement	Ionisation chamber	Calibration/correction factors	(see 6.5.5)
kVp selection	Selector on console/ 'Pre-reading' meter	Cable voltage drop; Rectifier voltage drop; mA regulation; Space-charge effects; Mains variation; Meter-reading errors	(see 10.8) (see 19.3.4) (see 16.3.3) (see 18.6) (see 17.7.1) (see 6.5.1)

Measurement/ procedure	Method	Potential sources of error	Comment
mA/mAs selection	Selector on console	Mains variation Gassy tube Worn filament	(see 17.7.1) mA increases & fluctuates Emission decreases
Exposure time	Timer/mAs selector	Inaccurate timer	e.g. clockwork timers on portables
H.V.T. estimate	Attenuation measurements through thin metal filters e.g. Al, Cu, Sn, Pb	Scatter reaching detector; Intensity fluctuating during measurements	(see 5.4)
TLD measurement of radiation dose	Heating TLD dosimeter and measuring the light emitted with a photomultiplier	Variation in sensitivity within same TLD batch; surface contamination; presence of oxygen; dependence on measurement time; ageing effects	(see 32.3.4)
'Isodose' line measurement of therapy beam	Small remotely-controlled probe in a water tank	Probe positional errors; probe size; fluctuating beam intensity; effect of tank depth on scatter contribution; error in '100%' value	A fixed reference probe may be used to reduce errors due to intensity fluctuations
Radionuclide Therapy	Drink of I131 as NaI; Injection of P32 or Y90 colloid	Dispensing errors; errors in measurement in ion-chamber due to calibration factors and sample volume; activity left in container/syringe after dose given	(see 39.4)
Interstitial/ Intacavitary Therapy	Ir192 wires; automatic or manual afterloaders; radium tubes and needles; Au198 grains	Estimate of activity; effect of radioactive decay over period of treatment; source positional errors; estimate of contribution of scatter to dose; errors in estimates of patient's treatment volume and position; movement during treatment; effect of dose rate on treatment	(see 34.3.1)
Measurement of radioactivity within an organ	Collimated scintillation detector	Incorrect positioning; insufficient counts; unknown organ depth	10 000 counts are required to give a 1% error (S.D.) (see Appendix V)

6.6 STATISTICS

In the preceeding sections it was described how repeated measurements of the same quantity reduce, but not eliminate, the errors of measurement associated with that quantity. This is the situation where a quantity (e.g. a length) has an exact value but where the measured values are clustered around the exact value.

There is another class of measurements which involves a cluster (or population) of values, and that is when measurements are made on different objects belonging to the same category. In this case, the errors of measurement on an individual object may be completely negligible when compared to the magnitude of the natural variation between the objects themselves. For example, the heights of all the radiographers within a given department will probably exhibit quite a large variation and certainly more than the errors involved in measuring the height of one radiographer.

The body of knowledge which concerns itself with the analysis of information ('data') obtained from observations is known as *statistics*. There are two types of statistics: *descriptive* and *inferential*. Descriptive statistics is concerned solely with such things as the organisation of the data, its graphical display, numerical calculations of means etc., while inferential statistics may be described as the science of making decisions in the face of uncertainty (i.e. on the basis of incomplete information). The latter is the situation frequently encountered in the field of medical statistics where complete information is rarely available.

A group of items belonging to the same category is known as a *population*. A population may be very large (e.g. the number of atoms in a radioactive sample) or small. Note that 'population' as used here does not necessarily imply that people are involved.

Where it is difficult or impossible to collect data on every member of a population, it is necessary only to select a representative sample of that population such that the smaller and more manageable sample has all the important characteristics of the population from which it was drawn, save that of size. This technique is known as 'random sampling', and is much used in public opinion polls, for example. If the sample were not 'random', then there would be a bias in the data collected which would not be present in the larger population and false conclusions may be drawn. To give a trivial example, an accurate figure for the average salary of people between the ages of, say, 25 and 30 years is not obtained if data from stockbrokers only is used.

6.6.1 Measures of location and deviation

The graphical representation of the data associated with a population is usually drawn with the measured values on the X-axis and the number of each measured value on the Y-axis. The position of the graph so obtained on the X-axis is known as the *location* of the population, and the width of the graph is its *deviation*. The statistical quantities (usually just called 'statistics') which are used to measure location are the mean, mode or median, while the statistic used to measure deviation is the 'standard deviation'. These are described below, together with some other statistical measures.

Mean, mode and median of a population

The mean value of a population is the same as the average, and is obtained by dividing the sum of all the data by the number of items in the population. This is shown by the formula:

$$\bar{X} = \frac{\sum_{i=1}^{n} X_i}{n}$$

Equation 6.7

Here, $\bar{X}$ is the mean value, X_i is the ith measured value of the population and n is the number of items. Hence i takes values between 1 and n. The term $\sum_{i=1}^{n} X_i$ means the sum of all the values of X from $i = 1$ to $i = n$, i.e. the sum of the values of all the measurements. Dividing by n produces a value which is somewhere between the minimum and maximum values of the data which forms the population. An alternative way of considering the mean is to subtract it from all the other values of X. When this is done, the positive values exactly cancel out the negative values.

The value which occurs most frequently in a given population is not necessarily the mean value, however. Figure 6.1a–6.1d shows that there are two other measures, or statistics, of curve location: the mode and the median. The *mode* is defined as the value which occurs most frequently, and the *median* is the middle value of all the measurements (e.g. in a series of measurements: 1, 2, 4, 4, 5, 6, 6, 6, 7 the median is 5 and the mode is 6). The figures show how these three statistics vary with asymmetrical distributions of values, for 'positive skewness' in Figure 6.1b and 'negative skewness' in Figure 6.1c.

The standard deviation is a measure of the variation in the values of a distribution, i.e. by how much the distribution deviates from the mean value. Two symmetrical distributions with the same mean but different standard deviations are shown in Figure 6.2. In a population of n samples and where the ith measured value (i varies from 1 to n) is x_i, either of the two formulae shown below may be used to calculate the standard deviation, σ, of the distribution:

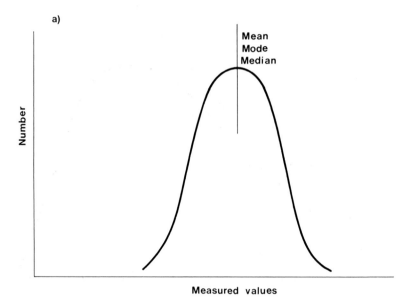

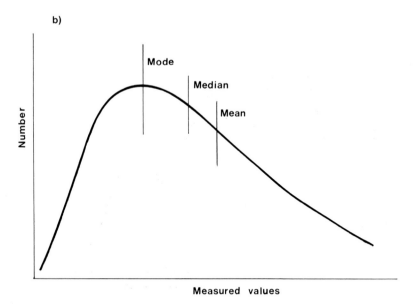

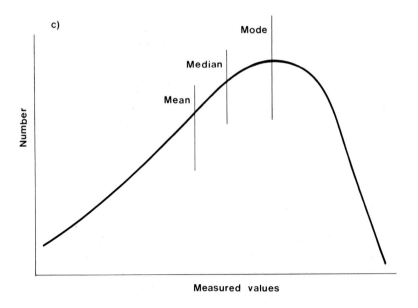

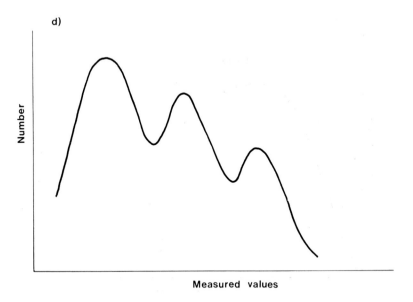

Fig. 6.1 Measures of location of a population: (a) symmetrical distribution, (b) positive skewness, (c) negative skewness, (d) multimodal distribution.

Standard deviation of a population

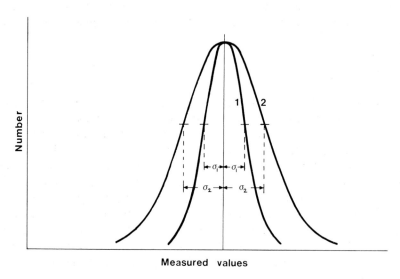

Measured values

Fig. 6.2 The standard deviations of two symmetrical populations 1 and 2, with both distributions having the same means.

$$\sigma = \sqrt{\dfrac{\displaystyle\sum_{i=1}^{n} (X_i - \bar{X})^2}{n-1}}$$

$$\sigma = \sqrt{\dfrac{\displaystyle\sum_{i=1}^{n} (X_i^2) - \dfrac{\left(\displaystyle\sum_{i=1}^{n} X_i\right)^2}{n}}{n-1}}$$

Equation 6.8

The second formula is particularly convenient when using a calculator or computer, since the mean need not be calculated first.

The *coefficient of variation* expresses the standard deviation as a percentage of the mean of a distribution and is equal to $100\sigma/\bar{x}\%$.

Standard error of the mean
There will inevitably be an uncertainty, even if small, in the practical measurement of a mean value due to the errors inherent in the original observations (6.5.2). This uncertainty may be expressed as the standard error of the mean, and is given by:

$$\text{S.E.} = \dfrac{\sigma}{\sqrt{n}}$$

Equation 6.9

It may be shown that it is 68% probable that the true value of the mean (ignoring systematic errors — 6.5.2) lies within one standard error above or below the measured mean. Notice that both the standard deviation and standard error of the mean become smaller as the number of measurements, n, increases.

6.6.2 Statistics and radiology

Statistical methods are used widely in all aspects of diagnostic imaging and radiotherapy, and this section touches upon a few examples.

The analysis of sizes and types of X-ray films used in different diagnostic investigations is a useful method for predicting future film requirements, and hence reducing waste. Similarly, the reasons for repeated investigations may be itemised and numbered, so leading to a clearer understanding of the commonest causes of faulty radiographs. From this analysis, steps may be taken to reduce the number of repeated investigations leading to reduced film wastage, better financial management, and a lower radiation dose to the patient. Neither of these two examples imposes a complex mathematical or statistical burden on a department, but there are real advantages to be gained in using them.

A rather more fundamental (and visible) example of statistics in X-ray imaging is the so-called 'quantum mottle' seen on a television monitor when screening a patient using an image intensification system. This mottle, or quantum noise, is particularly noticeable at low mA or when short-persistence phosphors are used in the intensification system. It is due to the statistical variation of the video signal, which in turn is caused by the random variation in the production of electrons from the faceplate of the intensifier. At the desired low doserates for screening, there is random variation in the mean values of the X-ray intensity transmitted through the patient, and hence in the production of electrons from the faceplate of the intensifier, the light emitted from the intensifier phosphor and reaching the television camera tube, and the generation of an electrical video signal from the target of the tube. The standard deviation of an average of N electrons produced per second is just $\sqrt{N}$, so that increasing the mA by a factor of 4 increases the mottle by an absolute factor of 2 (i.e. $\sqrt{4}$). However, the *relative* quantum mottle has been reduced from $\sqrt{N}/N = 1/\sqrt{N}$ to $\sqrt{4N}/4N = 1/2\sqrt{N}$, so that there has been a halving of the perceived 'noise' on the television monitor. Hence, the effect of quantum mottle on the image is reduced as the mA is increased. Obviously a balance must be struck between using such a low doserate that the picture obtained is not adequate for diagnostic purposes or using such a high doserate that the patient receives an unnecessarily high radiation dose. A high-output X-ray tube is required on a CT scanner, for example, in order to reduce the quantum noise in the reconstructed sectional image which otherwise would hide structural detail.

A measurement of the fetal biparietal diameter or the crown-rump distance may be used to estimate the age of the fetus. However, not all fetuses grow at the same rate, so a range of normal values for different fetal ages and ethnic groups is first determined by ultrasonic methods, and an unknown age may then be read from an appropriate graph. This is a simple technique, but how may we assess the accuracy of the age read from such a graph — is it within a day, a week or a month? Figure 6.3 shows a plot of the mean biparietal diameter (bpd) against age together with a pair of lines separated from the mean by 2 standard deviations. This means that at any given age, the bpd will be about 95% certain to lie somewhere between the -2σ line and the $+2\sigma$ line. A measured bpd may be used to estimate an age by drawing a horizontal line on the graph and reading the intersections of the three lines on the Age axis. We may then say that a normal fetus' age is 95% probable to lie between these three lines, with the most likely age given by the mean value. Note that the lines separate more as the age increases, so that there is more uncertainty closer to term than earlier. A typical age estimated by the graph will be accurate to within 1 to 2 weeks, and it is quite unrealistic to expect to be more accurate than this — not because the measurement technique needs improvement, but because of the natural variation in the population of bpds.

In radiotherapy, the absorbed radiation dose to a tumour volume is specified by the radiotherapist. However, in a practical situation, it may be known that the absorbed dose is not constant over the whole of the volume to be treated. The radiotherapist may therefore specify a particular dose to a given point, a mean dose or a modal dose depending upon the clinical situation. The mean or modal dose to a volume may be calculated from a computer printout of the dose distribution.

Statistical methods may be used to select between two different diagnostic or treatment regimes in order to discover which one gives better diagnostic information or treatment results. It is important to select appropriate

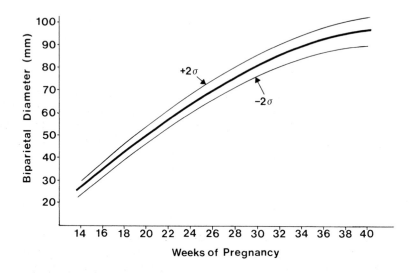

Fig. 6.3 Typical appearance of graph relating the age of a fetus to its mean biparietal diameter (bpd). Also shown are the 2 standard deviation limits on either side of the mean, within which 95% of normal values lie.

parameters to measure the relative performance of the two techniques. These may include the number of 'false positives' or 'false negatives' for a diagnostic test, or the '5-year survival rate' or suitably defined 'quality of life' for a therapeutic regime. In any event, a population of values will exist for each regime, and statistical tests of the differences between populations may be used to distinguish between the two techniques in question.

Finally, statistical methods are employed to find correlations between disease and the environment. This branch of study is known as *epidemiology* and is valuable in suggesting causal links between our way of life, or the pollution in our environment, and the diseases we suffer. This may be performed on a local, national or international level. Obvious examples include smoking and lung cancer or diet and heart disease.

Excercise 6.1

a.   What are the fractional and percentage errors in an mA value which is set to 20, but which is really 22?

b.   If a kVp setting is in error by $+5\%$, the mA by -1%, and the timer over-estimates by 2%, what is the percentage error in the Heat Units delivered during an exposure? (see Equation 6.4)

c.   Which condition results in a greater effect on the Intensity of an X-ray beam:

  (i)   an error of 10% in the mA
  (ii) an error of 10% in the kVp?
(Note: Intensity is proportional to mA $\times$ kVp^2 — see 28.2.2)

d.   A particular exposure-timer is always in error by 0.01 s. What is the percentage error in the actual exposure time for the following set times: 0.01 s, 0.02 s, 0.1 s, 0.5 s, 1.0 s?

e.   Find the mean and the median of the following samples:

  (i)   37, 34, 40, 35, 33, 36, 37
  (ii)   10, 4, 6, 11, 13, 8, 11
  (iii) 52, 70, 37, 55, 42, 31, 47

f.   The following readings are taken with a Balwin-Farmer dose-measuring system for a series of 1 minute exposures on a therapy machine: 69.92, 70.20, 69.95, 70.14, 70.14, 69.97, 70.02, 70.24, 70.10, 70.00. Calculate the mean, standard deviation and standard error of the mean of this population. State the range where 95% of all such readings would lie.

SUMMARY

1.   All measurements are based upon 'standard' units of seven independent quantities: mass, length, time, temperature, electric current, brightness and number of elementary particles in a body. In particular, mass, length and time are called the 'fundamental' units of measurements.

2.   The SI system of units is based upon the metre, kilogram and second for the measurement of length, mass and time respectively. The other 'base' units

are: kelvin (temperature), ampere (electric current), candela (brightness) and mole (number of particles in a body).

3.   'Derived' units are formed from combinations of the base units. Many derived units are sufficiently important to have special names, e.g. newton (force), joule (energy), watt (power). See Table 6.2 for the definitions of these and other derived units.

4.   There are additional types of unit which, although not strictly conforming to the SI system, are nevertheless of such great practical use that they are likely to be retained. Examples of these units in medicine include the measurement of blood pressure in mm of mercury (rather than newton per square metre), and in radiography the units of kV_p, mAs, keV and HU (see Table 6.3).

5.   Experimental measurements are always subject to errors, both random and systematic.

6.   The precision of a set of measurements is a measure of their repeatability, while their accuracy is how close they are to the exact result.

7.   Accuracy is improved by taking a large number of measurements and correcting for the sources of systematic errors.

8.   The fractional error is the error divided by the mean value.

9.   The fractional error in a product is obtained by adding the individual fractional errors of each term in the product, and the fractional error in a quotient by subtracting them. If the signs of the errors are unknown, they are added to obtain the 'worst case' error.

10.   The location of a distribution of measurements (a 'population') may be defined either by the mean, the mode or the median.

11.   A measure of the spread of a population is given by the standard deviation, where 68% of all values lie between -1 and $+1$ standard deviation from the mean, and 95% of values lie within -2 and $+2$ standard deviation.

7. Laws of physics (classical)

Direct or indirect reference is made to the basic laws of physics throughout this book, so that it is as well to review these laws here before going any further. However, the laws of 'modern' physics, which include concepts from Einstein's Relativity Theory (1905) and Quantum Theory (1900) will not concern us until Chapter 24 onwards, so that only 'Classical' physics will be discussed in this chapter. Modern physics is introduced in Chapter 23.

7.1 CONSERVATION OF MATTER (MASS)

Statement
Matter is neither created nor destroyed, but may change its chemical form.
form.

This law was propounded after discovering that the total mass after a chemical reaction was the same as the total mass of the ingredients before it.

7.2 CONSERVATION OF ENERGY

Statement
The total amount of energy in a system is constant.

Here, the total amount of energy is obtained by summing all the kinetic energies (KE) and potential energies (PE) of the system in question. This law implies that energy is never 'used up', but merely changes from one form to another.

Some of the common forms of energy are listed below:

Chemical	Kinetic
Gravitational	Sound
Electrical	Radiation
Nuclear	Heat

Can you think of an example of each and the ways in which energy in one form may be changed to others? (Use the production of X-rays as one of your examples.) These two classical laws on the conservation of mass and energy are combined into one law by modern physics (Ch. 23).

7.3 CONSERVATION OF MOMENTUM

Statement
The total linear or rotational momentum in a given system is constant.

This conservation law is as fundamental to physics as the law of conservation of energy. For example, there are two types of collisions which occur between bodies: elastic and inelastic. An *elastic* is one in which the total kinetic energy is conserved, as in the case of two 'perfect' billiard balls colliding, and an *inelastic* collision is one in which the total kinetic energy is not conserved. In both cases, however, the total momentum is conserved although the velocities of the bodies after impact will be different in the two cases. Consideration of the conservation of momentum in this book is mainly confined to the interactions of X-rays with matter (Ch. 30), although the law is universal.

7.4 NEWTON'S LAWS OF MOTION

Newton's Laws of Motion may be derived from the foregoing laws, but they are so useful as to merit a separate section. They are defined as follows:

Law 1: A body is at rest or has a constant velocity unless acted upon by a net external force.

Law 2: The rate of change of momentum of the body is proportional to the applied force.

Law 3: The action of one body on a second body is always accompanied by an equal and opposite action of the second body on the first.

The terms 'velocity' and 'momentum' in the first two laws imply *direction*, as they are both vector quantities (6.3.1).
If a body of mass m and velocity u has a force F applied to it, and the velocity has changed to v after a time t, then the mathematical equivalent of the second law is:

$$\frac{mv - mu}{t} \propto F \qquad \qquad \text{(see 1.7)}$$

i.e. $\quad \dfrac{m(v - u)}{t} \propto F$

Now $(v - u)/t$ is just the acceleration, a, of the body, from the definition of acceleration (6.3.2).
Hence, $ma \propto F$, or $F = kma$, where k is a constant of proportionality (1.7).

By suitable selection of units, k may be made equal to unity, and we have, finally:

$$F = ma \qquad\qquad \text{Equation 7.1}$$

This is the familiar equation of Newton's Second Law. In SI units, F is in newtons, m in kg and a in ms^{-2}. Equation 7.1 is used as the basis of the definition of the newton (6.3.3), i.e. 1 newton = 1 kg $\times$ 1 ms^{-2}

Insight

As an illustration of the use of this law, we are now in a position to calculate the kinetic energy as a body of mass m moving at a velocity v. If we apply a steady force F in the opposite direction to that of v, the body will slow down and eventually come to rest. The kinetic energy (E) of the body is just the work done by F in bringing the body to rest (6.3.6),

i.e. $\quad E = -F \times s \qquad\qquad \text{Equation 7.2}$

where s is the distance taken for the body to come to rest. (F is negative, since it acts in opposition to v — as does the acceleration a.) From Newton's Second Law, $F = ma$ so that the above equation becomes:

$$E = -m \times a \times s \qquad\qquad \text{Equation 7.3}$$

The acceleration, a, is the 'change in velocity per unit time'

i.e. $\quad -\dfrac{v}{t}$

and the time taken to stop is given by t = distance/average velocity

i.e. $\quad t = \dfrac{s}{\frac{1}{2}v} = \dfrac{2s}{v} \quad$ (see 6.3.1)

Thus,

$$a = -\frac{v}{t} = -\frac{v}{2s/v} = -\frac{v^2}{2s}, \quad \text{so that} \quad as = -\frac{1}{2}v^2,$$

which may be substituted into equation 7.3 to give:

$$E = \tfrac{1}{2}mv^2 \qquad\qquad \text{Equation 7.4}$$

Newton's Third Law is usually paraphrased as 'Action and reaction are equal and opposite'. There are many examples of this in everyday life such as the reaction on a gun produced by firing a bullet, a hammer hitting a nail, etc., but it is important to realise that there need not necessarily be any physical *contact* between the two bodies for their reactions one upon the other to be equal and opposite. For example, the gravitational force acting on the moon due to the earth is the same as that acting on the earth due to the moon. Similarly, electrostatic or magnetic forces between two bodies are equal and opposite as we shall see in later chapters.

7.5 AVOGADRO'S NUMBER AND THE MOLE

All substances consist of atoms or molecules, which may react chemically with the atoms and molecules of other substances. Molecules combine together in fixed proportions in order to produce a given chemical compound, and it is therefore possible to predict the number of molecules of the compound from a knowledge of the number of molecules in each of the original elements or compounds.

In the case of gases, *Avogadro's hypothesis*, first put forward in the early nineteenth century and abundantly verified by experiment thereafter, postulated that: 'equal volumes of gases at the same temperature and pressure contain equal numbers of molecules'.

This is just a special case of the more general statement that 'the number of molecules per *mole* is the same for any substance', where a mole is the SI unit of the 'amount of substance' and is defined as:

Definition

> The *mole* is the amount of substance which contains as many elementary particles as there are atoms in 0·012 kg of carbon-12.

Here carbon-12 is used as a standard as for technical experimental reasons. For all but the most accurate work the mole may be considered to be the same as the number of atoms in 0·001 kg (i.e. 1 g) of hydrogen, since each carbon atom is twelve times heavier than each hydrogen atom. Thus, if we have a substance whose molecular weight is 25, then 0·025 kg of it contains the same number of molecules as exist in 0·012 kg of carbon-12, which contain the same number of molecules in 0·002 kg of hydrogen gas (H_2). Each of these is a mole of that particular substance.

The number of molecules in a mole of any substance is very large indeed and has the value of 6×10^{23} (just over half a million million million million!). This number is known as *Avogadro's Number* (or Constant), and has further relevance to us only in the theory of the linear and mass attenuation coefficient of X-ray interaction with matter (Ch. 30). It has units of 'number per mole', i.e. $mole^{-1}$.

SUMMARY

1. The 'Classical' Conservation Laws are:

    a. *Matter* is neither created nor destroyed.
    b. Total *energy* is constant, but may change from one form to another.
    c. The total *momentum* of a given system is constant.

2. Newton's Laws of Motion are a consequence of the Conservation Laws, and are:

    a. Every body is at rest or has uniform motion unless acted upon by an external force.

   b.   The rate of change of momentum is proportional to the applied force.

   c.   Every action has an equal and opposite reaction.

3.   The kinetic energy of a body of mass m moving at velocity v is $\frac{1}{2}mv^2$.

4.   There are equal numbers of molecules in a mole of any substance. This number is Avogadro's Number, and has a value of 6×10^{23} mole^{-1}.

8. Heat

We are all familiar with the *feelings* of 'hot' and 'cold'; indeed we are crucially dependent upon our bodily warmth staying within a very limited range in order to be alive at all. Compared to the vast extremes of temperature existing in the Universe, from the near absolute zero of space to the millions of degrees within stars, our experience of 'hot' and 'cold' is very limited indeed. In fact, we are better at noticing 'hotter' and 'colder' than an absolute 'hot' or 'cold', as may be shown by the following simple experiment. If the left hand (say) is placed for a minute or so in a bowl of hot water, and the right hand in a bowl of cold water and then both transferred to a bowl of tepid water, two different sensations are experienced: the left hand feels cold and the right hand feels warm, although the tepid water cannot be both cold and warm at the same time! Again, the bodily readily adapts to central heating and only continues to *feel* warm if the temperature is gradually increased above the level of comfort for a visitor (who has had time to partially adapt to the outside environment).

In order to investigate heat further, we therefore must use a more objective measure of 'hot' and 'cold' as described in the following sections.

8.1 HEAT ENERGY AND TEMPERATURE

When heat is given to a body its atoms or molecules are given an increased energy of movement, i.e. kinetic energy. Conversely, a body whose molecules have a higher kinetic energy than another body is said to be 'hotter', or at a higher 'temperature'. In particular, if the two bodies are placed in contact, then energy will be transferred from the hot body to the cold body, since collisions between the two types of molecules will result in a more even distribution of energy. Thus, the body at the lower temperature receives a net increase in kinetic energy, and so its temperature rises, while that of the hotter body falls. This process continues until the temperatures of the two bodies are the same, or to express it differently, until there is no longer any net transfer of kinetic energy from one body to the other. This condition is known as 'thermal equilibrium', and is a state of dynamic (rather than static) equilibrium. If two bodies are able to transfer heat energy to each other, then the heat energy always flows from the body at the higher temperature to the body at the lower temperature, irrespective of the *size* of the bodies concerned. Likewise, the temperature existing at thermal equilibrium will always lie somewhere between the initial temperatures of the two bodies.

8.1.1 Temperature scales

There are only two temperature scales with which we need be concerned: kelvin and Celsius (also called Centigrade). The Celsius scale is defined as 0°C at the temperature of melting ice, and 100°C at the temperature of boiling water at an atmospheric pressure of 76 cm of mercury ($1 \cdot 01 \times 10^5$ newtons per square metre). On this scale, the temperature of absolute zero is approximately $-273 \cdot 15$°C, and corresponds to zero kinetic energy of the molecules of the body — i.e. the molecules have completely stopped moving. This is, of course, the lowest limit of movement, so that no lower temperatures than this can exist — hence 'absolute' zero. This temperature is taken as zero on the kelvin scale (0 K), while the temperature of melting ice is $273 \cdot 15$K — i.e. one Celsius degree is equivalent to one unit of kelvin. Note that a temperature on the kelvin scale does not have the degree symbol in front of the 'K'. It is a convenient approximation to consider that $0°C \equiv 273 \ K$, so that the following simple conversion formula may be used:

$$T°C \equiv (T + 273) \ K \qquad \qquad \text{Equation 8.1}$$

8.1.2 Units of heat energy and heat capacity

If heat energy is given to a body, then (by definition) its molecules are given a higher kinetic energy and its temperature will rise. Hence it is convenient to express a quantity of heat energy in terms of the temperature change it produces in a given body. Let us say that we wish to raise the temperature of a body by one kelvin unit. What factors influence the energy (Q) required? Well, there are two (ignoring changes of 'phase' — e.g. solid to liquid): the *mass* (m) of the material and the *type of material*. Similarly, we would expect that twice the energy is needed to raise the temperature by two kelvin units. Combining all these factors, we have:

$$Q = mc(T_2 - T_1) \qquad \qquad \text{Equation 8.2}$$

where Q is the heat energy required to raise a mass m of a material from a temperature T_1 to T_2. Q is expressed in the usual SI unit of energy, i.e. the joule, and m is in kg. The factor c is approximately constant for a particular material, and is known as the 'specific heat capacity' of that material.

Rearranging Equation 8.2, we have:

$$c = \frac{Q}{m(T_2 - T_1)}$$

so that c, the specific heat capacity, is in units of joules per kg per kelvin ($J \ kg^{-1} \ K^{-1}$), and may be defined in the following manner:

Definition

The *specific heat capacity* of a body is the heat energy in joule which is required to raise the temperature of 1 kg of the body by 1 kelvin unit.

The specific heat capacity is thus specific to a given substance, enabling the behaviour of the same mass of different substances to be compared.

Example

The specific heat capacity for water is about $4 \cdot 2$ kJ kg^{-1} K^{-1}. What heat energy is required to raise a mass of 10 g from 280 K to 285 K?

Writing down the values, we have:

$c = 4 \cdot 2 \times 10^3$ J kg^{-1} K^{-1}
$m = 10^{-2}$ kg
$(T_2 - T_1) = 5$
$Q = ?$

Substituting the known values in Equation 8.2, we have:

$Q = 10^{-2} \times 4 \cdot 2 \times 10^3 \times 5 = 21 \cdot 0 \times 10$

i.e. $Q = 210$ joule

(Note the importance of changing each quantity into the correct units, e.g. 10 g into 10^{-2} kg.)

Another unit of heat energy which is useful in practice is the 'heat capacity':

Definition

The *heat capacity* of a body is the heat energy in joule which is required to raise the temperature of the body by one kelvin unit.

Note that this definition differs from the previous one for 'specific' heat capacity in that no mention is made of 'unit mass', i.e. the heat capacity refers to the *whole* of a particular body, not 1 kg of it. However, the heat capacity is just the specific heat capacity, c, multiplied by the mass, m, and its units are simply joule per kelvin (JK^{-1}).

Exercise 8.1

A given quantity of heat energy is supplied to two bodies of equal mass, one with a small and one with a large specific heat capacity. Which body experiences the large increase of temperature?

Insight

The Calorie and the Mechanical Equivalent of Heat. Historically, it was not evident that mechanical work performed on a body was capable of producing a specific quantity of heat energy until the experiments of Joule. He showed that the heat energy produced, E, was proportional to the work performed, W, on the molecules of the body as in the relationship:

$W = JE$

where J is constant, called the 'Mechanical Equivalent of Heat'. J has a value of approximately $4 \cdot 2$ joules per calorie, where a *calorie* is a measure of heat energy and is defined as: 1 *calorie* is required to raise 1 g of water by 1 Celsius degree.

However, it is not necessary (or even desirable) to have a special unit of energy for heat, and the SI system measures heat energy in joules, as for all other forms of energy.

8.2 TRANSFER OF HEAT

What is it which causes the temperature of a body to increase, decrease or stay the same? In other words, under what circumstances can the molecules of a body be given a greater kinetic energy, a smaller kinetic energy or undergo no change? A little thought will confirm that it is the *environment* in which the body is situated which determines any subsequent changes of temperature, for if the environment is able to donate more heat energy to the body than it receives from the body (for example) then the net gain of heat energy by the body will increase its temperature. Similarly, its temperature may be kept constant either by isolating it from its environment (e.g. in a vacuum flask) or by allowing it to achieve equilibrium with its surroundings, in which there is no net gain or loss of heat from the body.

The mechanisms of heat transfer form an important part of the study of radiography, because large amounts of heat energy are produced over a small area on the anode of an X-ray tube. The mechanical stresses associated with the large temperature rises and the vaporisation (8.4) and pitting of the anode material make it possible to damage an X-ray tube quite easily. This is particularly true of small mobile or dental units which may not have any safety 'interlock' system to prevent such damaging exposures (or sequence of exposures) being undertaken. The anodes of all X-ray tubes must therefore be designed so as to transfer heat *away* from the focal spot as quickly as possible in order to minimise the temperature rise to this region. Obviously, this cannot be accomplished unless the mechanisms of heat loss are understood, so sections 8.2.1 to 8.2.4 discuss conduction, convection and radiation, before returning to their practical application to the design of X-ray tubes in section 8.5.

8.2.1 Conduction

Conduction is the transfer of heat between bodies by physical contact of those bodies, and results therefore in a transfer of kinetic energy by atomic collision. Thus, if a poker is pushed into a coal fire, the tip of the poker experiences a rapid rise of temperature as it receives copious supplies of kinetic energy (by conduction) from the very energetic molecules within the fire. Also, the energetic atoms in the tip of the poker influence their neighbours by collision, so that kinetic energy is gradually transferred along the length of the poker by the conduction process. This is equivalent to the statement that heat energy 'flows' along the poker by conduction, and may be perceived by the motion of the incandescent red band along it.

What affects the *rate* of flow of heat along such a conducting rod? If we call the rate of flow of heat q joule per sec (i.e. watt — see 6.3.7) then it is found that:

a. $q \propto A$, the cross-sectional area of the rod
b. $q \propto (T_1 - T_2)$, the temperature difference between the ends of the rod
c. $q \propto (1/l)$, where l is the length of the rod.
d. q depends on the *material* of the rod.

Combining all these factors, we have:

$$q = \frac{kA(T_1 - T_2)}{l}$$
Equation 8.3

Here k is introduced as a constant of proportionality (1.7), which is constant for a given material, and is therefore known as the *thermal conductivity* of that material. Note that the rate of flow of heat, q, may be increased by using a wider and shorter rod and increasing the temperature difference, all of which are intuitively reasonable. The quantity $(T_1 - T_2)/l$ is called the 'temperature gradient'.

Materials are conveniently classified as 'good' or 'bad' thermal conductors, or 'bad' and 'good' thermal insulators respectively, depending on the value of k, the thermal conductivity. Metals make good thermal conductors, while plastics and wood (for example) are poor thermal conductors.

Exercise 8.2
a.   Has a good conductor a higher or a lower value of k than a poor conductor?

b.   In what units would you expect k to be expressed? (Hint: arrange Equation 8.3 so that k is on its own on one side of the equation, as shown for Equation 8.2).

The values of the thermal conductivities of the materials commonly used in the construction of an X-ray anode are shown in Table 8.1.

Table 8.1 Thermal conductivity of materials

Material	Thermal conductivity $(W\ m^{-1}\ K^{-1})$	Comments
Copper	386	Excellent conductor — used as anode in stationary anode tube
Tungsten	202	Fairly good conductor — used as target in X-ray tubes
Molybdenum	147	Relatively poor conductor — used for anode stem in rotating anode tube (also for anode disk)
Glass	1·0 (approx.)	Poor thermal conductor — oil transfers heat from glass of X-ray tube by convection.
Rubber	0·05 (approx.)	Very poor conductor
Air	0·02	Very poor conductor — removes heat from X-ray shield by convection

8.2.2 Convection

Convection is the main agency by which heat is transferred in fluids (i.e. liquids and gases). It may be seen operating when an electric kettle is switched on, for example. The water near the hot element in heated by conduction, so that it expands, becomes less dense, and therefore rises as a result of hydrostatic pressure (similar to a bubble in a glass of water). Cold water is then drawn in from the sides and undergoes the same process. As the warmer water rises, it loses its excess heat to the surrounding water by conduction and therefore is able to sink and become reheated at a later stage. Thus, 'convection currents' are produced as illustrated in Fig. 8.1, the overall effect of which is to heat the whole volume of fluid — not just the region at which the heat is applied.

Two interesting points emerge from this:

    a. It is not possible to have convection currents without some conduction.

    b. It is necessary for there to be a gravitational field in order for the convection currents to be initiated, as the warm 'bubble' of fluid always moves in the opposite direction to the force of gravity, by hydrostatic pressure.

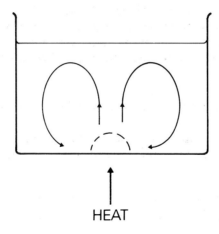

HEAT

Fig. 8.1 Principles of convection. Applied head causes the dotted region to expand, become less dense and rise, being replaced by cooler parts of the liquid and setting up convention currents.

8.2.3 Radiation

Radiation of heat is the only form of heat transfer which can take place through a *vacuum*. The most obvious and striking example is the heat we can feel from our Sun, where the radiation must pass through a nearly perfect vacuum for 93 million miles! Light and heat reach us from other stars, but we are able to discern only the light, as we are not sufficiently sensitive to heat (although the latter may be detected by appropriate sensors).

We are able to feel heat by radiation because it imparts kinetic energy to the molecules of our tissues, which we discern as an increase of temperature. Other radiations such as light and radio waves are not sensed in this way at normal intensities of radiation. Heat radiation occurs in the band just beyond the red part of the visible electromagnetic spectrum, i.e. infra-red (for a fuller discussion of the electromagnetic spectrum, see Ch. 24). All bodies radiate electromagnetic waves if their temperatures are above absolute zero (0 K). This does not necessarily mean that *we* can discern the radiations because, as mentioned above, we are most sensitive to a very narrow band of the electromagnetic spectrum, extending from blue light to the infra-red. Now, bodies of different colours and surface compositions radiate somewhat differently, so it is convenient to consider 'black-body' radiation in the next section.

8.2.4 Black-body radiation

A particular object looks black because very little of the light incident upon it is reflected or transmitted. A 'black body' is therefore defined as a body which absorbs 100% of all radiation at all frequencies incident upon it. If such a black body is imagined to be in thermal equilibrium (8.2) with its surroundings, then equal amounts of radiation must be absorbed and emitted per second. Hence the black body must radiate more energy than any other type of body, since no other body absorbs 100% of the radiation incident upon it. Thus we may summarise the foregoing arguments by the following statements:

a.   All bodies emit radiation.
b.   A black body absorbs 100% of all radiation incident upon it.
c.   A black body is the most efficient emitter of radiation of any body.

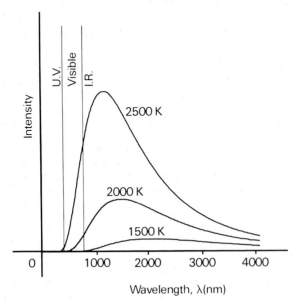

Fig. 8.2 The spectrum of electromagnetic radiation emitted by a 'black body' at different temperatures. The total intensity is a sensitive function of temperature ($I \propto T^4$).

We now need to know in more detail the spectrum of radiation emitted by a black body. Figure 8.2 illustrates the spectrum of radiation emitted by a black body, i.e. the intensity of radiation (4.1) at each wavelength of radiation. Important comments concerning this graph include:

a.   the wavelength corresponding to the peak radiation moves progressively to the left as the temperature of the body increases

b.   the height of the graph is very sensitive to changes in temperature.

c.   the spectrum of radiation is a smooth curve spanning a large variation in wavelength of which we perceive only a small band (visible and infra-red)

d.   the *total* intensity of radiation emitted by the body at a given temperature is just the sum of the intensities at all wavelengths and is therefore given by the *area* under each curve. It is found that the total intensity is proportional to the *fourth* power of the temperature (Stefan's Law), i.e. $I \propto T^4$

---

or $I = \sigma T^4$ Equation 8.4

---

where σ is 'Stefan's Constant'.

Thus, a doubling of the kelvin temperature results in the heat emitted by radiation being increased by a factor of $2^4 = 16$ times! Radiation therefore varies greatly with the temperature of a body.

A curve of emitted radiation at about 1000 K is equivalent to a poker being withdrawn after a short time and glowing a dull cherry red. As the temperature increases, the colour changes through light red to white, since an increasing amount of the blue end of the visible spectrum is emitted along with the longer 'red' wavelengths (2000 K to 2500 K in the figure). An electric light, for example, operates at such a 'white hot' temperature. Objects which are even hotter than our own Sun (i.e. some other stars) extend even more into the short wavelengths and therefore appear bluish in colour. Similarly, the rotating anode of an X-ray tube becomes 'white hot' during powerful exposures, and its temperature may exceed 2000 K.

Insight

The mechanism of the emission of radiation is the acceleration and deceleration of the charged particles which make up the atoms and molecules of a body. An example particularly relevant to radiography is the sudden deceleration of electrons when they strike the anode of an X-ray tube — the 'Bremsstrahlung' or 'braking' radiation, where some (or all) of the kinetic energy of an electron is transformed into an X-ray photon (Ch. 28). Another example is the production of radio waves, where electrons are forced to oscillate at high frequencies in a transmitter aerial, producing radio waves at the same frequency. Thus, the interaction of energetic atoms (or plasma, in stars) produces a broad band of emitted quanta of electromagnetic radiation because of the range of interactions possible. The radiation forms part of the electromagnetic spectrum, and that narrow range of frequencies (infra-red) which is capable of being efficiently absorbed by whole atoms and molecules (as opposed to the nuclei or electron shells) gives them kinetic energy and is therefore 'heat' as we know it subjectively. Higher frequencies of radiation interact with the electron orbits of atoms, and very high frequencies interact with the nuclei of atoms.

8.3 THERMAL EXPANSION

Most substances expand when heated, owing to the increased kinetic energy of the atoms. The 'linear expansivity' is a measure of this thermal expansion and is defined as 'the fractional change in length per unit change in kelvin temperature'. The thermal expansion of different materials is an important consideration in the design of X-ray tubes, since the latter are subjected to large temperature changes throughout their working life. The expansions and contractions so caused may produce mechanical stresses between dissimilar materials of sufficient magnitude to cause a fracture and destroy the vacuum within the tube. A particularly weak point in this respect is the re-entrant glass/anode seal because of the wide fluctuations of temperature at this point. Thus, a glass material is chosen (e.g. pyrex) whose linear expansivity is very similar to that of the copper anode, so that they both expand by the same amounts and hence reduce the thermally produced mechanical stresses.

8.4 EVAPORATION AND VAPORISATION

We are all familiar with the evaporation of liquids which occurs when heat energy is supplied to them. Obvious examples of such evaporation include boiling kettles, the 'steaming' of frost from the early morning sun, and the cooling action of our own perspiration in the mid-day sun. Evaporation is caused by the loss of *whole atoms* from the surface of the liquid (unlike 'thermionic emission', where *electrons* are liberated — see Ch. 18). The most energetic atoms are able to escape from the forces of attraction of their neighbouring atoms near the surface of the liquid, and produce a 'vapour' in the air or vacuum above the surface.

Whole atoms may also be liberated from the surfaces of *solid* materials under the action of heat. This is more difficult to accomplish than is the case for liquids, of course, because of the stronger forces of attraction between the atoms of a solid compared to those of a liquid. Thus, the atoms have to be given a high kinetic energy at the surface of a solid in order to 'break free' of these forces, i.e. the solid must be subjected to a *high temperature*. The name for this process is *vaporisation* and occurs both from the filament and anode of an X-ray tube since both are subjected to high temperatures. The tungsten vapour so produced (particularly from the anode) condenses to form a thin solid layer of tungsten on the inside of the glass of the X-ray tube. This has a small filtration (Ch. 29) effect on the beam, but its major effect is to reduce the electrical insulation between the anode and cathode of the tube, thereby increasing the chances of electrical breakdown and consequent damage to the X-ray tube. However, in normal use this is a slow process because tungsten has a low 'vapour pressure', i.e. it does not vaporise easily at its normal working temperature (1000 to 2000°C).

8.5 HEAT LOSS FROM AN X-RAY TUBE

The mechanisms of heat transfer discussed in section 8.2 will now be discussed in relation to the heat loss from the anode of both a stationary anode and a rotating anode X-ray tube. In both cases, the reason for desiring an efficient heat loss from the anode is to protect it from damage and/or to allow shorter exposures of higher X-ray intensity.

8.5.1 Stationary anode tube

Figure 8.3 shows the construction of a typical stationary anode (A), together with the tube itself and casing (or 'housing'). Superimposed on the figure are arrows originating from the focal spot which represents the paths taken by the heat energy away from this small region of high temperature. The arrows marked (R) represent heat loss by radiation, while those labelled (C) represent conduction and (CV) represent convection. The sequence of events is as follows:

   a. An exposure is taken, resulting in a considerable amount of energy being deposited on the focal spot of the tungsten target. This energy must be quickly dispersed, or damage may occur.

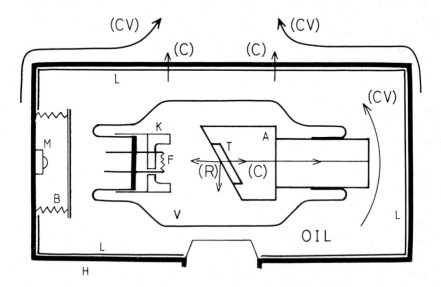

Fig. 8.3 Stationary anode tube and shield (housing). Heat is lost from the target mainly by conduction (see text). Key to parts: H — housing, L — lead foil, M — microswitch, B — bellows, V — vacuum within glass tube, K — cathode, F — filament, T — tungsten target, A — copper anode.

b.   Heat radiation from the focal spot passes through the vacuum of the tube, to be absorbed by the glass envelope and the oil.

c.   Conduction takes place through the tungsten 'target' into the copper anode block, and then along the anode stem.

d.   The end of the anode stem is in contact with the oil surrounding the tube, and so sets up convection currents and warms the whole oil. The oil expands, compresses the bellows and may actuate the microswitch (M in the figure) which prevents further exposures.

e.   Heat from the oil passes through the metal casing by conduction.

f.   The warm casing sets up convection currents in the air of the room. Radiation from the casing also helps to remove its excess heat.

Thus, all the three processes of conduction, convection and radiation are involved in the removal of heat from the focal spot. Notice that there are two fluids involved; oil and air, and both these remove heat by convection (as would be expected from 8.2.2) and that radiation passes through the vacuum (which neither of the other processes can accomplish, of course). However, the stationary anode X-ray tube is designed to lose the majority of heat by *conduction* into and through the anode block. How is this to be made as efficient as possible? In (8.2.1) it was shown that conduction depends upon the type of material, the cross-sectional area and the temperature gradient (see Equation 8.3). To maximise heat transfer by conduction, therefore, a material of high thermal conductivity is chosen (i.e. copper), a sufficiently large cross-sectional area of anode block is used, and the far end of the anode stem is kept as cool as possible by immersing it in oil. The tungsten insert itself has reasonably good thermal conductivity (although not as good as copper — Table 8.1), is thin and has an appreciable cross-sectional area so that heat flow into the copper block is rapid. One further point is that the large copper block also serves to keep the temperature increase it experiences within safe limits, i.e. it has a large 'heat capacity' (8.1.2). This also helps to 'draw' heat from the tungsten target by maintaining a high temperature gradient between the faces of the tungsten insert. The melting point of copper is 1083°C, and this imposes a practical limit to the amount of heat which may be deposited on the anode, or the melting point of copper will be reached. This is not the case for the rotating anode tube where the anode is made of solid tungsten (melting point 3380°C) or molybdenum (melting point 2620°C), as described below.

8.5.2 Rotating anode X-ray tube

The heat loss from the focal spot of a rotating anode follows the same pathways as those of the stationary anode X-ray tube, except that the main mechanism of heat loss is that of *radiation*, not conduction.

Figure 8.4 illustrates the main points of construction of a rotating anode X-ray tube. The tungsten anode disc reaches a high temperature, and may become incandescent at 'white heat'. However, heat is inhibited from flowing along the molybdenum stem by (a) the low thermal conductivity of molybdenum and (b) its relatively small cross-sectional area.

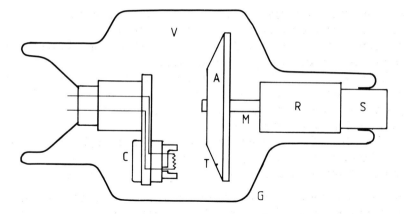

Fig. 8.4 Rotating anode tube. Heat is lost from the target mainly by radiation (see text). Key to parts: G — glass envelope, V — vacuum, C — cathode assembly, T — target area, A — anode disk, M — anode stem, R — rotor, S — rotor support.

Hence, the main agency of heat loss is by radiation, since conduction is inhibited and convection is impossible in the vacuum within the tube. Now radiation becomes greater at high temperatures (Stefan's Law, 8.2.4), so the rotating anode X-ray tube is most efficient when running at a high temperature. Thermal equilibrium (8.1) may be achieved during longer exposures if the rate of heat loss balances the rate at which heat is being deposited. The anode cools rapidly when the exposure is terminated; the higher the anode temperature the more rapid is the initial cooling, because of the fourth power in Stefan's Law (8.2.4).

The radiation emitted from the anode is absorbed by the glass envelope of the tube and the oil surrounding the tube, setting up convection currents in the oil. Heat is then conducted through the casing and convected in the air of the room, as in the case of the stationary anode X-ray tube.

Overheating of the anode may result in damage to the bevelled surface of the anode, a 'drooping' of the anode stem, or damage to the bearings of the copper rotor. For a fuller treatment of the construction of a rotating anode tube, see (21.2).

Exercise 8.3

a. Name and describe the three processes of heat transfer. How is each of these processes involved in the removal of heat from the anode of an X-ray tube (stationary or rotating).

b. What factors determine the rate at which heat is removed from the focal spot of a stationary anode X-ray tube to the end of the anode stem?

c. What is meant by 'black-body radiation'? What does this radiation have in common with X-rays?

SUMMARY

1. Heat is a form of energy produced by the movement of atoms (kinetic energy) — measured in joule.
2. The greater the kinetic energy of the atoms, the higher the *temperature* and vice versa.
3. 'Absolute zero' temperature corresponds to zero atomic kinetic energy and has a temperature of 0 kelvin (K).
4. On the kelvin scale, the temperature of melting ice is approximately 273 K.
5. The temperature of a body is constant if it loses as much heat energy per second as it gains — it is then said to be in thermal equilibrium with its surroundings.
6. Heat may be transferred from one point to another by conduction (solid bodies), convection (fluids) and radiation (may travel through a vacuum, and forms part of the electromagnetic spectrum).
7. Heat must be transferred quickly from the focal spot of an X-ray tube if damage to the anode is to be avoided.
8. For a stationary anode tube, *conduction* is the main mechanism of heat loss — therefore copper anode of large cross-section is used.
9. For a rotating anode tube, *radiation* is the main mechanism of heat loss. Higher anode temperatures are possible resulting in efficient heat loss by radiation (Stefan's Law: Intensity $\propto$ T^4). Conduction is inhibited.

9. Electrostatics

Electrostatics is the term given to the study of static electrical charges. Many examples of the effects of electrostatics in our ordinary lives may be cited, from the sparks which may occur (from clothes) while undressing, to the destructive discharges of lightning during storms and the unruly behaviour of recently washed hair! It was discovered by experiment that there are *two* types of electric charge, one of which was called 'positive' and one 'negative', the selection of these terms being a mathematical convenience which in no way describes what a 'charge' actually *is*. Fortunately, however, it is not necessary to possess this knowledge in order to predict the behaviour of electrical charges; we need to know only their general properties as described in the next section. It is now known that, for example, electrons possess a negative charge, and protons a positive charge. Many other particles encountered in atomic and nuclear physics also possess charge.

9.1 PROPERTIES OF ELECTRICAL CHARGES

The general properties of electrical charges are as follows:

1. Charges are of two types: positive and negative.

2. The smallest unit of electrical charge is that possessed by an electron (for negative charges) or a proton (for positive charges). These two charges are of equal magnitude, although opposite in sign. (Modern nuclear physics predicts the existence of particles called 'quarks' which may possess $\frac{1}{3}$ or $\frac{2}{3}$ of the charge of an electron.)

3. Electric charges exert forces on each other, even when separated by a vacuum. The forces are mutual, and equal and opposite, as expected from Newton's Third Law (7.4).

4. Like charges repel each other and unlike charges attract each other, i.e. two positive or two negative charges each experience a force tending to push the charges further apart, while a positive and negative charge each experience a force tending to pull the charges closer together.

5. The magnitude of the mutual forces between charges is influenced by the medium in which they are embedded, being greatest when that medium is a vacuum.

6. Electrical charges may be *induced* in a body by the proximity of a

charged body, leading to a force of attraction between the two bodies.

7. Electrical charges may flow easily in some materials ('electrical conductors'), but with difficulty through others ('electrical insulators'). Nevertheless, both types of material are capable of having charges induced in them (see 6).

In addition, moving electrical charges produce a magnetic field. This is discussed in more detail in Chapter 12.

The above list constitutes a general account of the properties of electrical charges which will concern us in the following sections of this chapter and the book as a whole.

9.2 FORCE BETWEEN TWO ELECTRICAL CHARGES IN A VACUUM

Consider two charges of magnitude q_1 and q_2 separated by a distance d in a vacuum, as shown in Figure 9.1. Then, assuming that both charges are positive (say), charge

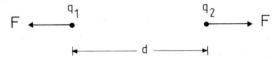

Fig. 9.1 The forces between two electric charges are equal and opposite.

q_1 will exert a force of repulsion (F) on q_2, and q_2 will exert the same force of repulsion on q_1. It may be shown by experiment that:

  a. $F \propto q_1$
  b. $F \propto q_2$
  c. $F \propto 1/d^2$ (i.e. another example of the Inverse Square Law — Ch. 4).

Thus F is proportional to the magnitude of each charge and to the inverse square of the distance of separation between the charges. These facts may be grasped intuitively if it is assumed that electrical 'lines of force' emanate from charges in straight lines (analogous to light or X-rays from a source of radiation — obeying the Inverse Square Law), and that the number of such lines of force is proportional to the magnitude of the charge (analogous to the 'brightness' of the source). This is shown diagrammatically in Figure 9.2,

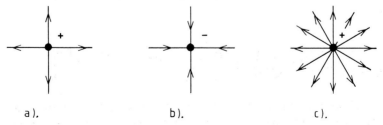

    a).   b).   c).

Fig. 9.2 Electric 'lines of force' associated with (a) a weak positive charge, (b) a weak negative charge, (c) a strong positive charge.

where the arrows point in the direction of the force experienced by a positive charge if placed at that point. Lines of force are discussed further in (9.4).

Combining the factors in (a), (b) and (c) above, we have:

$$F \propto \frac{q_1 q_2}{d^2}$$

Equation 9.1

If q_1 and q_2 are both positive or both negative quantities, then F is positive (Rule 1, Ch. 1) and represents a mutual force of repulsion. If, however, q_1 and q_2 are of opposite sign, then F is negative and represents a mutual force of attraction.

In (1.7) it is shown that a proportional sign may be replaced by an equals sign if a 'constant of proportionality' is introduced. Applying this fact to equation 9.1 we have:

$$F = \frac{q_1 q_2}{4\pi\varepsilon_0 \cdot d^2}$$

Equation 9.2

This equation is often referred to as the 'Coulomb Law' of force between two charges, and has particular relevance to the forces between charged particles in atomic physics (e.g. Ch. 26 and 28).

Here, the constant of proportionality is $1/4\pi\varepsilon_0$, where ε_0 is called the 'permittivity of free space' (i.e. vacuum), and has a value of 8.85×10^{-12} farads/metre (see 9.7.1 for the meaning of a farad). The charges q_1 and q_2 are expressed in *coulombs*, the distance of separation, d, in metres, and the force F in newtons. A charge of 1 coulomb (1 C) corresponds approximately to the total charge carried by 6×10^{18} electrons (or protons). Alternatively, 1 coulomb may be defined from Equation 9.2 as follows:

Definition

A charge of 1 *coulomb* is possessed by a point if, when placed 1 metre away from an equal charge in a vacuum, a force of repulsion of $1/4\pi\varepsilon_0$ newton is experienced.

This definition is obtained simply from Equation 9.2 by substituting $q_1 = q_2 = d = 1$ unit, when $F = 1/4\pi\varepsilon_0$. However, it is equally acceptable for our purposes to consider that 1 coulomb is equivalent to 6×10^{18} elementary charges.

9.3 PERMITTIVITY AND RELATIVE PERMITTIVITY (DIELECTRIC CONSTANT)

Equation 9.2 holds true only when the charges are within a vacuum, where ε_0 is the 'permittivity of free space'. In any other medium, the equation is modified to:

$$F = \frac{q_1 q_2}{4\pi\varepsilon d^2}$$ Equation 9.3

where ε is the 'permittivity' of the medium.

It is often convenient, however, to compare the permittivity of a medium relative to that of a vacuum. For example, if the permittivity of the medium is twice the value of that of a vacuum, then the 'relative permittivity', K, is 2 and may be obtained by the following simple formula:

$$K = \varepsilon/\varepsilon_0$$

or, cross-multiplying,

$$\varepsilon = \varepsilon_0 K$$ Equation 9.4

so that equation 9.3 may be rewritten as

$$F = \frac{q_1 q_2}{4\pi\varepsilon_0 K d^2}$$ Equation 9.5

K is also known as the 'dielectric constant' of the medium, so that relative permittivity and dielectric constant are the same. It is just a number, and therefore does not possess any units. K is discussed further in the section on capacity (9.7).

9.4 ELECTRIC FIELD STRENGTH (INTENSITY)

We have seen that an electric charge is capable of influencing other charges at a distance from it. This 'influence at a distance' is known as a 'field' and, for the purpose of comparison of different electric fields, is measured by its force on a unit positive charge. This is the same principle as measuring the gravitational field of the Earth by its force on a body of unit mass, i.e. 1 kg. The electric intensity (or electric field strength), E, is therefore measured in units of newton/coulomb, since it is defined as the force exerted on a unit charge. To take the example of the electric field around a point charge, if we wish to know the value of the electric field strength at a point, then we simply place a unit charge at that point and measure the magnitude ad direction of the force exerted upon it. However, we already know both these facts from Equation 9.5 if we substitute a value of $q_2 = 1$ (i.e. q_2 is the unit charge which is measuring the electric field strength of q_1).

Thus, for a point charge,

$$E = \frac{q_1 \times 1}{4\pi\varepsilon_0 K d^2}$$

i.e. $E = \dfrac{q_1}{4\pi\varepsilon_0 K d^2}$

Figure 9.2 illustrates the electric field existing around a point charge, where the arrows represent the direction of the force on a unit positive charge placed at a point, and the closeness of the lines of force represents the intensity of the electric field.

9.5 ELECTROSTATIC INDUCTION OF CHARGE

9.5.1 Induction of a conductor

If an electrical charge is placed near an electrical conductor, as shown in Figure 9.3, then it is found that charges are *induced* on the body as shown in the figure. Notice that the opposite sign of charge is induced on the surface of the body closest to the inducing charge, and the same sign of charge is induced on the opposite side of the body. Also, equal numbers of both positive and negative charges are induced. These conditions result in a net force of attraction between the inducing charge and the induced charges on the body since the unlike charges are closer together than the like charges. Now an electrical conductor is a material in which only electrons are able to flow, since the positive charges on the protons in the atomic nuclei are fixed in position in the solid material and unable to take part in the conduction process. Thus, it is the *electrons* in body A (in the figure) which are attracted to the charged body, 'leaving behind' a net positive charge as they move. Thus, for every electron which is displaced, a positive charge is revealed, so that it is easy to see why electrostatic induction results in the formation of equal numbers of positive and negative charges. Why do not all of the electrons of the body A reach the surface closest to the inducing charge? Well, an equilibrium of charge distribution is reached such that the force of attraction towards the inducing charge on any electron in A is balanced by the force of attraction by the positive charges revealed on the opposite side of A. No more net electron flow is then possible. Withdrawal of the charged body results in a uniform distribution in A once more.

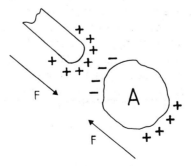

Fig. 9.3 Induction of charges on a conducting body A, resulting in a force of attraction (F) with the inducing body.

9.5.2 Induction of an insulator (dielectric)

If the above experiment is repeated with an electrical insulator rather than an electrical conductor, positive and negative charges are induced on the insulator and a force of attraction results. This may be readily demonstrated by charging a comb or piece of plastic by friction on a cloth and placing it close to a small piece of paper, which promptly jumps towards and clings to the charged body. This is really a somewhat surprising result, since electrons are not able to move through the body (unlike an electrical conductor) and impart a charge to one side or the other. The insulator is given the general term 'dielectric' to describe this process of induced charge since two (di-) types of charge are produced by the induction. Some dielectrics are more efficient at producing induced charges, and this is measured by the value of the 'dielectric constant' (9.3). There are two mechanisms of the actions of a dielectric: molecular distortion and the rotation of 'polar molecules'.

Molecular distortion
A body is composed of many millions of atomic particles of either sign, and is electrically neutral only if there are equal numbers of positive and negative charges which are distributed uniformly throughout the body. The presence of an external charge, however, influences every charged particle (i.e. electron or proton) within the body such that the electrons experience a force in the opposite direction to that on the protons of the atomic nuclei (Ch. 25). If the electrons are tightly bound to the nuclei (as is the case for a dielectric), then these opposing forces produce atomic and molecular distortions of the paths of the orbiting electrons.

Figure 9.4(a) illustrates the self-cancelling action of the positive and negative charges on a simplified atom. The electron orbit is spherical and so the *average position* (mathematically) is the centre of its orbit, which coincides with the position of the positive nucleus. Thus, the practical effect is the same as having equal positive and negative charges at the same point, i.e. the body behaves as though it were neutral. When the atom is subjected to an electric

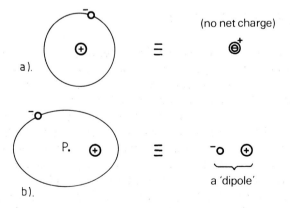

Fig. 9.4 Atomic 'polarisation' caused by an externally applied electric field E.

field, however, the electron orbit is displaced relative to the atomic nucleus as shown in Figure 9.4(b). The average position of the electron is now displaced to one side of the nucleus (point P in the figure), so that the atoms (or molecules, on a larger scale) have become 'polarised' into 'electric dipoles'.

Polar molecules

Some molecules exist for which the average position of the electrons is not coincident with that of the nuclei. Thus, even when such a molecule is not subjected to an electric field, it is polarised. The effect of an externally applied electric field is to *rotate* these polarised molecules such that they tend to become aligned with the field. Practical dielectrics use such materials since they produce a much stronger effect than molecular distortion alone.

Figure 9.5 summarises the effect of both of these mechanisms in the induction of charge on a dielectric. The elementary dipoles all tend to 'line up' with the direction of the externally applied electric field, E, so that positive charges occur on one side and negative charges occur on the other. *Within* the body, however, the dipoles are so close together that the positive and negative ends of adjacent dipoles cancel each other's effects (as far as the external world is concerned).

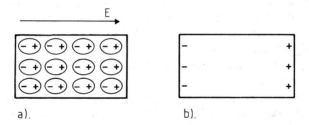

a).   b).

Fig. 9.5 Induction of charges on an insulator (dielectric): (a) alignment of polarised molecules within dielectric, (b) net effect of surface charges only.

9.6 ELECTRIC POTENTIAL

There is a close parallel between electric potential energy and other forms of potential energy (6.3.6), e.g. gravitational potential energy. If a body of mass m is at a height h above a particular reference level (the 'zero' level) then its potential energy is defined as the work which has to be performed in lifting it from the reference level to that height. The work done is the 'force times the distance' and is therefore mgh (6.3.6). It is immaterial whether the mass is lifted straight up or by some circuitous path, as shown in Figure 9.6. Also, the *position* of the mass on the plane given by the height h is unimportant — the only factors affecting the potential energy being m, g and h. Thus, the plane at h above the 'zero' level is called an 'equipotential' surface, since a body placed anywhere on this surface has an equal gravitational potential energy.

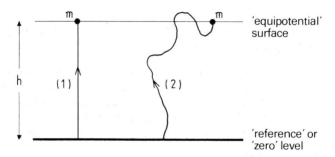

Fig. 9.6 Gravitational potential energy.

To return to the concept of electric potential energy, we require (by analogy) the following:

a. A 'reference' or 'zero' level, from which all electrical potential energies are to be measured.

b. A knowledge of the work done in moving a 'test object' from the agreed zero level to a particular point relative to the electrically charged object in question. The magnitude of this work is then defined as the 'electrical potential' of the charged object at that point.

These concepts are explored in the following sections.

9.6.1 Zero electrical potential

What point may be chosen as a reference, or zero, point from which all electrical potentials may be measured? The most convenient point is that at which the force exerted by the charged body on the 'test' charge (i.e. a unit positive charge) is zero, and that point is at *infinity*, no matter what the size, shape and charge of the body whose potential is being measured. Thus, the reference, or zero, level is at infinity, and all work performed on the unit charge is measured from there. Obviously, infinity is chosen for its mathematical convenience rather than its practicality!

It is often stated that 'the earth is at zero potential', but how does this agree with the selection of infinity as being the point of zero potential? To answer this, we have only to ask what work needs to be performed on the unit charge in bringing it from infinity to some arbitrary point relative to the earth. Now the earth is assumed to be exactly electrically neutral, i.e. it contains equal numbers of equally distributed positive and negative charges. Thus, there is no force between the neutral earth and the unit charge, so no effort is needed to move the latter towards the earth. Hence, no work is done, and the electrical potential of the Earth, or any other neutral body, is therefore zero.

9.6.2 Potential and potential difference (PD)

To summarise the above discussion, we may define electric potential formally as follows:

Definition

The *electric potential* at a point P is the work done in moving a unit positive charge from infinity to that point.

It is often convenient in practice to compare the potential at one point relative to another, rather than to know its absolute value. If the potential at a point A is V_A, and is V_B at point B, then the 'potential difference' (PD) between A and B is simple $V_A - V_B$, and represents the difference in work done on a unit charge when moved from infinity to the points A and B in turn. This leads to the following definition of PD:

Definition

The *potential difference* between two points is the work done on a unit charge in moving it from one point to the other.

The next section defines the SI unit of electric potential and potential difference before examining some specific examples of how they may each be calculated.

9.6.3 The volt

The volt is the SI unit (Ch. 6) of potential, and is encountered both in static and flowing electricity, and is defined as:

Definition

1 volt of *potential* exists at a point if 1 joule of work is performed in moving 1 coulomb of charge from infinity to that point.

Similarly, for potential difference, we have:

Definition

1 volt of *potential difference* exists if 1 joule of work is performed in moving 1 coulomb of charge from one pont to the other.

We may summarise these definitions by relating the units in the following manner:

$$\text{volts} = \frac{\text{joules}}{\text{coulombs}} \qquad \text{Equation 9.6}$$

This equation merely expresses in particular units what is meant by electric potential or potential difference and that is the 'work done per unit charge'. We shall use this relationship of 'volts equals joules per coulomb' when introducing the concept of electrical power in the next chapter (10.6).

9.6.4 Electric potential due to a point charge

Consider a point charge Q, as shown in Figure 9.7, where a unit charge has

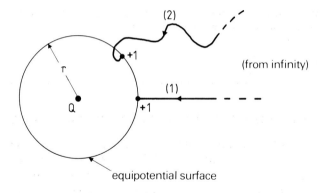

Fig. 9.7 Electrical potential energy of a point charge Q.

been moved from infinity to a distance r from Q. The nearer the unit charge comes to Q, the greater is the force of repulsion (if Q is positive) or attraction (if Q is negative), so that the potential is *positive if* Q *is positive* and *negative if* Q *is negative*, since the potential is defined as the 'work done *on*' (rather than *by*) a unit charge. From considerations of symmetry it is clear that the 'equipotential surfaces' (see Fig. 9.6) will be concentric spheres with Q as the centre. Also, as in the example of gravitational potential energy, the particular path chosen is of no importance, so that paths 1 and 2 in Figure 9.7 give exactly the same value of electrical potential.

Electrical potential is usually given the symbol V, where, for this example:

$$V = \frac{Q}{4\pi\varepsilon_0 r}$$

Equation 9.7

where r is in metres, Q is in coulombs, and V is in volts.

The electric potential due to a point charge is often given the term 'Coulomb' potential, and the force between two charges is the 'Coulomb' force (see 9.2).

Insight

The force on a unit charge at a distance r from Q (Fig. 9.7) is

$$F = \frac{Q \times 1}{4\pi\varepsilon_0 r^2}$$

To move the unit charge towards Q a force $-F$ must be applied. If this force is applied over a distance dr, then the work done is $-F.\,dr$ (force × distance).

The total work done in moving the unit charge from infinity to a distance r is thus

$$V = \int_{\infty}^{r} -F\,dr = \int_{\infty}^{r} -\frac{Q}{4\pi\varepsilon_0} \cdot \frac{1}{r^2} \cdot dr = \frac{Q}{4\pi\varepsilon_0} \left[\frac{1}{r} \right]_{\infty}^{r}$$

i.e. $V = \dfrac{Q}{4\pi\varepsilon_0 r}$,

in agreement with Equation 9.7. Similarly, the potential difference between two points at distances r_1, r_2 from Q is

$$V = \frac{Q}{4\pi\varepsilon_0} \cdot \left[\frac{1}{r_1} - \frac{1}{r_2} \right]$$

9.6.5 Electrical potential due to conducting sphere

If a charge Q is given to a conducting sphere, then it becomes distributed on the *surface* of the sphere, by mutual repulsion of the elementary charges which constitute Q, as shown in Figure 9.8. Hence, it is immaterial whether the sphere is solid or hollow. In general, whatever the shape of the body, the charge becomes distributed in such a way that the whole of the body is at a *constant potential*. This is equivalent to the statement that no potential difference occurs between any two points on or within the body. Now, assuming that a potential difference *does* exist between two points then there will be a net force on the charges between these points and they will be forced to flow until this PD is zero. Thus, the sphere in Figure 9.8 has a constant potential for all points within and on its surface, but what is the potential for points outside the sphere? It may be shown mathematically that, for points outside the sphere, the sphere behaves as though all the charge Q is placed at its centre, so that the results of the previous section may be used.

Hence, Equation 9.7 applies to such points, and the graph in Figure 9.8 illustrates how the potential is constant within the sphere and falls outside it.

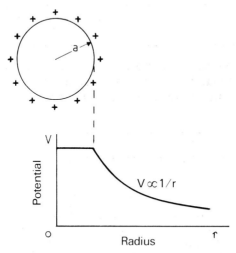

Fig. 9.8 Electric potential of a conducting sphere. The potential is constant within the sphere and reduces outside it.

9.7 ELECTRICAL CAPACITY

The previous sections of this chapter have shown that whenever a body has a net positive or negative charge it also possesses an electrical potential, because work must be performed in moving a unit charge from infinity to that body. This potential is positive if the charge on the body is positive, and negative if the charge is negative. The 'electrical capacity' (or just 'capacity'), C, of a body (the 'capacitor') relates these two quantities of charge and potential in a very simple way:

$$\text{Capacity} = \frac{\text{Charge}}{\text{Potential (or PD)}}$$

or, $C = \dfrac{Q}{V}$ 　　　　　　　　　　　　　　　Equation 9.8

This is a very important equation and should be committed to memory.

9.7.1 Definitions and unit of capacity (farad)

The following definition applies to a body consisting of one surface only (e.g. a sphere):

Definition
> The *electrical capacity* of a body is the ratio of the total charge on the body to its potential.

In the case of two surfaces being brought close together, we must consider the potential *difference* (9.6.2) between the surfaces rather than the potentials of each. This consideration leads to the following alternative definition of capacity:

Definition
> The *electrical capacity* of a body is the ratio of the total charge of one sign on the body to the potential difference between its surfaces.

It is important to remember that the capacity involves both the charge *and* the potential (or PD) of a body, since it is often erroneously stated that 'capacity is the amount of charge a body can hold'. The addition of the phrase 'per unit potential difference' is required to make the definition correct.

The SI unit of capacity is the *farad*, and may be defined as:

Definition
> An electrical system has a capacity of one *farad* if a charge of 1 coulomb held by the body results in a potential (or potential difference) of 1 volt.

Equation 9.8 thus may be expressed as:

$$\text{farads} = \frac{\text{coulombs}}{\text{volts}}$$
　　　　　　　　　　　　　　　　　Equation 9.9

Insight

An alternative definition of the electrical capacity is the *change* of charge divided by the corresponding *change* of potential difference.

If a capacitor starts with a charge Q and potential difference V then, by definition, $C = Q/V$.

If an extra charge, ΔQ, is added to the plates and an extra potential difference of ΔV results, then

$$C = \frac{Q + \Delta Q}{V + \Delta V}$$

(i.e. total charge/total PD).

Cross-multiplying, we have $CV + C\Delta V = Q + \Delta Q$

But $CV = Q$ and so may be cancelled, leaving $C\Delta V = \Delta Q$

i.e. $C = \dfrac{\Delta Q}{\Delta V}$

in accordance with the alternative definition of capacity given above.

This equation is sometimes useful in numerical exercises (eg. in capacitor discharge circuits — see example in 9.11.1).

A farad (F) is a rather large unit of capacity in practice, and it is more usual to express capacity in units of microfarads (μF) or picofarads (pF), where:

$1 \, \mu\text{F} = 10^{-6} \, \text{F}$

and $1 \, \text{pF} = 10^{-12} \, \text{F}$

Examples of the use of these definitions are given in the following section for clarification.

9.7.2 Capacity of an isolated sphere

In (9.6.5) it was shown that a charge of Q coulombs on an isolated conducting sphere produced a potential, V, of $Q/(4\pi\varepsilon_0 r)$ volt on the sphere. Thus, the capacity C, given by $C = Q/V$, is simply:

$$C = \frac{Q}{V} = \frac{Q}{Q/(4\pi\varepsilon_0 r)}$$

i.e. $C = 4\pi\varepsilon_0 r$ farad

Thus, the capacity of an isolated sphere is proportional to its radius, r. However, the values of capacity obtainable from such a capacitor are very low. For example, the earth may be regarded as a very large conducting sphere, and its capacity is about 10^{-3} farad! Also, of course, completely isolated conducting spheres are difficult to achieve in practice, and would be of very inconvenient shape and size to use within an electric circuit.

Higher values of capacity may be achieved by using two conducting surfaces placed close together, as outlined below.

9.7.3 Capacity of two concentric spheres

Figure 9.9 illustrates two concentric spheres, the inner one of which has been given a charge of $+Q$ coulombs, and the outer one which has been connected to 'earth', and is so at 'earth potential', i.e. zero potential (9.6.1).

The presence of the positive charges on the inner sphere induces (9.5.1) an equal and opposite number of negative charges on the inside of the outer sphere. (Electrons flow from earth to the outside of the outside sphere, where they cancel the positive charges which would otherwise exist there.)

In calculating the capacity, we have only to know two things: the total charge of one sign and the potential difference between the surfaces. We know that the former is Q, and we must therefore calculate the latter. Since the potential of the outer space is zero, we thus have only to calculate the potential of the inner sphere, V. Now, V is contributed to by both spheres in the following manner:

   a. Potential of inner sphere due to $+Q$ on inner sphere only

$$= \frac{Q}{4\pi\varepsilon_0 a} \quad \text{(see 9.7.2)}$$

   b. Potential of inner sphere due to $-Q$ on outer sphere only

$$= -\frac{Q}{4\pi\varepsilon_0 b},$$

since the potential *within* a sphere (solid or hollow) is the same as at its surface (9.6.5). V is just the sum of the separate contributions of the two spheres, so that:

$$V = \frac{Q}{4\pi\varepsilon_0 a} - \frac{Q}{4\pi\varepsilon_0 b} = \frac{Q}{4\pi\varepsilon_0} \cdot \left[\frac{1}{a} - \frac{1}{b} \right]$$

i.e. $\quad V = \frac{Q}{4\pi\varepsilon_0} \cdot \left[\frac{b - a}{ab} \right]$

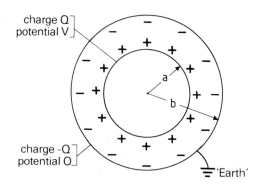

charge Q
potential V

charge -Q
potential O

'Earth'

Fig. 9.9 Two concentric spheres — the inner sphere is given a charge Q and the outer sphere is 'earthed' at 0 volt.

From our definition of the capacity C,

$$C = \frac{Q}{V} = \frac{Q}{\dfrac{Q}{4\pi\varepsilon_0}\left[\dfrac{b-a}{ab}\right]}$$

i.e. $C = 4\pi\varepsilon_0\left[\dfrac{ab}{b-a}\right]$

Equation 9.10

C may now be altered by the selection of the radii a and b. In particular, if a and b are made very similar, so that $(b - a)$ is small, then equation 9.10 shows that C may be made very large. However, concentric spheres are not very practicable, unlike the following example of a capacitor made from two *parallel* conducting plates.

9.7.4 Parallel-plate capacitor

Figure 9.10 shows two parallel plates of equal area, A, separated by a distance d. The plates are made of electrically conducting material so that charge may flow in and out of each plate. If the capacitor is 'charged' (e.g. by connecting its ends across a battery), then a charge of $+Q$ will exist on one plate and a charge of $-Q$ on the other. If the battery is disconnected, both charges will continue to be 'stored' on the plates of the capacitor under the action of the mutual attraction of the charges on opposite plates. This is why a capacitor is often described as a device for storing electric charge. (A large capacitor must be treated with great respect for this very reason, since a severe electric shock may be experienced from it even when the electrical supply is disconnected!)

A potential difference (equal to that of the battery) exists across the plates, since work would have to be done in order to move a unit positive charge from the negative plate across the gap to the positive plate. Thus, the capacity of the parallel-plate capacitor is, by definition, given by $C = Q/V$, and if V is calculated in the same way as the previous example, it may be shown (see Insight below) that:

$$C = \frac{\varepsilon_0 KA}{d}$$

Equation 9.11

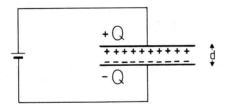

Fig. 9.10 A parallel-plate capacitor charged by a battery.

This is a very useful equation, and one which may be explained from basic principles by the effect of changing the following quantities:

Area of plates

If the area of the plates is increased, then more charge will be able to flow into the plates from the battery until the charge per unit area is the same as before. V remains unaltered, since it is always equal to the potential difference of the battery, which is constant. Hence Q has increased in proportion to the area of the plates while V is unaltered, so that C is also proportional to the area of the plates, since $C = Q/V$. For example, if the area A has been doubled, then twice the charge may be stored so that C has also been doubled.

Thus, $C \propto A$.

Separation of plates

If, everything else being equal, the plates are brought closer together, then there is a greater force of attraction between the charges on opposite plates, so 'drawing out' more charge from the battery onto the plates. The potential difference is unaltered, being the same as that of the battery. Therefore, Q is *inversely* related to plate separation (i.e. Q increases as d decreases) so that C also has an inverse relationship with d. Halving the separation of the plates doubles the charge which is able to be stored at the same potential difference, resulting in a doubling of the capacity.

Thus, $C \propto \dfrac{1}{d}$.

Dielectric constant

Placing a slab of a dielectric material between the plates results in charges being induced on its faces (9.5.2), as shown in Figure 9.11. The close proximity of the charges on the plates and on the dielectric surfaces results in some 'cancellation' of charges (as shown ringed). The work done in moving a unit positive charge from the negatively charged plate to the positively charged plate is therefore less, i.e. the potential difference across the capacitor is reduced. The capacity has therefore increased, since the ratio Q/V is greater than without the dielectric. In fact, a battery connected across the capacitor will be able to store more charge on the plates after the dielectric has been inserted.

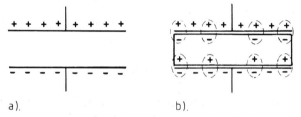

a).   b).

Fig. 9.11 The action of a dielectric in a parallel-plate capacitor. The induction of charge in the dielectric cancels some of the charge stored on the plates (as shown ringed) so that the PD between the plates is reduced.

From Equation 9.11, the capacity of a parallel-plate capacitor without a dielectric is: $C_{air} = \varepsilon_0 A/d$, since the dielectric constant (9.3) of air is 1. Thus, the *ratio* of the capacity in the presence of a dielectric to that in its absence is $\varepsilon_0 KA/d : \varepsilon_0 A/d$, i.e. K, the dielectric constant. This leads to the following useful definition of dielectric constant:

Definition

The *dielectric constant* of a material is the ratio:

$$\frac{\text{Capacity with a dielectric}}{\text{Capacity without a dielectric}}.$$

The choice of the dielectric is one of the major factors in determining the performance of practical capacitors (9.12).

Insight

The capacity of a parallel-plate capacitor may be calculated more easily by extending the calculations for the capacity of concentric spheres (9.7.3), as given by equation 9.10:

$$C = 4\pi\varepsilon_0 \left[\frac{ab}{b - a} \right]$$

Now the separation between the surfaces $(b - a)$ may be denoted by d. If we now assume that the radii of the two concentric spheres increases to a very large value, while keeping d constant, then radii a and b become almost equal, such that $a \cdot b$ is approximately equal to a^2. Also, the surface of the sphere, A, is given by $A = 4\pi a^2$

i.e. $a^2 = A/4\pi$

Thus, the above equation becomes:

$$C = 4\pi\varepsilon_0 \cdot \frac{a^2}{d} = 4\pi\varepsilon_0 \cdot \frac{A}{4\pi d}$$

i.e. $C = \frac{\varepsilon_0 A}{d}$

If now a dielectric is introduced between the plates, then,

$$C = \frac{\varepsilon_0 KA}{d},$$

in agreement with Equation 9.11. An infinite radius is the same as a flat surface, so that this applies to flat plates of area A.

9.8 CAPACITORS IN PARALLEL

If three capacitors (say) are connected in parallel, then they behave together like *one* capacitor of a particular value, as shown in Figure 9.12. The value of this capacitor is known as the 'total' or 'equivalent' capacity and may be calculated as follows.

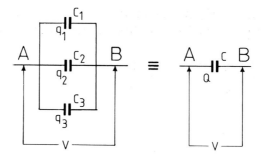

Fig. 9.12 Capacitors in parallel. The capacitor C is equivalent to the effect of C_1, C_2, C_3 connected together.

The total capacity, C, is defined as $C = Q/V$. The total charge Q is just the sum of the charges on the individual capacitors (q_1, q_2, etc.), while the potential difference is that across each individual capacitor, i.e. V.

Thus, $C = \dfrac{Q}{V} = \dfrac{q_1 + q_2 + q_3}{V} = \dfrac{q_1}{V} + \dfrac{q_2}{V} + \dfrac{q_3}{V}$

But $C_1 = \dfrac{q_1}{V}$; $C_2 = \dfrac{q_2}{V}$; $C_3 = \dfrac{q_3}{V}$

$$\therefore \quad C = C_1 + C_2 + C_3 + \ldots \qquad \qquad \text{Equation 9.12}$$

Thus, the total capacity is obtained by summing the individual capacities. Note that the total capacity must always be greater than the largest value of individual capacity.

9.9 CAPACITORS IN SERIES

Connecting three capacitors in series produces a 'total' or 'equivalent' capacity which is different from that obtained by connecting the same capacitors in parallel.

Establishing a potential difference V across the three capacitors results in charges of $+q$ and $-q$ on the plates of each individual capacitor, since they

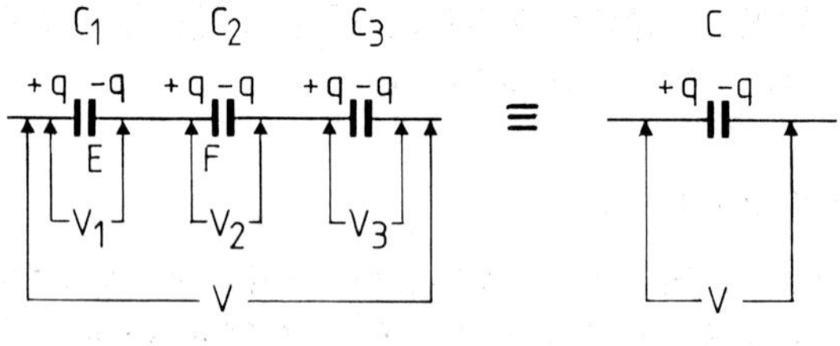

Fig. 9.13 Capacitors in series.

were originally electrically neutral. For example, electrons equivalent to a charge of $-q$ flow into plate E leaving behind $+q$ charge on plate F (Fig. 9.13).
Now,

$$\frac{1}{C} = \frac{V}{Q} = \frac{V_1 + V_2 + V_3}{q} = \frac{V_1}{q} + \frac{V_2}{q} + \frac{V_1}{q}$$

But,

$$\frac{V_1}{q} = \frac{1}{C_1}; \frac{V_2}{q} = \frac{1}{C_2}; \frac{V_3}{q} = \frac{1}{C_3}$$

$$\therefore \quad \frac{1}{C} = \frac{1}{C_1} + \frac{1}{C_2} + \frac{1}{C_3} + \dots \qquad \qquad \text{Equation 9.13}$$

In this case, the total capacity C is always less than the smallest value of the individual capacities, as shown in the examples below.

Examples

a. What is the total capacity when $3\mu F$, $4\mu F$ and $6\mu F$ capacitors are joined in parallel?
Using $C = C_1 + C_2 + C_3 + \dots$, we have
$C = 3 + 4 + 6 = 13\mu F$.

b. What is the total capacity when the above capacities are joined in series?

Using $\dfrac{1}{C} = \dfrac{1}{C_1} + \dfrac{1}{C_2} + \dfrac{1}{C_3} + \dots$, we have

$$\frac{1}{C} = \frac{1}{3} + \frac{1}{4} + \frac{1}{6} = \frac{9}{12}$$

i.e. $\dfrac{1}{C} = \dfrac{3}{4}$.

Turning both sides upside-down,
$C = \frac{4}{3} = 1\frac{1}{3} \, \mu F$.

Notice that this is less than any of the individual capacities, whereas the first example gave a total capacity greater than any of the individual capacities.

9.10 CHARGING AND DISCHARGING A CAPACITOR THROUGH A RESISTOR

9.10.1 Direct current

Consider the situation illustrated in Figure 9.14(a) where a battery (a source of constant potential difference) is connected across a resistor R and a capacitor C in series. When the switch S_1 is closed, electrons flow into one of the plates of the capacitor and away from the other plate, as shown illustrated. The potential difference across the capacitor, V_c, due to the charge on the plates, therefore increases. However, it does not increase indefinitely, but settles to a value which is the same as (but opposite to) that of the battery, V_B. To explain this, consider an electron at point P. When S_1 is closed, a complete circuit is made, and the force exerted on the electron due to the presence of the battery is able to move the electron towards the plate of the capacitor. However, as soon as the plate starts to build up electric charge, it in turn creates a force on an electron at P in the opposite direction, which slows down the rate of flow of charge into the plate. Eventually, of course, the two opposing forces on the electron become equal and there is no further movement of electrons on either side of the circuit. Thus, no further work is performed on the electrons, and the potential difference across the capacitor is equal and opposite to that of the battery.

The graph shown in Figure 9.14(b) illustrates these points. It is seen that there is an initial rapid rise of V_C when S_1 is closed, but that this slows down and approaches V_B relatively slowly. The effect of the resistance R is to limit the electron flow rate so that V_B is approached more slowly for large values of R than for small values of R, as shown on the graph.

If the battery is now disconnected, the capacitor will retain its charge and potential difference by the forces of mutual attraction of opposite charges. It is said to be 'storing charge'. Closing switch S_2 (Fig. 9.14(c)) 'discharges' the capacitor through R, i.e. electrons are able to travel from the negative plate towards the positive plate through the resistance R. Hence the charge on the plates (and therefore V_C) reduces so that the rate of electron flow is correspondingly reduced, and the variation of V_C with time is as shown in

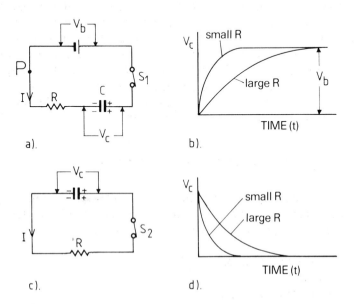

Fig. 9.14 Charging, (a) and (b), and discharging, (c) and (d), a capacitor through a resistor.

Figure 9.14(d). Eventually the capacitor is completely discharged so that the charge and potential difference are both zero. Again, the effect of R is to slow down the 'collapse' of V_C.

The first example of charging a capacitor demonstrates that, colloquially speaking, 'A CAPACITOR DOES NOT PASS D.C.', for, after the short time required to charge the plates of the capacitor, all further electron movement ceases.

Both of the above experiments are examples of the exponential law (Ch. 5). This is most striking from the comparison of many of the graphs in Chapter 5 to Figure 9.14(d) which obeys the formula:

$$V_C = V_0 e^{-t/RC}$$

(Note the similarity of this equation to $N_t = N_0 e^{-\lambda t}$ for the exponential decay of radioactivity and $I_x = I_0 e^{-\mu x}$ for the exponential attenuation of X-rays through matter.)

The quantity RC is called the *time-constant* of the circuit. If R is in ohm and C is in farad, then RC is in seconds. After a discharge time of one time-constant, i.e. after t = RC, then the potential difference across the capacitor has dropped to $1/e$ of its initial value, i.e. 0·37 or 37%. Thus if the original potential difference is 6v, the value after 1 time-constant is 0·37 × 6 = 2·2v. A further time-constant later, the potential difference will be reduced by another factor of 0·37, i.e. 0·37 × 2·2 = 0·8v. Note that this is very similar to the concept of half-life (5.2.2), since both are examples of an exponential decay.

9.10.2 Alternating current

The previous section has shown that a capacitor will eventually possess the same potential difference as the electrical supply connected across it. If the potential difference of the supply is changed, therefore, a new equilibrium will become established where, again, the two values of potential difference are equal. In this sense, the potential difference across the capacitor 'follows' that of the supply if the latter varies with time so that if an alternating current (Ch. 15) supply is connected across a capacitor, therefore, it may be said that 'A CAPACITOR PASSES A.C.' since the charge and PD on the capacitor are continually changing in sympathy with the supply.

9.11 CAPACITORS IN RADIOGRAPHY

The ability to store electrical energy on the plates of capacitors has important practical consequences in their use in radiography. Some of the uses to which capacitors have been put may be summarised as follows:

  a. Capacitor discharge circuits.
  b. Electronic timers.
  c. High tension smoothing.
  d. Compensation circuitry.

e. Phase-splitting for anode induction motor.
f. Integrating dosemeters.
g. Arc-suppression on contactors and relays.
h. Ionisation chambers (e.g. 'thimble').
i. Voltage doubling circuits.

There is insufficient space here to digress too far into the realms of radiographic equipment. However, in order to show how the physical principles of the action of capacitors are put to good practical use, the first two of the examples listed above will be discussed here briefly. The third example of high tension smoothing is examined in (20.4.1).

9.11.1 Capacitor discharge circuit

The capacitor discharge circuit is a useful application of capacitors for small low-power units where the electrical supply is somewhat variable, or where batteries must be used, as in some remote locations.

A capacitor or bank of capacitors, is first charged so that the PD across it is the same as that of the supply (9.10.1) whereupon the supply is disconnected. When a radiographic exposure is required, the capacitor is connected across the X-ray tube as shown in Figure 9.15.

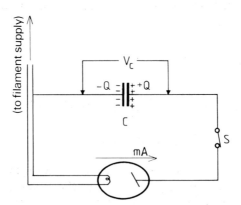

Fig. 9.15 Capacitor discharge circuit.

On closing switch S, electrons are able to flow from the negative plate of the capacitor towards and through the X-ray tube and onto the positive plate. This forms the radiographic exposure. Here, the X-ray tube is acting as a 'resistance' to the electron flow and so the situation is identical to that illustrated by Figure 9.14(d), i.e. a capacitor discharging through a resistor.

Example
A capacitor of $0.5\,\mu F$ is charged to a potential of 90 kV. What is the charge on its plates? It is connected to an X-ray tube and an exposure of 25 mAs is made. What is (a) the charge on the plates, (b) the PD across the capacitor, (c) the PD across the X-ray tube after the exposure?

This problem may look very difficult at first sight, but is in fact very easy. Its solution relies on two pieces of information: (i) $C = Q/C$ and (ii) mAs is the same as millicoulombs (6.4.2). Thus, initially we have the following conditions:

   a. $C = 0.5\,\mu\text{F} = 0.5 \times 10^{-6}\,\text{F}$
   b. $V = 90\,\text{kV} = 90 \times 10^3\,\text{V}$
   c. $Q = ?$

Now $C = \dfrac{Q}{V}$, so that $Q = VC = 90 \times 10^3 \times 0.5 \times 10^{-6}$

   i.e. $Q = 45 \times 10^{-3}$ coulombs
         $Q = 45$ millicoulombs (mC)
(Note that C must be in farads, V in volts and Q in coulombs).

An exposure of 25 mAs is made, i.e. 25 mC flows through the X-ray tube, and has come from the total charge stored on the capacitor. Thus, the charge on the plates of the capacitor is *reduced* by 25 mC, i.e. there is 20 mC of charge on each plate after the exposure. The PD across the X-ray tube is the same as that across the capacitor, of course, since they are joined in parallel, and may be calculated from another application of $C = Q/V$, where

   a. $C = 0.5\,\mu\text{F} = 0.5 \times 10^{-6}\,\text{F}$
   b. $Q = 20\,\text{mC} = 20 \times 10^{-3}\,\text{C}$
   c. $V = ?$

Since $C = \dfrac{Q}{V}, \; V = \dfrac{Q}{C} = \dfrac{20 \times 10^{-3}}{0.5 \times 10^{-6}} = 40 \times 10^3$

   i.e. $V = 40\,\text{kV}$ after the exposure

Alternatively, use may be made of the relationship $C = \Delta Q/\Delta V$ (see Insight in 9.7.1) where ΔQ and ΔV are the changes in the charge and potential difference respectively. Using the same argument as before, we know that 25 mC has been removed from the plates of the capacitor

   i.e. $\Delta Q = 25\,\text{mC} = 25 \times 10^{-3}\,\text{C}$, so that $\Delta V = \Delta Q/C = \dfrac{25 \times 10^{-3}}{0.5 \times 10^{-6}}$

   i.e. $\Delta V = 50 \times 10^3\,V = 50\,\text{kV}$.

This change in the PD, ΔV, is thus 50 kV, so that the final PD must be $90 - 50 = 40$ kV, in agreement with the first method of solution.

Either of these two methods may be used, and an exercise involving this type of question is included in Exercise 9.1 at the end of this chapter.

9.11.2 Capacitor-controlled timers

An exposure-timer employing the charging rate of an RC circuit is illustrated in Figure 9.16, where switch S is normally in position B, which keeps the capacitor C discharged through the variable resistor R. When the exposure is initiated, S is made to move to A and a constant DC supply (represented by the battery C) is able to charge C through R (9.10.1). The increasing potential difference across the capacitor, V_C, is applied to a special electronic circuit

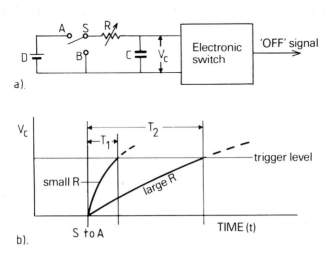

Fig. 9.16 Simplified construction and operation of a capacitor-controlled timer.

which switches power to an output circuit when V_C reaches a precise value (the 'trigger level'). By selecting different values of R, this may occur at different times from the initiation of the exposure, as shown illustrated in Figure 9.16(b). The output from the electronic switch is used to terminate the exposure, so that a particular exposure time results. The selection of the value of R determines the exposure time T, and the knob used to select different values of R on the X-ray operating panel is suitably calibrated for the appropriate exposure times.

The equation expressing the build-up of voltage across the capacitor is:

$$V_C = V_0 (1 - e^{-t/RC})$$

where, as in (9.10.1), RC is the *time-constant*. After one time-constant, when t = RC, the term in the bracket will be $1 - 1/e$, which is 0·63, so that the potential difference will have risen to 63% of its final value.

Exercise 9.1

a. Show that RC has units of seconds, using the relationships $R = V/I$, $I = Q/t$, $C = Q/V$.

b. What will be the potential difference after two time-constants for the capacitor charging circuit if the supply EMF is 240v?

9.12 TYPES OF CAPACITOR

Different types of capacitor are manufactured for different applications. In selecting a particular capacitor the user must be aware of various factors influencing his choice:

a. Voltage rating, i.e. what maximum value of PD the capacitor must be able to withstand (this is influenced by the *dielectric strength* of the dielectric, expressed in volt/metre)
b. the 'leakage' of the capacitor, i.e. how effective an electrical insulator is the dielectric
c. whether it is to be used for DC or AC
d. physical size
e. price

The types of capacitor available include:

a. variable multiplate 'air' capacitors
b. waxed paper dielectric
c. electrolytic
d. tantalum
e. polystyrene
f. ceramic
g. polycarbonate
h. plastic film
i. mica

where the name of each type refers to the dielectric material used in each case.

It is beyond the scope of this textbook to discuss these further or to compare one with another. However, the construction of the first three types only is shown briefly in the following section.

9.12.1 Variable multiplate 'air' capacitor

Figure 9.17(a) shows the basic construction of this type of capacitor, which is widely found in radio 'tuning' circuits, for example. Two sets of metal leaves are able to rotate with respect to each other, so that the area which they have in common may be changed. Now, since the capacity is proportional to the area of the plates (9.7.4), the system comprises a *variable* capacitor with air as the dielectric.

9.12.2 Waxed paper capacitor

Figure 9.17(b) and (c) show the construction of a capacitor having waxed paper as the dielectric (dielectric constant about 6). The conducting plates (aluminium) are thin, so that the plates and the dielectric may be 'rolled up' as a spiral, with an extra layer of waxed paper to avoid opposite plates in the spiral being in electrical contact and to increase the effect of the dielectric on the val-

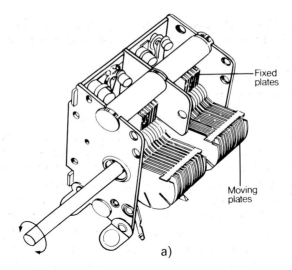

Fig. 9.17 (a) Variable multiplate 'air' capacitor.

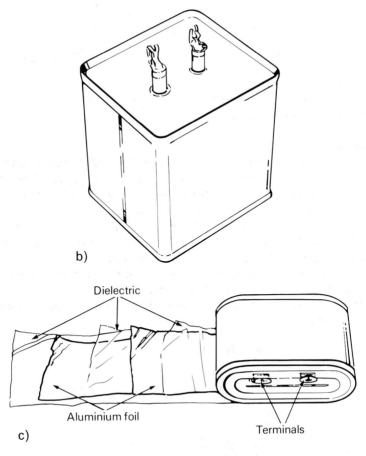

Fig. 9.17 (b) and (c) Capacitors using waxed paper as a dielectric.

ue of the capacity. Such capacitors are very common, being relatively cheap and suitable for general purpose use, although somewhat bulky for the larger values of capacity.

9.12.3 Electrolytic capacitor

The dielectric used in electrolytic capacitors is formed from thin layers of chemicals (e.g. aluminium oxide) which are deposited on the plates by electrolytic means, i.e. by immersing the plates in a suitable liquid and passing a current through them. Very thin layers of dielectric may be deposited on the plates, resulting in high values of capacity for a relatively small overall size of capacitor. This is because the capacity is inversely proportional to the plate separation (9.7.4). However, such capacitors are suitable for unidirectional current flow (i.e. not AC), as the dielectric loses its insulating properties if the current flows in the opposite direction. Such capacitors, therefore, are coded (by colour or symbol) as to which end is which, as shown in Figure 9.17(d).

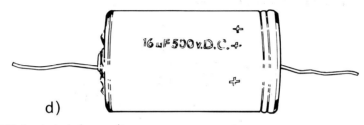

d)

Fig. 9.17(d) An electrolytic capacitor.

Exercise 9.2

a.   Explain what is meant by the terms 'electrical charge' and 'electric potential difference'. Hence explain the term 'electric capacity' of a body.

Define the SI units of charge, potential difference and capacity. (Note that *explain* and *define* require different answers.)

b.   A body of $50\mu F$ capacity is connected across a 1000-volt electrical supply. What is the charge on the plates of the capacitor? If the supply is disconnected what charge remains stored on the capacitor?

c.   How would you connect three capacitors in order to obtain (a) the greatest, and (b) the least value of total capacity?

d.   What is the total capacity produced by the following arrangement of individual capacitors:

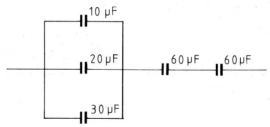

(*Hint:* first calculate the total capacity of the capacitors in parallel.)

e. What are the factors upon which the capacity of a parallel-plate capacitor depend? Explain the effect on the capacity produced by varying these factors.

f. What is the effect on the capacity of a body of:

(i) altering the charge on the plates
(ii) altering the PD across the plates
(iii) making the plates out of an electrically insulating material.
(iv) making the dielectric between the plates of an electrically conducting material?

g. A capacitor of value $8\mu F$ has a potential difference of 60kV applied to it. It is then connected across an X-ray tube and an exposure of 32 mAs made.

What is: (i) the original charge on the plates
(ii) the final charge on the plates
(iii) the final potential difference across the plates
(iv) the final potential difference across the X-ray tube?

SUMMARY

1. There are two types of electric charge, i.e. 'positive' and 'negative'. Negative charge is carried by an electron, and a positive charge is carried by a proton.

2. Like charges repel; unlike charges attract.

3. Electric charges may be *induced* in both conductors and insulators (dielectrics).

4. An 'electric field' at a point due to a body containing an electric charge is defined as the force exerted on a unit positive charge placed at that point.

5. A unit charge is 1 coulomb, and may be defined as the charge carried by 6×10^{18} electrons or protons.

6. A body containing a charge always possesses an *electric potential*, measured in volts. This is defined as the work done (joules) in moving a unit positive charge (coulomb) from infinity to the body (i.e. Volts = Joules/Coulomb). The electric potential on and within a conductor is constant.

7. The electric 'potential difference' (PD) between two points is also measured in volts, and is the work done in taking a unit positive charge from one point to the other.

8. The electric 'Capacity', C, of a body given by $C = Q/V$, where Q is the charge in coulombs held by the body, and V is its potential or potential difference in volts. The unit of capacity is the *farad*, but may often be quoted in terms of microfarad (μF) where $1 \ \mu F = 10^{-6} F$.

9. C is *independent* of either Q or V, for a particular capacitor, because Q and V vary in proportion to each other, leaving their *ratio* unchanged.

10. The 'properties' of capacitors may be summarised as follows:

a. Capacitors are capable of 'holding' or 'storing' a charge by the action of the mutual attraction of opposite charges on the plates of the capacitor.

b.   There are equal numbers of positive and negative charges on opposite plates.

c.   There is potential difference between the plates (see 7).

d.   Capacitors do not 'pass' DC, but do 'pass' AC.

e.   The joining together of capacitors results in the formation of a total capacity, C, given by:

$$C = C_1 + C_2 + C_3 + \ldots \text{ (in parallel)}$$

$$\frac{1}{C} = \frac{1}{C_1} + \frac{1}{C_2} + \frac{1}{C_3} + \ldots \text{ (in series).}$$

9.   The capacity of a parallel-plate capacitor is given by:

$$C = \frac{\varepsilon_0 K A}{d}$$

i.e. $C \propto K$, the dielectric constant between the plates

$C \propto A$, the area of plates

$C \propto \dfrac{1}{d}$, where d is the separation of the plates.

10. Electricity (DC)

The previous chapter was concerned with static electric charges; this chapter discusses the behaviour of moving electric charges, i.e. electricity. In a vacuum, gas or liquid, both positive and negative charges may move relatively freely and so may take part in the production of an electric *current* — the negative charges (electrons) flowing in the opposite direction to the positive charges. Both of these types of charge are called 'ions'. An air ionisation chamber (32.3.1) and a car battery both contain positive and negative ions moving in opposite directions, for example. However, in a *solid* material the atomic nuclei (Ch. 25) are unable to break free of the forces confining them relative to their immediate neighbours, and can therefore take no part in the electrical flow. Thus, it is the way in which the orbiting *electrons* behave which determines the electrical properties of a particular solid substance. This leads us to consider the electrical properties of materials in terms of the electron theory of conduction.

10.1 SIMPLE ELECTRON THEORY OF CONDUCTION

In order to explain the fact that some materials (e.g. metals) are good electrical conductors while other materials (e.g. plastics, rubber) are poor electrical conductors, we must look a little closer into the structure of the atom. This section anticipates to some degree the fuller treatment of the structure of the atom as described in Chapter 25. However, we only require to know that electrons orbiting the atomic nuclei are allowed to adopt particular orbits — the so-called 'discrete' energy levels — all other orbits being forbidden. When atoms are brought close together, as in a solid material, the orbits of the electrons are strongly influenced by the proximity of the neighbouring atoms and the discrete levels of allowable electron orbits are broadened into 'bands' of permitted energy levels, as illustrated in Figure 10.1 (a) and (b).

Two bands of permitted energy levels are of interest to us: the 'valence band' and the 'conduction band'. The *valence* band is that band which contains the outermost electrons of the atom, and may be partially or completely full of its permitted maximum number of electrons. The valence band therefore determines the *chemical* properties of the atom, i.e. its ability to form 'bonds' with other atoms. Bands of lower energy than that of the valence band are normally completely full. The *conduction* band is populated by electrons which have, for whatever reason, become free of their original atoms. This situation

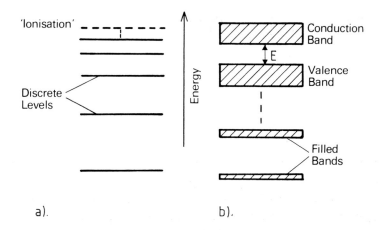

Fig. 10.1 (a) Electron levels in a solitary atom, and (b) electron bands in a solid.

corresponds to the ionisation of a single atom (Fig. 10.1 (a)) where an electron is completely removed from the atom. The essential point is that once an electron is in the conduction band of a solid it is able to move relatively freely and hence may take part in electrical conduction through the material. Thus, if no electrons are in the conduction band, the material shows zero conduction (or is a 'perfect insulator'). Similarly, a material with a large number of electrons in the conduction band is a good conductor of electricity, or poor insulator.

What determines the number of electrons in the conduction band of a particular material, and hence its electrical properties? The energy difference, E, between the top of the valence band and the bottom of the conduction band (Fig. 10.1(b)) is what distinguishes insulators, conductors and semiconductors. Figure 10.2 shows how this energy gap is large for insulators, small for semiconductors and may overlap for conductors.

Here we have to mention briefly the effect of *temperature* on conduction. At low temperatures, the atoms are vibrating at a relatively low kinetic energy (8.1) and so the effect of inter-atomic collisions on the orbiting electrons is small, and they occupy their lowest possible states, i.e., all the lower energy bands are full, and the remaining electrons exist within the valence band. This means that no electrons exist in the conduction band (e.g. in Fig. 10.2(a)) since they cannot gain enough energy to 'jump' over the forbidden band between the valence and conduction bands. As the temperature increases, the effect of the inter-atomic collision is to impart sufficient energy to some of the electrons to enable them to jump up into the conduction band, where they are essentially 'free' and able to take part in the conduction process. Some of these electrons will lose energy by collision and promptly 'fall back' to the valence band. Thus, at a given temperature, there is an approximately constant number of electrons in the conduction band, since an equal number of electrons per second fall back as are raised to the conduction band (i.e. a 'dynamic' equilibrium). We would therefore expect the conduction of an *insulator* to increase as the temperature is increased.

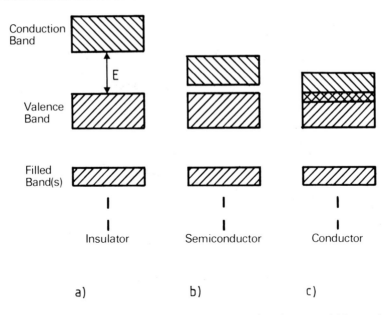

Fig. 10.2 Electron energy bands for (a) an insulator, (b) a semiconductor, and (c) a conductor.

A semiconductor (e.g. silicon) has a much lower energy gap, E, so that electrons are more easily raised from the valence to the conduction band than in the case of the insulator. (The effect of carefully controlled amounts of 'impurities' in the semiconductor materials is discussed in Ch. 19.) Again, we would expect the conduction to increase as the temperature of the semi-conductor is raised, since correspondingly more electrons will exist in the conduction band. A semiconductor shows a conduction between that of conductors and insulators — hence the prefix 'semi'.

A metallic conductor (e.g. copper) possesses conduction bands and valence bands which overlap, so that a very large number of electrons always exist in the conduction band, *whatever the temperature*. The conduction of such a material is therefore very much better than either a semiconductor or insulator. The main mechanism impeding the flow of electrons is the collision of such 'free' electrons with the atoms along their path. An increase of temperature therefore has the effect of impeding the flow of free electrons still further so that the conduction *decreases* for a metallic conductor. The effect of temperature on the 'resistance of electron flow' (defined in 10.4). is illustrated in Figure 10.3 (not to scale).

To summarise this section on the electron theory of conduction, we may note that insulators keep a tight grip on their electrons (i.e. very few electrons are able to break free into the conduction band), and so are unable to take part in flow through the material. However, conductors have electrons in their outer orbits which are very loosely held by their respective atoms and so are virtually 'free' to flow through the material already. On the energy band model, this is equivalent to the valence and conduction bands overlapping.

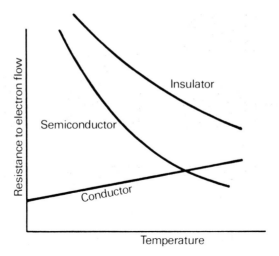

Fig. 10.3 The effect of temperature on electrical conduction.

10.2 ELECTRIC CURRENT

Electricity is the flow of electrons in a material, the rate of flow of electrons being a measure of the electric current. However, two essential conditions must be satisfied in order to produce a continuous current, and these are:

a.   There must be a source of electric *potential difference* (see 9.6.2).

b.   There must be a *complete circuit* around which the electrons are able to pass.

These two points are illustrated in Figure 10.4 The battery B is a source of constant potential difference, but if the switch S is open (as in Fig. 10.4(a)) then no electrons flow and the bulb does not light up. When the switch S is closed (as in Fig. 10.4(b)) a complete, or continuous, circuit is made around

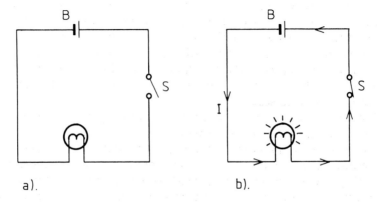

Fig. 10.4 A continuous circuit is necessary for an electric current to flow.

which the electrons are able to flow indefinitely, and the blub lights. The potential difference may thus be thought of as the 'driving force' which causes the electrons to flow, while the current is the rate of flow of the electrons, i.e. the number of electrons passing a given point per second.

Definition

An *electric current of 1 ampere* (A) flows at a point if a charge of 1 coulomb (C) of charge flows past that point per second.

Mathematically, therefore,

1 ampere = 1 coulomb/second	Equation 10.1

From Section 9.2 we know that a charge of 1 coulomb is equivalent to approximately 6×10^{18} electrons, so that 1 ampere is just this number of electrons passing a point in one second. (The precise modern definition of the ampere involves the 'motor principle' and in explained in 13.3.1).

Insight

It is interesting to discover the typical average velocity of the electrons flowing in a circuit, as it is very much less than might be expected at about 0·5 mm/second! Why then does the bulb in Figure 10.4 light up well before electrons from the battery could reach it? It is because the effect of electrons moving in one part of the circuit affects the electrons in all other parts of the circuit, so that they all start to flow virtually instantaneously.

10.2.1 mA, mAs and millicoulombs

The electric current flowing through an X-ray tube is measured in milliamperes (mA), where $1 \text{ mA} = 10^{-3} \text{ A}$. This unit measures the *rate* of flow of electrons through the tube. The unit which measures the *total number* of electrons which have travelled through the X-ray tube for a given radiographic exposure is the *milliampere-second* (mAs), and is obtained by *multiplying* the mA by the exposure time in seconds, i.e.

mAs = mA × seconds	Equation 10.2

(See 6.4.2 for an example of an exposure of 60 mAs.) Now the total number of electrons which flow in a circuit is just a measure of *charge*. The unit of electrical charge at the 'milli-' level is the millicoulomb, which may be expressed in terms of the mA by using Equation 10.1:

millicoulombs = mA × seconds   Equation 10.3

The similarity of the above two equations shows that:

1 mAs = 1 millicoulomb	Equation 10.4

10.3 POTENTIAL DIFFERENCE AND EMF

For a detailed description of electric potential and potential difference (PD), the reader is referred to (9.6.2). In summary, the definition of potential difference outlined in that section also applies to this section, i.e.

Definition
> The potential difference in volts is equal to the work done in joules in moving 1 coulomb of charge from one point to another, or

---

volts = joules/coulomb   Equation 10.5

However, in electricity we are concerned with moving charges, and it is here that, as mentioned previously, the potential may be regarded as the 'driving force' causing the electrons to flow, rather like the difference in gravitational levels causing a ball to roll down a slope.

'Electromotive Force' (EMF) is also expressed in volts and is measure of the difference of electrical potential energy developed across a *source* of electricity (e.g. a battery or generator). Thus the EMF is the 'driving force' behind the electron flow in a circuit. However, the potential difference measured across the terminals of a battery, for example, is less than the EMF when a current flows because of the internal resistance of the battery. This effect is known as 'regulation' and is explained in more detail in Chapter 16.

It is therefore possible to speak of the potential difference across any part of an electrical circuit, including the source of the electricity, but the 'EMF' is reserved solely for the latter, so that one would not, for example, use the term 'EMF across a resistor'. A resistor is not a source of electricity, and so the term 'potential difference' is appropriate.

10.4 RESISTANCE

The elementary electron theory of the conduction of electricity (10.1) refers to two mechanisms impeding the flow of electrons in a material: lack of 'free' electrons (as in an insulator) and collision of the flowing electrons with the vibrating atoms of the material. This 'resistance to flow' is called simply 'electrical resistance' or 'resistance' and is measured in ohms, as defined in (10.5). Obviously, insulators will have very much higher values of resistance than a metal of the same shape and size. However, equal volumes of the *same* material may have more markedly different resistances, depending on their shape, as outlined below.

10.4.1 Factors affecting resistance

The following list collates the quantities previously discussed which affect the electrical resistance of a substance:

a.   the *shape* of the substance
b.   the *type* of the substance
c.   the *temperature* of the substance

Note that this list does *not* include either the potential difference across the substance or the current flowing through it (see 10.5). Taking the above list in turn:

Shape
Obviously a body may take an infinite variety of sizes and shapes, so we shall restrict our attention to straight bodies of constant cross-section, since these are amenable to simple mathematical treatment.

Figure 10.5 illustrates such a body and the effect on the resistance R of altering its length l, and cross-sectional area A.

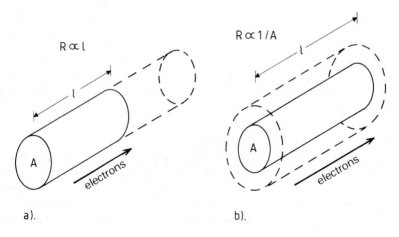

Fig. 10.5 The variation of resistance with length and cross-sectional area.

It is easy to see why the resistance of the body should be proportional to the length (i.e. $R \propto l$), since if the length is doubled (say) then there are twice as many vibrating atoms for each electron to get past! The means that the resistance will also be doubled. The effect of the cross-sectional area is perhaps less clear intuitively. However, if the cross-sectional area doubles, then twice as many electrons are capable of taking part in conduction, while the number of atoms which *each* electron must circumnavigate is the same. Thus, the resistance to flow halves, since the current is doubled. This situation is analogous to water flowing in a large diameter pipe compared to a small diameter pipe, where the larger area allows a faster flow rate of water. Resistance is thus inversely proportional (1.7) to area, i.e. $R \propto 1/A$.

Type of substance
Good electrical conductors will show a lower resistance than electrical insulators, by definition. However, as we have seen above, the shape of the substance also affects its resistance, so that a standard size and shape must be

used when comparing the resistances of different materials. The standard used is a cube of side 1 metre, and the resistance is measured when passing an electric current through opposing faces of the cube. (In practice, of course, a 1 cm cube may be used (for example) and the resistance for a 1 metre cube calculated.) The value of the resistance so obtained is called the 'resistivity' or 'specific resistance' and is measured in units of ohm-metres. Resistivity is often given the symbol ρ (Greek 'rho'), and it is clear that the resistance of a substance is directly proportional to its resistivity, i.e. $R \propto \rho$.

Combining all the above factors, we have:

$$R \propto \frac{\rho l}{A}$$ Equation 10.6

In SI units, ρ is defined so as to make the 'constant of proportionality' of the above equation equal to unity, so that we obtain finally:

$$R = \frac{\rho l}{A}$$ Equation 10.7

The specific resistances of insulators are about a million times greater than those of semiconductors which in turn are about a million times greater than those of metallic conductors.

Temperature
As described in (10.1), the effect of temperature on the resistance of a body differs depending upon whether the body is a conductor or an insulator. Figure 10.3 shows that the resistance of insulators decreases with temperature (because of more electrons in the conduction band) and the resistance of conductors increases in a linear manner with temperature (because of increased collisions with energetic atoms). Thus we would expect the resistivity to vary with temperature, which is why it is usually quoted at a particular temperature (e.g. 20°C). The *temperature coefficient of resistance*, $\propto$, is defined as the 'fractional change of resistance (or resistivity) per unit temperature change', i.e.

$$\propto = \frac{\text{change in resistivity}}{\text{original resistivity}} \Big/ \text{temperature change}$$

$\propto$ has a value of about 0·004 for copper and 0·00001 for manganin (an alloy), so that the resistivity changes less for a given temperature change for manganin than copper.

Exercise 10.1
   a.   Explain what is meant by the terms 'electrical conductor' and 'electrical insulator' and show how their electrical behaviour may be described by the elementary electron theory of conduction.
   b.   List the factors upon which the resistance of a conductor depends.
   1 metre of wire of a given cross-sectional area is found to have the same resistance as a length of wire of the same material but of double the cross-

sectional area. How long is the second wire? (*Hint:* Use equation 10.7 for each wire.)

10.5 OHM'S LAW

Ohm's Law applies to metallic conductors and combines, in a particularly simple and elegant way, the relationship between current, potential difference and resistance. It is found experimentally that the current flowing through such a conductor increases *in proportion* to the potential difference applied across it (i.e. as the 'driving force' on the electrons is increased). Thus, if a potential difference of two volts (say) causes a current of one ampere to flow through a particular conductor, then four volts causes a current of two amperes and so on. This is Ohm's Law, and may be stated more formally as:

Ohm's Law
The current flowing through a metallic conductor is proportional to the potential difference which exists across it provided that all physical conditions remain constant.

The main 'physical condition' which must remain constant is *temperature*, for temperature affects the passage of electrons through the material (Sections 10.1 to 10.4).

Mathematically, Ohm's Law is just:

$$I \propto V \hspace{4cm} \text{Equation 10.8}$$

where I and V are the magnitude of current and potential difference respectively.

Note that Ohm's Law does not mention the word 'resistance' at all. The resistance of the body is introduced into Equation 10.8 as a constant of proportionality (1.7), i.e. as a means of relating the units of I and V so that an equals sign may be used.

Now $V \propto I$ (rewriting 10.8), so that $V = R \cdot I$

where R is a constant for a given body. Thus, we have the rather more useful mathematical expression of Ohm's Law:

$$V = I \cdot R \hspace{4cm} \text{Equation 10.9}$$

It cannot be over-emphasised at this point that R is a *constant* for a given body at a given temperature and therefore *does not depend* upon V or I.

R is measured in ohm (Ω), such that if $V = 1$ volt and $I = 1$ ampere, then Equation 10.9 produces $1 = I \cdot R$, i.e. $R = 1$ ohm, leading to the following definition of an ohm:

Definition

A body is said to have an electrical resistance of *1 ohm* if a potential difference of 1 volt across it produces an electrical current through it of 1 ampere.

(Note that a potential difference always occurs 'across' a body, *never* 'through' it. Likewise, an electric current always flows 'through' a body, it does not exist 'across' it.)

Although Ohm's Law is so simple in formulation, it has far-reaching implications in the field of electrics and electronics. Some of the practical examples of this law are given in the following sections, and the reader is advised to study them and to try the later exercises.

10.5.1 Resistors in series

If we join three resistors 'end-to-end' (i.e. in 'series') and apply a potential difference V volts across the two ends, then a particular current I flows, as illustrated in Figure 10.6. Note that the same current flows through each resistor, since electrons are not lost or gained within any part of the circuit. We wish to calculate the value of resistance, R, which would behave in exactly the same way as the three resistors, i.e. a PD of V producing a current I through R. This value of R is known as the 'total' or 'effective' resistance, and may be calculated using Ohm's Law.

If a PD of V_1, V_2, V_3, exists across R_1, R_2, R_3 respectively, we may apply Ohm's Law in turn:

$$V_1 = IR_1; V_2 = IR_2; V_3 = IR_3$$

In addition, we know that V is composed of the sum of the three individual potential differences (analogous to a run of three waterfalls), i.e.

$$V = V_1 + V_2 + V_3$$
$$\therefore \quad V = IR_1 + IR_2 + IR_3$$
$$\text{Thus } V = I(R_1 + R_2 + R_3)$$
$$\therefore \quad \frac{V}{I} = R_1 + R_2 + R_3$$

Applying Ohm's Law to the total resistance, R, we have $V = IR$

$$\text{i.e.} \quad \frac{V}{I} = R$$

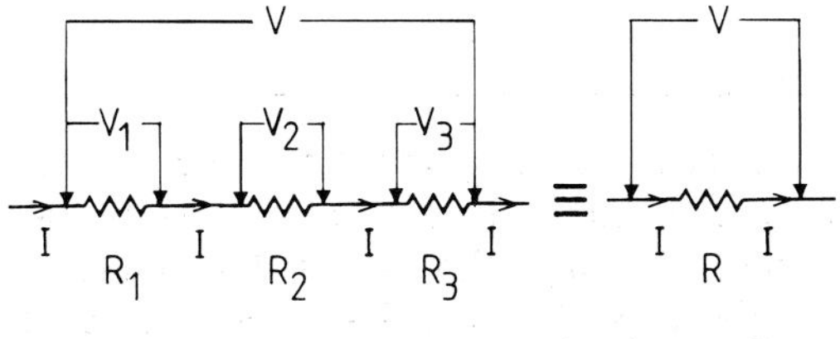

Fig. 10.6 Combining resistors in series to produce a total resistance R.

From comparison of the above two equations, it is clear that:

$$R = R_1 + R_2 + R_3 + \text{etc.}$$ Equation 10.10

Thus the total resistance is obtained simply by adding together the value of the separate resistances.

10.5.2 Resistors in parallel

A potential difference V exist across points A and B in Figure 10.7, and since each resistor is connected to A and B the potential difference across *each resistor* is V also. Electrons flow in the circuit until point A is reached, when a choice of three different pathways is available. However, since electrons are neither gained nor lost at any part of the circuit, the total electron flow through the three resistors is the same as I.

i.e. $I = i_1 + i_2 + i_3$ Equation 10.11

Equally, of course i_1, i_2, i_3, combined at B to produce I once more.

Applying Ohm's Law to each of the resistors we have

$$V = i_1 R_1; \; V = i_2 R_2; \; V = i_3 R_3$$

or $i_1 = V/R_1; i_2 = V/R_2; i_3 = V/R_3$

so that, by Equation 10.11,

$$I = V\left(\frac{1}{R_1} + \frac{1}{R_2} + \frac{1}{R_3}\right)$$

or

$$\frac{I}{V} = \frac{1}{R_1} + \frac{1}{R_2} + \frac{1}{R_3}$$

Ohm's Law applied to the resistor R gives:

$$V = I \cdot R$$

or

$$\frac{I}{V} = \frac{1}{R}$$

Comparing these equations, we have finally:

$$\frac{1}{R} = \frac{1}{R_1} + \frac{1}{R_2} + \frac{1}{R_3} + \text{etc.}$$ Equation 10.12

In this case, the total resistance R is always *reduced* by joining resistors in parallel. Numerical examples are given in the next section.

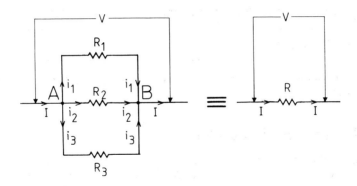

Fig. 10.7 Combining resistors in parallel to produce a total resistance R.

10.5.3 Further examples of Ohm's Law

a.   A 10 volt battery is connected across a 30 Ω resistor. What current flows in the circuit?

From Ohm's Law: $I = V/R$

i.e. $I = \frac{10}{30} = \frac{1}{3}$ A.

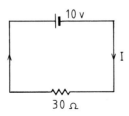

b.   A 6 volt battery is connected across a 10 Ω and a 20 Ω resistor connected in series. What current flows in the circuit, and what is the potential difference across each resistor?

Total resistance $= 20 + 10 = 30\ \Omega$.
From Ohm's Law, $I = V/R = \frac{6}{30} = \frac{1}{5}$ A.

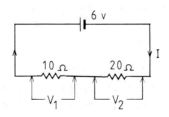

Applying Ohm's Law to each resistor,

$$V_1 = \tfrac{1}{5} . 10 = 2 \text{ volts}; V_2 = \tfrac{1}{5} . 20 = 4 \text{ volts}.$$

Note that (i) the *same current* flows through each resistor and
(ii) $V_1 + V_2 = 2 + 4 = 6$ volts, i.e. the same as the battery voltage, as would
be expected.

   c.   A 6 volt battery is connected across 10Ω and 20Ω resistors connected
in parallel. What is the current flowing in each resistor and in the whole of the
circuit?

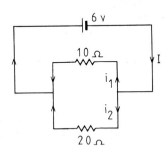

The potential difference across *each* resistor in this circuit is that of the
battery, i.e. 6 volts. Applying Ohm's Law to each resistor:

$$i_1 = \tfrac{6}{10} = 0.6 \text{ A}; i_2 = \tfrac{6}{20} = 0.3 \text{ A}$$

Thus, the current flowing in the whole circuit is

$$(i_1 + i_2) - \text{i.e. } 0.9 \text{ A}.$$

10.6 ELECTRICAL ENERGY AND POWER

When an electric current flows through a conductor, the electrons must be
'driven' by the difference in electric potential across the conductor. As
described earlier, the moving electrons suffer collisions with the atoms of the
conductor which therefore produces a 'resistance' to flow of the electrons. This
is analogous to pushing an object along the top of a table, where a constant
velocity is obtained when the force applied to the object is equal and opposite
to the frictional force between the object and the table, i.e. work is continually
being done on the object (see 6.3.6) in order to maintain its movement. This
work manifests itself as heat produced between the two frictional surfaces.
Exactly the same argument applies to the flow of electrons through a
conductor, i.e. work is continually performed on the electrons to keep them all
moving in the same direction, and the consequence of this work is that heat is
produced, because the atoms gain energy from the electrons by collision. The
fact the heat is produced by the flow of electric current is no great surprise, of
course, in view of the action of electric fires, for example!

10.6.1 The joule

The joule is the SI unit of energy (6.3.6), in terms of which all forms of energy may be expressed (e.g. mechanical, electrical etc.). The key to the method of calculation of electrical energy lies in the meaning of 'potential difference'. It was shown in Section 9.6.3 that the potential difference (volts) is defined in terms of the work done (joules) in taking a unit charge (1 coulomb) between two points. Thus, the PD is already related to energy by:

volts = joules/coulomb   Equation 10.13

i.e. PD is the 'work done (energy) per unit charge'.
   Re-arranging this equation, we have

joules = volts × coulombs   Equation 10.14

Example
   A total electric charge of five coulombs flows in a conductor across a potential difference of 10 volts. What is the total electrical energy expended?
   From the above equation, we have simply:

energy = 10 × 5 = 50 joule.

This energy is transformed into heat energy, of course, so that it is possible to calculate the temperature increase of the conductor if its heat capacity is known (8.1.2).

10.6.2 The watt

The watt is the SI unit of *power*, defined as the *rate* of doing work (6.3.7), where 1 watt = 1 joule per second. Thus, if we divide both sides of Equation 10.14 by time, we have

$$\frac{\text{joules}}{\text{second}} = \text{volts} \times \frac{\text{coulombs}}{\text{second}}$$

Now joules/second = watts, and coulombs/second = amperes (10.2), so the above equation reduces to:

watts = volts × amperes   Equation 10.15

This is a general equation used in the calculation of electrical power which applies to any electrical system, whether a source of electricity (e.g. a battery) or the power generated in a current-carrying material (whether it obeys Ohm's law or not). However, it is particularly useful to apply this formula to a metallic conductor, which obeys Ohm's Law (10.5).

10.6.3 Power in a resistor

Consider a current I passing through a metallic conductor of resistance R, across which a potential difference of V is applied, as shown in Figure 10.8.

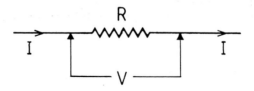

Fig. 10.8 Power produced in a resistor.

We may use the general Equation 10.15 for the electrical power being expended:

i.e. $W = V \times I$.

However, we know that the resistor also obeys Ohm's Law: $V = I \cdot R$ so that we may substitute this last value of V into the first equation, i.e.

$$W = I \cdot R \times I$$
i.e. $W = I^2 R$

Similarly, we may substitute $I = V/R$ into the first equation, obtaining

$$W = V \times \frac{V}{R} = \frac{V^2}{R}$$

Thus, the following three equations for electrical power in a resistor may be used:

$$
\begin{aligned}
W &= VI \\
W &= I^2 R \\
W &= V^2/R
\end{aligned}
\qquad\qquad \text{Equation 10.16}
$$

The second equation is of more interest to us than the third, and occurs in other places in subsequent chapters (e.g. in AC transformer losses and power losses in cables — 10.7). Some worked examples may clarify the use of these equations:

Examples

a.   10 amps flows through a 2Ω resistor. What power is generated in the resistor?
   Using $W = I^2 R$, $W = 100 \times 2 = 200$ watts.
   Alternatively we may first calculate V from Ohm's Law ($V = IR = 20$ volts) and substitute into $W = VI = 20 \times 100 = 200$ watts, to give the same answer.

b.   In the above example, what is the total electrical energy if the current flows for five minutes?

Now, watts = joules/seconds

∴   joules = watts × seconds

$= 200 \times 5 \times 60$

∴   Energy is 60 000 J or 60 kJ.

c.   A 6 volt battery is connected to a 60 Ω resistor. What current flows, and what power is (i) generated by the battery, (ii) generated in the resistor?

From Ohm's Law $I = V/R = \frac{6}{60} = 0{\cdot}1$ amps.

Power from the battery $= V \times I = 6 \times 0{\cdot}1 = 0{\cdot}6$ watt.

Power in the resistor $= I^2 R = 0{\cdot}1^2 \times 60 = 0{\cdot}6$ watt.

Thus the power from the battery is the same as that generated in the resistor, as would be expected from the Principle of Conservation of Energy (7.2).

10.6.4 The kilowatt-hour (kWh)

Another measure of electrical energy is the kilowatt-hour (kWh), which is used to determine the energy used by all consumers of electricity, whether domestic, industrial or in hospitals. The kilowatt is just 10^3 watts and is a unit of power, so that kilowatts × time is a measure of energy.

Now, as we have seen previously 1 watt × 1 sec = 1 joule so that $1 \text{ kW} \times 1 \text{ h} = 10^3 \times 60 \times 60$ joules, i.e.,

$$1 \text{ kWh} = 3{\cdot}6 \text{ MJ}$$

The kilowatt-hour is thus seen to represent a large amount of energy.

10.7 POWER LOSS IN CABLES

Consider the situation where an electrical generating station (coal, oil or nuclear) is remotely situated from a centre of population. The electricity so generated is connected to the town (for example) by means of the thick conducting cables on 'pylons', which have small, but definite, electrical resistances (the 'cable resistance'). As we have seen in the previous section, a current flowing through a resistance generates power in that resistance which is manifested as heat. Thus, the electrical power available to the town is reduced by just that amount of power produced (or 'lost') in the cables. This term 'lost' does not imply any breaking of the Principles of Conservation of Energy; it is being used in a purely colloquial sense of power being 'lost', or 'not available', to the user. It is obviously desirable to reduce this 'lost' power to a relatively insignificant value, and the purpose of this section is to describe the ways in which this is managed.

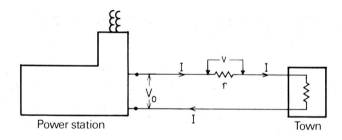

Fig. 10.9 Simplified diagram of a power station supplying electrical power to a town. Some of the power is 'lost' owing to the resistance, r, of the cables.

Figure 10.9 illustrates the situation described above, where it is mathematically convenient to show the cable resistance as a separate resistor of value r connected to perfectly conducting cables.

The power produced by the station is $V_0 \times I$ (Equation 10.15). The power generated in the cable resistance is $I^2 r$ (Equation 10.16). Hence the power loss in the cable is reduced if $I^2 r$ is reduced. This may be accomplished in two ways:

a.   reducing r, the cable resistance, i.e. using thick cables of good conducting material (10.4.1);

b.   reducing I, the current flowing through the cable.

There is a commercial and engineering limit to the thickness of cable which may be used in practice, and some optimum value is chosen. However, the greater improvement is obtained by reducing I, since the power loss is proportional to I^2. Thus, it is desirable to use as low a value of current as possible, but the voltage from the power station V_0, must be made correspondingly higher (132 000 volts on the National Grid) so that the power from the station ($V_0 I$), is also as great as it was before reducing I. A simple numerical example will clarify this point:

Example

a.   If $V_0 = 100$ volts; $I = 1$ amp; $r = 10\,\Omega$, then the power from the station $= V_0 I = 100$ watt and the power 'lost' in the cable $= I^2 r = 1^2 \cdot 10 = 10$ watt; i.e. 10% of the power generated is 'lost' in the cable.

However, if $V_0 = 1000$ volts; $I = 0{\cdot}1$ amps; $r = 10\,\Omega$, then the power from the station $= V_0 I = 100$ watts, as before, but the power 'lost' in the cable $= I^2 r = 0{\cdot}1^2 \cdot 10 = 0{\cdot}1$ watt; i.e. $0{\cdot}1\%$ of the power of the generator.

Thus, a current reduction by a factor of 10 makes a 'power loss' reduction by a factor of 100.

To summarise, therefore, electrical power is transmitted over long distances at *high voltages* and *low currents* in order to minimise the power loss in the cables.

10.8 MAINS CABLE RESISTANCE AND X-RAY EXPOSURES

As the previous section has shown, the effect of the resistance of the cables connecting the source of power to the electrical load is to produce a reduction in the electrical potential difference developed across the load. This section considers the effect of the resistance of the mains cables leading to the X-ray units within a hospital.

If the total cable resistance of all the cables connecting the generator to the hospital is R_g, and R_h is the resistance of the cables within the hospital connecting to a given X-ray unit, then the potential difference, V, available to the unit is just the E.M.F. minus the total potential difference developed across the cables, i.e.

$$V = E - I (R_g + R_h)$$ Equation 10.17

In this equation, E is the EMF applied by the generator, and I is the current drawn from the mains supply for a given X-ray exposure. Note that this current is not the same as the mA, since the mA is the current flowing in the *secondary* of the high-tension transformer. Obviously, the term $I(R_g + R_h)$ represents the 'volts-drop' across the cables, as given by Ohm's Law. The practical effect of this is to reduce both the kV_p and mA to the unit since the potential difference applied to the high-tension and filament transformers has been reduced (to a value of V/E times their nominal values).

Equation 10.17 produces two important conclusions:

a.   as the current I increases, V is reduced (see 16.3.3 on regulation)
b.   the full EMF of the generator can be applied across the X-ray unit only if either $I = 0$ or $R_g + R_h = 0$, since then $V = E$. Neither of these possibilities is a practicable solution, so the cable voltage drop is reduced to as small a value as possible by reducing the cable resistance by the appropriate selection of cable material and diameter (10.4).

In a fixed installation, the mains cables within the hospital may be very thick to provide the necessary low voltage drop, but this is not the case with portable units since such thick cables would make the equipment unmanageable. The thinner cables used with portable sets will therefore have a significant resistance, and the longer cables running to the mains outlets at the top of the hospital will have a higher resistance than those shorter cables used for the ground floor. This situation would lead to films of variable optical density, with the 'thinner' films being produced on the higher floors. However, there is a simple way of standardising the X-ray exposure factors so that the same settings may be used at every location of the portable within the hospital, and that is to always use the 'worst-case' cable resistance, i.e. that of the longest cable. In practice, this means selecting resistances within the portable unit such that the sum of these 'ballast' resistances and the individual cable resistances is constant. A typical method is to have the socket outlets coded in some way (numerically or by colour, for example) so that a switch on the console may be set to the same code in order to select the correct ballast resistor.

Insight

New techniques may make the problem of power loss in cables obsolete. For example, 'superconductors' have a resistance of zero at low temperatures so that the power loss is zero also (I^2r, where r is zero). However, practical difficulties make this an uncertain commercial possibility at present.

Orbiting space stations which collect solar energy and beam it to Earth via microwaves (24.2) are a serious possibility for the future. Cables are not required, of course, between the satellite and Earth, but will be required from the receiver to the towns it serves, so that cable loss is important here also.

Exercise 10.2

a. Define and explain Ohm's Law. Hence define the unit of resistance (ohm). What is the effect on the resistance of a conductor of:

  (i) increasing the current through it
  (ii) decreasing the potential difference across it.
  (iii) increasing its temperature.

b. What total resistance is obtained if resistances of 10Ω, 20Ω, 40Ω are placed (i) in series and (ii) in parallel.

c. Calculate I, i_1, i_2, V_1, V_2 in the following circuit.

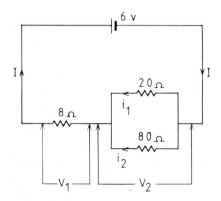

d. Explain what the following electrical units represent:

  (i) the coulomb
  (ii) the ampere
  (iii) the volt
  (iv) the ohm
  (v) the joule
  (vi) the watt
  (vii) the milliampere-second (mAs)

Write down as many mathematical relationships between these units as you can, *then* compared with the Summary (point 11).

e.   Explain why large amounts of electrical power are transmitted over long distances at a high potential difference.

SUMMARY

1.   An electric current in a solid is just the flow of electrons within the solid — the positive charges (nuclei) being unable to travel through the solid.

2.   Solid matter is composed of three types of material: insulators, conductors and semiconductors.

3.   A conductor contains 'free' electrons, i.e. electrons which are not tightly bound to the nuclei. An insulator has tightly bound electrons.

4.   On the energy-band model, free electrons inhabit the conduction band. Metallic conductors have conduction bands and valence bands overlapping, while insulators have widely separated conduction and valence bands.

5.   An increase of temperature increases the resistance of conductors (by electron collision) and decreases the resistance of insulators (more electrons jump into the conduction band).

6.   Resistance $\propto$ specific resistance, ρ

$$\propto \text{ length of conductor, } l$$

$$\propto \frac{1}{A} \text{ where } A \text{ is the cross-section area.}$$

i.e. $R = \rho l / A$.

7.   Ohm's Law: Current $\propto$ PD at constant temperature.

8.   Resistance defined by $R = V/I$ (Ohm's Law) such that 1 volt across 1 Ω causes 1 amp.

9. $R = R_1 + R_2 + R_3 + \ldots$ (resistors in series)

$$\frac{1}{R} + \frac{1}{R_1} + \frac{1}{R_2} + \frac{1}{R_3} + \ldots \text{ (resistors in parallel).}$$

10.   Power loss in cables reduced by (a) reducing cable resistance, (b) reducing I(loss $\propto I^2$). Therefore, power transmitted at high voltage and low currents.

11.   Resistance of mains cables both inside the hospital and to the generator results in the potential difference to the X-ray unit being reduced. This is particularly important for portable units, where variable exposures may be produced unless 'ballast' resistors appropriate to each mains socket are selected by the radiographer prior to exposure.

12.   Relationships between units:
   a.   volts = joules/coulomb (definition)
   b.   1 ampere = 1 coulomb/second (definition)
   c. $V = IR$ (Ohm's Law)
   d. $W = VI$ (general expression for power)
   e. $W = I^2 R$ (power in a resistor)
   f.   Energy = power $\times$ time = $W \times t$ (definition)
      or $V \times I \times t$
      or $V \times C$ (since $C = It$).
   g.   1 mAs = 1 millicoulomb.

11. Magnetism

11.1 MAGNETIC POLES

We are all familiar with the behaviour of a magnetic compass, in aligning itself in a North–South direction. Such a compass is an example of a 'permanent' bar magnet, each end of which has a magnetic 'pole'. The 'north-seeking' end of the magnet is called a 'north pole' and the 'south-seeking' end is called the 'south pole'. Thus, there are two types of magnetic pole (north and south), just as there are two types of electric charge (positive and negative)—see 9.1. Many other properties of magnetism are similar to those of electrical charges, as may be seen by comparison of this chapter with Chapter 9. However, there is one fundamental difference between magnetic poles and electric charges: charges

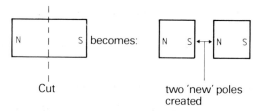

Cut   becomes: two 'new' poles created

Fig. 11.1 The effect of cutting a bar magnet on two. Magnetic poles always exist in pairs.

may exist in *isolation* (e.g. as a solitary electron) whereas poles always exist in *pairs*. Consider for example, the situation in Figure 11.1, where an attempt has been made to separate the north and south poles of a permanent magnet by cutting it in two.

As shown in the figure, the only consequence of this action is that two further poles are revealed as soon as the two parts of the magnet are separated.

Further subdivisions of the magnet always produce smaller and smaller bar magnets no matter how small the individual pieces. Thus, we would expect that the individual *atoms* of the material are also magnetised (i.e. each atom possesses a north and a south pole) in order to explain this phenomenon, and such is the case. As we shall see later (Chapter 12), magnetism is actually caused by moving electrical charges (i.e. electric currents), so magnetic atoms are produced by the circulating orbits of the charged electrons of the atoms. If the orbits of the electrons of an atom tend to be in the same direction, then the total effect is to produce a very magnetic atom (e.g. iron) whereas if the orbits tend to cancel each other's magnetic effect then a weak or even non-existent magnetic atom results.

11.2 FORCE BETWEEN TWO POLES

The effect of two poles upon each other may be described in qualitative terms as:

'like poles repel; unlike poles attract'

This is very similar to the case of two charges (9.2). The calculation of the magnitude of the force between two poles in a vacuum likewise follows a similar argument to that between two charges. Mathematically, a north pole is

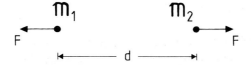

Fig 11.2 The mutual force of repulsion between two similar poles.

considered to be positive and a south pole negative. This enables the following simple equations to be written. If poles of strength m_1 and m_2 are separated by a distance d (Fig. 11.2), then a mutual force F exists between them, where:

$$F \propto m_1 m_2 / d^2 \qquad \text{Equation 11.1}$$

In the SI system of units the constant of proportionality (1.7) of this equation is $1/4\pi\mu_0$ such that

$$F = \frac{m_1 m_2}{4\pi\mu_0 d^2} \qquad \text{Equation 11.2}$$

where F is in the newtons, d in metres and m_1, m_2 are in webers (Wb). μ_0 is the 'permeability of free space', and has a value of $4\pi \times 10^{-7}$ henry per metre (H m^{-1}). The henry is discussed further in (14.6).

Note the similarity between Equation 11.2 and Equation 9.2 for the electrostatic case. This similarity is extended to the case where the poles are embedded in a medium:

$$F = \frac{m_1 m_2}{4\pi\mu d^2} \qquad \text{Equation 11.3}$$

where μ is the 'permeability' of the medium. The d^2 term in the above equation shows that the force between magnetic poles obeys the Inverse Square Law (Ch. 4).

11.3 MAGNETIC FIELDS

A magnetic field may be said to exist at a point if a force would be experienced by a magnetic pole if it were placed at that point. Thus, the term 'magnetic

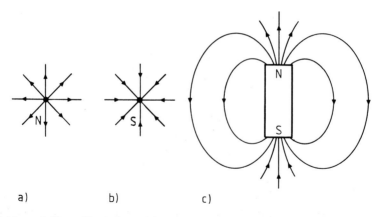

Fig. 11.3 Magnetic lines of force due to (a) a north pole, (b) a south pole, (c) a bar magnet. In each case, the arrows point in the direction a north pole would move if placed at a point.

field' is used to indicate the extent of the magnetic effect around (and within) a magnetised body.

Figure 11.3 illustrates the concept of magnetic lines of force by reference to a hypothetical single north pole, a single south pole and a bar magnet. The arrows on the lines of force indicate the direction of force exerted on a north pole placed at that point. The north pole would therefore travel along the line of force if it were free to move. Obviously, the lines of force cannot cross each other as the pole cannot travel in two directions at once! The total number of lines of force is referred to as the 'magnetic flux', as explained in the following section.

Insight

There is one fundamental difference between electric and magnetic lines of force, for electric lines of force always begin on a positive charge and end on a negative charge, whereas magnetic lines of force are *continuous*, as illustrated by the accompanying diagrams

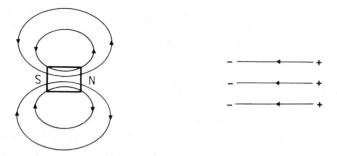

11.4 MAGNETIC FLUX AND FLUX DENSITY

The total number of lines of force passing through the area A shown in Figure 11.4 is defined as the *magnetic flux* (N) passing through A (or 'linked with' A).

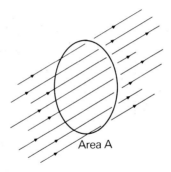

Fig 11.4 Magnetic flux through an area A.

The magnetic flux density (B) at a point is just the magnetic flux in a *unit area* placed at right-angles to the lines of force. In Figure 11.4 the flux density is assumed constant and the plane of area A is perpendicular to the lines of assumed constant and the plane of area A is perpendicular to the lines of force. We therefore have the following simple relationship between magnetic flux, magnetic flux density and area:

$B = N/A$ Equation 11.4

---

i.e.
   magnetic flux density = magnetic flux per unit area.

We shall have occasion to utilise the concepts of magnetic flux and magnetic flux 'linkage' with a conductor later in this book, particularly when discussing electro-magnetic induction (Chapter 14).

   The SI system of units relates magnetic and electric units together by the definition of the unit of magnetic flux density through the Motor Principle (sometimes called the Motor Effect — Chapter 13). As discussed previously (11.1), magnetism is just a consequence of electrical currents, so that current and magnetic flux density are intimately related. The unit of magnetic flux is the weber (WB) and the unit of magnetic flux density is the tesla (T), where 1 T = 1 WB m^{-2} (i.e. 1 weber per square metre).

11.5 MAGNETIC INDUCTION

Magnetism may be *induced* in a material, as may electric charges (9.5). This may be accomplished in a variety of ways, including mechanical and electrical methods. However, the principle of inducing magnetism in a substance is to subject it to a *magnetising force* (H), i.e. to place it within a magnetic field. The atoms of the sample will then tend to rotate in line with the direction of the magnetising force, provided that the atoms are magnetic. Different substances will respond to different extents, as shown later (11.6). Figure 11.5 illustrates the principle of magnetic induction, where an unmagnetised sample (Fig. 11.5(a)) containing atoms pointing in random directions is subjected to a

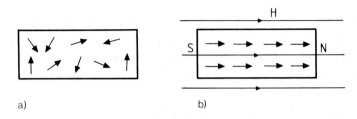

Fig. 115. Inducing magnetism in a sample. The elementary atomic magnets align themselves with the magnetising field.

magnetic field. The atoms then tend to 'line-up' with the direction of the applied magnetic field, just like a compass 'lines-up' with the Earth's magnetic field. This process produces a north pole at one end of the sample and a south pole at the other as a consequence of the alignment of the atoms, and magnetism is said to have been 'induced' in the sample.

The effect of the aligned atoms is to produce a total flux density, B, within the sample which is greater than that in air alone, such that:

$$B = \mu H \qquad \text{Equation 11.5}$$

where μ is the permeability of the medium (11.2). Here, the magnetising force, H, is to be regarded as the *cause* of the total magnetic flux density, B, in the medium of permeability μ.

A sample containing very magnetic atoms has a large value of μ so that, once the whole sample is magnetised, a correspondingly large magnetic flux density results. Table 11.1 shows some values of *relative* permeabilities for some

Table 11.1 Relative permeabilities of materials

Material	Relative permeability (μ_r)	Comments
Vacuum	1·0	(by definition)
Air	1·0000004	usually taken as 1·0
Water	0·99999	Diamagnetic
Bismuth	0·999985	Diamagnetic
Platinum	1·0001	Paramagnetic
Iron	5500	Ferromagnetic
Nickel	600	Ferromagnetic
Cobalt	240	Ferromagnetic
Stalloy	6700	Ferromagnetic alloy
Mumetal	80 000	Ferromagnetic alloy

common materials, i.e. permeabilities relative to that of a vacuum. The relative permeability (μ_r) of a substance is given by the simple formula:

$$\mu_r = \frac{\mu}{\mu_0} \qquad \text{Equation 11.6}$$

where μ_0 is the permeability of a vacuum (11.2).

As may be seen from the Table, there is a very wide variation of relative permeabilities in different substances, ranging from just under unity for bismuth (a 'diamagnetic' material — see 11.6.1) to 80 000 for mumetal, a metallic alloy which is therefore very easily and strongly magnetised.

11.5.1 Intensity of magnetisation

The total magnetic flux density, B, obtained by applying a magnetising force, H, to a substance is composed of two factors: that due to the air ($\mu_0 H$) and that due to the induced magnetism within the material. The total flux density is given by $B=\mu H$ (as shown in Equation 11.5). However, it is sometimes desirable to separate these two factors so that the magnetisation induced in the sample may be considered separately. This is known as the *intensity of magnetisation*, I, of the sample and measures the degree to which the sample itself has become magnetised.

Insight

Intensity of magnetisation is defined as the magnetic moment per unit volume of the magnetised sample. If a pole strength p per unit area is induced in a sample of constant cross-sectional area A and length l, then the magnetic moment (the turning force to a unit field perpendicular to its axis) is pAl.

Thus, intensity of magnetisation= magnetic moment/volume = $pAl/Al = p$; i.e. the intensity of magnetisation is equal to the induced pole strength per unit area (in Wb m^{-2}).

11.6 TYPES OF MAGNETIC MATERIALS

It is a matter of common experience that some materials are very easily and strongly magnetised while others appear to be unaffected by the presence of an external magnetic field. Thus we may confidently expect to pick up some steel pins with one end of a bar magnet, but would not expect to be able to pick up wooden matches by this means! Such differences in magnetic behaviour between materials is a result of there being three basic types of magnetic substance. These are called 'diamagnetics', 'paramagnetics' and 'ferromagnetics'. In radiography it is the ferromagnetic materials which are put to practical use (in transformers and electromagnetic relays and contactors), so the present section will concentrated mainly on this class of material. However, two brief sections of diamagnetic and paramagnetic materials follow first, in order that the differences in the three types of substance may be understood.

11.6.1 Diamagnetism

Diamagnetism is the term which is given to the influence of the applied magnetic field on the electrons orbiting the nuclei within any substance. As described later (14.3) Lenz's Law of electromagnetic induction describes the opposing effect between the induced currents and varying magnetic field when the latter is applied to a conductor. Electrons orbiting the nuclei of atoms may be considered as conductors with zero electrical resistance, and suffer changes in their orbits when the external magnetic field is applied. As a result of the magnetic field interacting with the moving electrons, the orbits change in such a way as to oppose the external field (i.e. Lenz's Law) and remain in that condition until the magnetic field is removed, when they revert to their original orbits. Thus, two conclusions follow:

a. *All* materials are diamagnetic.

b. Magnetic induction within the sample is produced which *opposes* the direction of the magnetising field, so that the relative permeability is less than unity. Bismuth is an example of a diamagnetic material (Table 11.1) and has a relative permeability of 0·999985, i.e. very slightly less than unity, so that diamagnetisation is a very weak phenomenon and is normally completely obscured by the other types of magnetic induction: paramagnetism and ferromagnetism when these exist in a material. Diamagnetism is unaffected by temperature variations.

11.6.2 Paramagnetism

The cause of the magnetism of individual atoms is the spinning and orbiting electrons around their nuclei. If the effect of the individual electrons is to cancel each others' contribution then the material is a diamagnetic, as outlined in the previous section. However, if there is a resultant atomic magnetic effect, so that each atom may be considered to be an elementary bar magnet, then the material is a 'paramagnetic,' and Section 11.5 of this chapter applies here also, i.e. an 'unmagnetised' sample is just one in which the atoms take up random orientations, and a 'magnetised' sample is one in which an externally applied field produces some order in the sample (see Figure 11.5).

Temperature is a measure of the kinetic energy of vibration of atoms (8.1) and so is a factor which tends to destroy the ordered alignment of atoms within the sample. Thus, a paramagnetic sample becomes demagnetised very quickly after the external magnetic field is removed as a result of the disrupting effect of the collisions between the atoms. Also, the higher the temperature becomes, the more difficult it is to magnetise the paramagnetic sample, and there is a point at which it may not be possible to magnetise the sample at all, and it is then solely a diamagnetic (since diamagnetism is unaffected by temperature).

An example of a paramagnetic material is platinum which has a relative permeability of 1·0001 (Table 11.1) — the figure being composed of a 'positive' effect due to paramagnetism only and a 'negative' effect due to diamagnetism only.

11.6.3 Ferromagnetism

Diamagnetism and paramagnetism are extremely weak magnetic phenomena compared to ferromagnetism. Ferromagnetic materials possess relative permeabilities up to several thousand, or even tens of thousands, as shown in Table 11.1 Thus the magnetic flux density of magnetised ferromagnetic materials may be very large and hence may be put to a variety of practical uses. Some of the applications of ferromagnetic materials are discussed below.

The reason for the strong magnetic induction experienced by ferromagnetic materials lies in the behaviour of the so-called 'magnetic domains' within them. Such a domain is a small volume (less than one cubic millimetre) within a ferromagnetic material in which all the atoms are pointing in the same direction. This is shown for an unmagnetised sample in Figure 11.6(a), where the atomic magnets within each domain are aligned, but there is no particular order in the orientation of the domains on a large scale, so that the sample is unmagnetised as a whole.

An externally applied magnetic field creates a rotating force on each domain, however, and the atoms within a domain rotate together until, if the magnetising field is strong enough, all the domains are pointing in the same direction (Fig. 11.6(b)). In this condition, the sample is said to have reached 'magnetic saturation' since no further magnetisation is possible.

It is because of the alignment of the atoms within each domain that the sample exhibits such a strong induced magnetisation to an applied magnetic field. Atoms within paramagnetic materials behave as individual magnets, rather than domains of aligned magnets, and so are much more difficult to align with a magnetising field owing to the disrupting effect of atomic collisions. Ferromagnetic materials also change their properties with temperature. At a particular temperature, known as the *Curie temperature*, the atoms can no longer overcome the disrupting effect of the kinetic energy of the atoms and the domains disappear. Thus, below the Curie temperature the material is a ferromagnetic and above the Curie temperature the material is a paramagnetic, in which state the relative permeability is greatly reduced as a consequence of the transition from atomic order to disorder.

Examples of ferromagnetic elements are iron, cobalt and nickel whose relative permeabilities are shown in Table 11.1. The Curie temperature for iron is 1043 K (770°C).

We shall now investigate the magnetisation of a ferromagnetic sample in more detail.

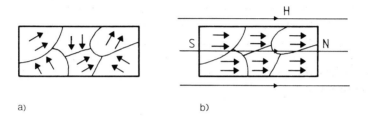

a)   b)

Fig. 11.6 The 'domains' within a ferromagnetic material. (The arrows represent the 'north' end of each magnetic atom.)

11.7 HYSTERESIS

For diamagnetic and paramagnetic materials, the intensity of magnetisation of the sample (11.5.1), is directly proportional (1.7) to the magnetising force, H. Thus, if H is doubled then I is doubled and so on. However, this is not the case with ferromagnetic materials owing to the effect of the domains upon each other. There is both an 'elastic' or 'reversible' force, and a 'frictional' or 'non-reversible' force between the domains. The reversible forces correspond to the movement of the domain boundaries (i.e. some domains become larger at the expense of others) when an external magnetic field is applied, and the 'irreversible forces' correspond to the rotation of the domains as they attempt to align themselves with the external field in a series of minute 'jerks'. This jerking movement between the domains means that the applied magnetic field increases before some of the domains can respond to it by rotation. This is analogous to frictional forces between a book and a table-top, for example, where the applied force must exceed the frictional force before any movement can occur. Thus, the orientation of the domains (and therefore the induced magnetism) *lags behind* the magnetising force. This effect is known as *hysteresis*, which means 'lagging behind', and is shown in graphical form in Figure 11.7. The figure shows a complete cycle of magnetisation, which means that the sample is taken to magnetic saturation in one direction, then to

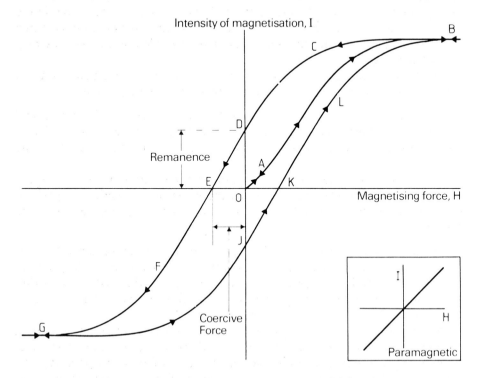

Fig. 11.7 A hysteresis loop for a ferromagnetic sample. A paramagnetic sample shows no hysteresis (inset in figure).

magnetic saturation in the opposite direction and so on — a 'cycle' being one complete journey around the *hysteresis loop* given by BCDEFGJKLB.

If the ferromagnetic sample is initially unmagnetised (i.e. the domains are pointing in random directions), then the graph will start at the origin O. As the magnetising force, H, is increased so the induced magnetism in the samples is increased along OA. If H is now reduced to zero, then the path OA is retraced and the sample becomes unmagnetised again — thus the path OA is 'reversible'. However, if H is increased beyond this point, the domains start to rotate in the direction of H and will not revert to their original positions if H is removed. As H is increased, so the domains become more closely aligned with the direction of the applied magnetic field until they are all pointing in that direction — B on the graph. Increasing H beyond this value can now have no effect on the induced magnetism within the sample, i.e. I cannot increase further since all the domains are already pointing in the same direction, and so a horizontal line appears on the graph. This region of the graph is known as *magnetic saturation*.

If now the magnetising force H is gradually reduced the curve BCD is produced, i.e. the graph follows a different path down to demagnetisation (BCDE) from that which it took to magnetisation (OAB). If H is made to increase in a negative direction (i.e. the magnetising force applied to the sample is in the opposite direction) then an argument similar to the above accounts for the magnetic saturation in the opposite direction, since all the domains will point in the same direction as H (path EFG). If H is altered in the positive direction, the path GJKLB results. Note that this does not coincide with OAB since the starting conditions of the sample are different (demagnetised at O, fully magnetised at G).

Two terms which are used in describing the effects of hysteresis in a given substance are *coercive force* and *remanence* (or *retentivity*), where:

   a.   Coercive force is given by the value of H equal to OK or OE, and represents the magnitude of the magnetising force which must be applied to completely demagnetise the sample (i.e. to make $I = 0$) once it has been fully magnetised.

   b.   Remanence (or retentivity or residual magnetism) is given by the value of I equal to OD or OJ, and represents the value of the residual magnetism once the sample has been fully magnetised and the magnetising field removed (i.e. $H = 0$).

The *area of the loop* is another important quantity and represents the *work done* in taking the sample around a complete hysteresis cycle. In practical terms, the greater the work done, the greater the energy liberated as *heat* within the sample (see Ch. 16 on transformers, where this effect is also known as 'hysteresis loss').

By way of comparison, the inset in Figure 11.7 shows the corresponding graph obtained for a paramagnetic sample. As is evident from the straight-line graph there is no remanence, coercive force or area of loop for a paramagnetic material — all of these quantities being a result of the hysteresis present only in ferromagnetic materials.

11.7.1 Soft Iron and Steel

Figure 11.8 illustrates the differences in appearance between the hysteresis loops obtained for materials suitable for permanent magnets (steel) and temporary magnets (soft iron).
The differences in the two hysteresis curves may be summarised as follows:

a.   the saturation of soft iron occurs at much lower values of H than the saturation of steel
b.   the value of the coercive force (11.7) is much greater for steel than soft iron
c.   the area of the hysteresis loop is much greater for steel than for soft iron.

Soft iron is therefore suitable for those applications where a strong induced magnetism is required with the minimum expenditure of energy, and where the induced magnetism may be switched off at will. Suitable applications of soft iron therefore include its use in electromagnetic relays (12.5) and transformers (Ch. 16). Note that, although the remanence (11.7) is greater for soft iron than steel, the coercive force is so low that even slight mechanical agitation of the sample is sufficient to demagnetise the sample.
Steel is a suitable material to use for permanent magnets, since it is much more difficult to demagnetise than soft iron, i.e. it has a high coercive force. It would thus be unsuitable for use as an electromagnet or as a transformer core.

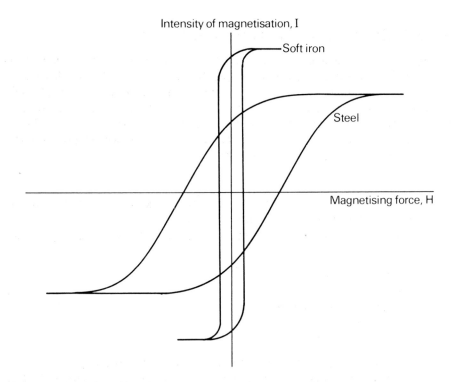

Fig. 11.8 A comparison of the hysteresis loops of soft iron and steel.

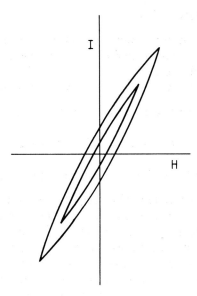

Fig. 11.9 Subsidiary hysteresis loops, where the ferromagnetic sample is not taken to magnetic saturation.

11.7.2 Subsidiary hysteresis loops

It is not necessary to take a ferromagnetic sample around a *complete* hysteresis loop, i.e. from saturation one way to saturation the other. If this not done, then 'subsidiary' hysteresis loops result, as shown in Figure 11.9. For example, only a special type of transformer (the 'constant voltage' transformer) takes its core to saturation — all other types make use of subsidiary hysteresis loops. However, an electromagnet or electromagnetic relay may well saturate the soft iron so as to ensure the maximum magnetic effect.

Exercise 11.1

a.   Explain what is meant by a north pole, and state why it is always accompanied by a south pole of equal strength.

b.   Define, as precisely as you can, what is meant by the following terms:

   (i) magnetic field
   (ii) magnetic line of force
   (iii) magnetic flux
   (iv) magnetic flux density
   (v) permeability
   (vi) relative permeability

c.   What is meant by the 'magnetic induction' of a substance?

d.   Discuss the similarities and differences between the magnetic induction of diamagnetic, paramagnetic and ferromagnetic substances.

e. Use the concepts of 'magnetic domains' to account for the high permeabilities and the hysteresis of ferromagnetic materials.

f. What is meant by 'hysteresis loss'? Compare the hysteresis loss of soft iron and steel with the help of a hysteresis diagram.

g. Define 'remanence' (or 'retentivity') and 'coercive force' and discuss their relevance for materials used for (i) permanent magnets and (ii) transformer cores.

SUMMARY

1. Magnetic poles always exist in *pairs* because the atoms of a magnetic substance behave like a small bar magnet.

2. The force between two poles is:

$$F = \frac{m_1 m_2}{4 \pi \mu d^2}$$

where F is in newtons

m_1, m_2 are in webers

d is in metres

μ (the 'permeability') is in henry per metre.

3. If μ_0 is the permeability of a vacuum, and μ is the permeability of a substance, then the 'relative permeability' μ_r is given by:

$$\mu_r = \mu / \mu_0$$

4. A 'magnetic field' exists at a point if a force would exist on a magnetic pole placed at that point.

5. The 'magnetic force' H is the magnitude of the magnetic field (also called the 'magnetic field strength') and has units of ampere per metre (A m^{-1}). It is independent of the medium through which it passes.

6. The magnetic flux density, B, is the magnetic flux per unit area, i.e. $B = N/A$, and is measured in weber m^{-2} and has the special unit of the tesla (T), where 1 T $= 1$ Wb m^{-2}. It is dependent upon the medium through which it passes.

7. The relationship between magnetising force, H, and magnetic flux density, B, is:

$$B = \mu H$$

where μ is the permeability of the medium. (Alternatively, $B = \mu_0 \mu_r H$ — see 3 above.)

B. If: μ_r is less than unity, the material is diamagnetic

is just greater than unity, it is paramagnetic

is much greater than unity, it is ferromagnetic.

9. All materials are diamagnetic, but the effect is usually negligible in comparison to paramagnetism or ferromagnetism in the same sample.

10. Paramagnetics become diamagnetics if the temperature is high enough, and ferromagnetics become paramagnetics above the 'Curie temperature'.

11. The reason for the very high relative permeabilities of ferromagnetics (Table 11.1) is the internal ordered arrangement of atoms into 'magnetic domains'. Within each domain, the atoms are pointing the same way, but this direction may vary from one domain to another. Domains pointing in random directions result in no overall magnetisation of the sample.

12. The application of a magnetising force, H, to a ferromagnetic material results in two types of force:

(a) one which allows the expansion of some domains at the expense of others (this is reversible when H is removed)

(b) one which rotates the domains in the same direction as H (this is not reversed exactly when H is removed).

13. The 'sticky' domains result in the magnetisation of the sample lagging behind the applied field — 'hysteresis'.

14. 'Remanence' is the residual magnetism when H is reduced to zero; 'coercive force' is the value of H which must be applied to demagnetise the sample (i.e. bring I to zero).

15. The area of the hysteresis loop is a measure of the work done in taking the sample through one complete hysteresis cycle — this manifests itself as heat within the sample. This is also known as 'hysteresis loss'.

16. Soft iron has a high permeability, a low coercive force and a small area of hysteresis loop and so is suitable for electromagnets and transformer cores.

17. Steel has a high permeability and a large coercive force, making it suitable for permanent magnets.

12. Electromagnetism

In the previous chapter it was shown that magnetism is a phenomenon associated with atoms, and is due to the spinning and orbiting of electrons around those atoms. Electrons are negatively charged particles (9.1), and so we may conclude that magnetism is caused by moving electric charges. It is thus reasonable to ask whether an electric current in a wire (for example) may also produce a magnetic field, since an electric current is just the flow of electrons in a conductor (10.1). This is found to be so in practice and the term 'electromagnetism' is used to describe this effect (i.e. 'electricity' producing 'magnetism').

12.1 ELECTRON FLOW AND 'CONVENTIONAL' CURRENT

When electricity was first discovered, it was assumed that it was the *positive* charges which flow in a conductor, and not the negative charges. This concept is now known as the 'conventional' current. However, it was discovered later that the positive charges in a solid material do not have any net movement (although they vibrate with heat energy — Ch. 8), since they form the protons in the nuclei of atoms (Ch. 25). Thus it is the *electrons* which move in a solid, as explained by the elementary electron theory of conduction (10.1).

In gas or liquid, any positive and negative charges present may take part in current flow, since the positive charges are free to move, unlike in a solid. In radiography and many other subjects, however, it is the *electron* flow in conductors which is most frequently under consideration, and herein lies a difficulty, for many rules (or conventions) in electromagnetism and electromagnetic induction (Ch. 14) are based upon the totally erroneous assumption of the 'conventional' current, which in a mathematical sense is supposed to flow in the opposite direction to that of the electrons.

This and further chapters will therefore discuss both electromagnetism and electromagnetic induction on the basis of electron flow *only*, in an attempt to eliminate much of the confusion which undoubtedly exists at present in many people's minds. Some caution is therefore required when studying these subjects from other books, as they may invoke the 'conventional' current for their rules. Differences in the two approaches are explained in the 'Insights' where appropriate.

12.2 MAGNETIC FIELD DUE TO A STRAIGHT WIRE

Historically, the presence of a magnetic field around a current-carrying conductor was first discovered by Oersted when passing a current through a straight wire placed near a magnetic compass, as illustrated in Fig. 12.1.

If the wire is aligned in a north–south direction (i.e. along the direction of the compass needle), then an electric current through the wire causes

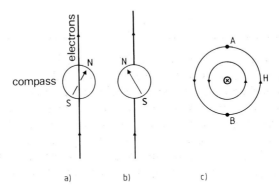

a)   b)   c)

Fig. 12.1 (a) and (b) show the effect of the magnetic field produced by the electrons flowing in the wire upon a magnetic compass, (c) shows the direction of the magnetic field around the wire is anticlockwise, as seen when looking along the direction of electron motion. ('⊗' means away from the eye of the observer, and '⊙' means towards the eye of the observer.)

deflections of the compass as shown: clockwise when the wire is above the compass, and anti-clockwise when the compass is above the wire. This is possible only if the lines of magnetic force (11.3) are circular and in an anti-clockwise direction when viewed along the same direction as the flowing electrons. We may therefore use the following convention:

Convention
Each moving electron produces an *anti-clockwise* magnetic field about itself when viewed along the direction of its motion.

A moving *positive* charge would produce a *clockwise* magnetic field, of course. This convention is illustrated in Figure 12.1(c), where the symbol '⊗' means that electron flow is away from the eye ('⊙' is towards the eye.) The arrows on the lines of force are in an anti-clockwise direction, in accordance with our convention, and give the direction in which a north pole would move if placed in that position (11.3). Thus, a weightless north pole would, if released, travel round and round the wire indefinitely in an anti-clockwise circle.

Exercise 12.1
Check that the convention described above agrees with the direction of rotation of the compass when placed above and below the wire — points A and B respectively.

12.3 MAGNETIC FIELD DUE TO A CIRCULAR COIL OF WIRE

Figure 12.2(a) shows a circular coil of wire in which an electric current is made to flow. Now, each individual moving electron produces anti-clockwise magnetic lines of force about itself (12.2) as illustrated in Figure 12.2(a). The closeness of the lines of force to each other represents the total magnetic effect, i.e. the magnetic flux density, as described in (11.4). The addition at a point of all the magnetic flux densities represented by the lines of force produces the total magnetic flux density at that point. Note that, within the coil, the lines of force all tend to be in the direction C to D, while outside the coil, they are from D to C. A top view of the coil (Fig. 12.2(b)) shows the pattern of the overall lines of force so obtained. It is interesting to note the similarity of these lines of force to those of a short bar magnet, where they emerge from the north pole end and travel around the magnet to the south pole end and back again (11.3). Here we have the reason for the 'atomic magnets', where (on a tiny scale) the coil would be equivalent to the net flow of electrons around a particular atomic nucleus, producing lines of force as in Figure 12.2(b) and hence the magnetised atom.

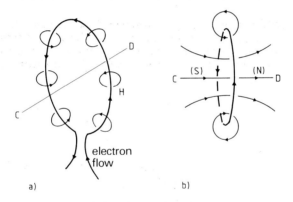

Fig. 12.2 The magnetic field around a coil of wire. Note the similarity to a small bar magnet.

12.4 MAGNETIC FIELD DUE TO A SOLENOID

A solenoid consists of several coils joined together, and so produces magnetic lines of force similar to a bar magnet, as shown in Figure 12.3(a). The effect of a piece of soft iron within the solenoid is to increase the magnetic flux density many times because of the induced magnetism within the soft iron (11.5 and 11.6.3). This effect is reflected by an increase in the number of lines of force compared to Figure 12.3(a). The combination of solenoid and soft iron in this manner is known as an electromagnet.

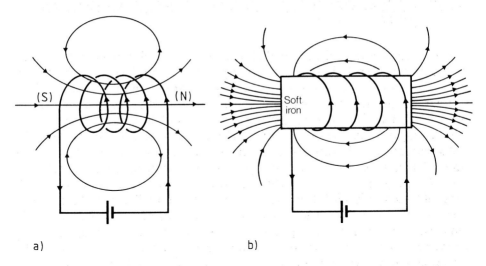

Fig. 12.3 (a) The magnetic field produced by a current-carrying solenoid, (b) shows the large increase in the magnetic field strength obtained when using a soft-iron 'core'.

Insight

A general method of calculating the magnetic flux from any general shape of current-carrying conductor is due to Biot and Savart. The formula shown in Figure 12.4 may be used to calculate the magnetic flux density from any general shape of wire. (Table 12.1 shows some of these examples.)

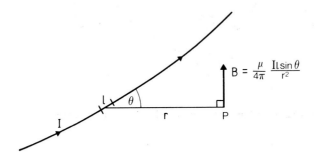

Fig. 12.4 Biot and Savart's Law for determining the magnetic flux density due to any shape of current-carrying conductor.

Now, $B = \mu H$ from (11.5)

$$\therefore H = \frac{B}{\mu} = \text{constant} \times \frac{Il}{r^2} \text{ (from re-arranging the equation in the figure)}$$

so that the units of the magnetic field strength (or magnetising force) H are in ampere/metre.

Conductor	Magnetic flux density, B. (Tesla)
Infinite straight wire	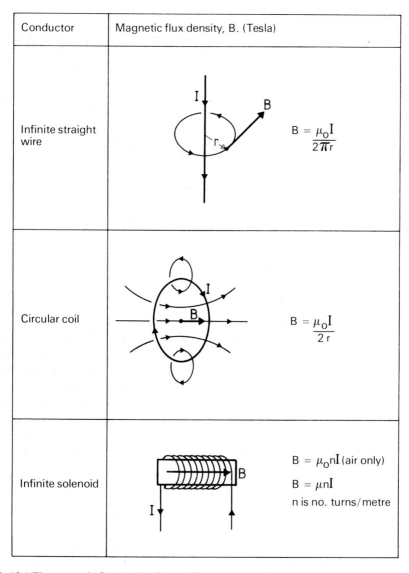 $B = \dfrac{\mu_0 I}{2\pi r}$
Circular coil	$B = \dfrac{\mu_0 I}{2 r}$
Infinite solenoid	$B = \mu_0 n I$ (air only) $B = \mu n I$ n is no. turns/metre

Table 12.1 The magnetic flux density from different shapes of current-carrying conductors.

12.5 THE ELECTROMAGNETIC RELAY

The electromagnetic relay is a very useful electrical device for switching electrical circuits on and off by remote control. It makes possible the switching of large currents and/or voltages to remote devices (e.g. an X-ray tube) by the application of a small current to the solenoid of the electromagnetic relay. The great advantage of the use of an electromagnetic relay for this purpose lies in the increased safety factor to the operator, since no large voltages or currents need to be connected to any of the controls on the operating console. Such controls on the X-ray panel (e.g. 'exposure prepare') supply power to electromagnets which switch on the appropriate part of the X-ray electrical circuit. This may be verified by hearing the 'clonking' noises which occur as different relays are actuated when various controls on the X-ray panel are used!

The general structure of the electromagnetic relay is as shown in Figure 12.5.

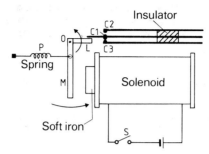

Fig. 12.5 The electromagnetic relay (see text for operation).

Operation

When switch S is open, no current flows through the solenoid and so the soft iron piece M is held in the position shown by the spring P. Contacts C_1 and C_3 are in contact, while C_1 and C_2 are 'open'. When S is closed, the current passing through the solenoid magnetises the soft iron core (11.5) which attracts M by induced magnetism. M pivots about O so that the arm L lifts C_1 away from C_3 and into contact to C_2. Thus, if the external circuit is joined between C_1 and C_2, it is 'made' (i.e. connected). Opening S reduces the current in the solenoid to zero and hence reverts the system to its original condition, since M (being soft iron with a low coercive force — 11.7) loses its magnetism and is pulled quickly away under the action of the spring P.

Exercise 12.2

a. Compare the similarities between the atomic magnets within a bar magnet and the magnetic field produced by an electric current in a coil of wire.

b. Why does a piece of soft iron within a solenoid increase the magnetic effect of the solenoid when an electric current is passed through it? Explain why this increase does not continue indefinitely as the current through the solenoid is increased. (*Hint:* See 11.7.)

c. What is an electromagnetic relay? Draw a simple diagram of its construction and hence explain how it operates. Discover as many applications as you can of the use of the electromagnetic relay in X-ray circuits, stating why it is used in each case.

SUMMARY

1. Atomic magnetism is caused by electrons orbiting atomic nuclei. Electromagnetism is caused by 'isolated' *moving* particles (e.g. 'free' electrons).

2. Circular magnetic fields exist around moving charges:

   a. anti-clockwise around negative charges
   b. clockwise around positive charges

when viewed along the direction of motion.

3. Negative and positive charges may flow in a vacuum, gas or liquid, but only negative charges (electrons) may flow in a solid. This is because the atomic nuclei (which contain the positively charged protons) are not free to move in a solid.

4. The magnetic flux density due to a current-carrying solenoid may be increased many times by inserting within it a material of high permeability, e.g. soft iron, since $B = \mu H$ (see Table 11.1). The magnetic domains become aligned with the direction of H, so adding to the overall magnetic flux density.

5. The electromagnetic relay is a device used for switching a circuit on and off under remote control, depending upon whether a solenoid is energised or not. The advantage of such a system is that a low current may be used to switch a high current or voltage at a remote location, thus increasing the safety factor against electrical shock for the operators of the equipment.

13. The motor principle

13.1 INTRODUCTION AND DEFINITION OF THE MOTOR PRINCIPLE

Chapter 12 described the production of a magnetic field from an electric current, i.e. electromagnetism. This short but important chapter considers what happens when an electromagnetic field is created *in the presence of* another magnetic field (which may be due to a nearby bar magnet, for example). To take a simple analogy: two bar magnets exert a strong force of repulsion or attraction when brought close together. If now one of the bar magnets is replaced by a *solenoid* (12.4), we would expect a force between the solenoid and the bar magnet when an electric current is passed through the solenoid, since it behaves like a bar magnet in such circumstances. The force acting upon the solenoid will cause it to move if it is free to do so. (The force is zero if the current is switched off, of course.) This interaction between electromagnetism and the magnetic field due to another magnetic system (which may itself also be electromagnetic) is known as the Motor Principle (or Effect) and may be formally stated as:

The Motor Principle
A current-carrying conductor will experience a force when placed within a magnetic field.

The principle of the electric motor is that it converts electrical energy into kinetic energy through the interaction of the magnetic fields produced within it. This is the same sequence of events as in the definition above, i.e. electrical energy to interaction of magnetic fields to energy of movement; hence the term Motor Principle to describe the effect.

13.2 DIRECTION AND MAGNITUDE OF FORCE ON CONDUCTOR

Consider a length l of straight wire which is carrying an electric current I, the whole wire being placed in a uniform magnetic field of magnetic flux density B (11.4), as shown in Figure 13.1. In the figure it is assumed that the direction of B and of the wire are both in the plane of the paper. Experimentally, the following results are observed:

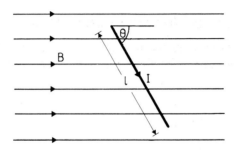

Fig. 13.1 The interaction of B and the magnetic field due to the wire produces a force on the wire — the Motor Principle.

    a. the *direction* of the force on the wire is always either into or out of the paper, i.e. at *right-angles* both to the direction of *B* and to *I*

    b. the direction of the force on the wire is reversed if *I* is reversed

    c. the *magnitude* of the force is proportional to:

        (i) the magnetic flux density, *B*

        (ii) The electric current, *I*

        (iii) the length of wire, *l*.

        (iv) the sine of the angle between the directions of B and *I*, i.e. $\sin \theta$ in Figure 13.1. Thus the force on the wire is maximum when the wire is at right-angles to the field ($\sin 90° = 1$) and *zero* when the wire is parallel to the field ($\sin 0 = 0$).

Combining the factors in (c) above we have:

    $F = BIl \sin \theta$ Equation 13.1

where *F* is in newton, *B* in tesla and *l* in metre.

    These findings may be used to define the unit of the tesla as follows:

Definition

    A magnetic flux density of 1 tesla (T) exists if the force on a straight wire of length 1 metre is 1 newton when the wire carries a current of 1 ampere and is placed at right-angles to the direction of the magnetic flux.

(Substituting these values in Equation 13.1 gives $1 = 1 . 1 . 1 . 1$, which is obviously correct.)

    The *direction* of the force on the current-carrying conductor may be obtained by the use of an appropriate rule, or 'convention'. The most frequent convention used is that which invokes 'Fleming's Right (or Left) Hand Rule' depending upon whether 'conventional' current (12.1) or electron flow is considered. This chapter considers only electron flow, as in previous chapters, and it is the author's experience that students become very confused with the practical application of Fleming's Hand Rules. This system is therefore described in Appendix I for those who wish to use it, and a different convention is offered below in the hope that it will prove easier to use in practice and also result in fewer arguments and sprained wrists!

13.2.1 Convention for direction of force

Consider the situation depicted in Figure 13.2(a), where a wire is carrying an electric current such that the electrons are flowing away from the eye of the

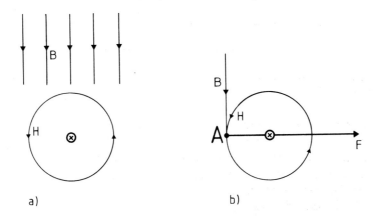

a)   b)

Fig. 13.2 Convention for establishing the direction of force on the conductor. Find a point A, where both fields are parallel, and draw a line from A through the conductor. This gives the direction of the force on the wire, F.

observer, i.e. into the paper. The magnetic field produced by this current is in an anti-clockwise direction (12.2) as shown. If now an external magnetic field B, is applied to the wire as shown, it is found that the wire experiences a force which pushes it to the right. Figure 13.2(b) illustrates the convention suggested here to determine the direction of the force. This may be outlined as follows.

Convention
>   Align one of the externally applied magnetic lines of force to be parallel with and touching one of the magnetic lines of force produced by the current. The direction from this common point to the conductor gives the direction of force on the conductor.

This procedure is shown in Figure 13.2(b) where the lines of force are parallel at point A. Joining the point A to the wire by an imaginary line establishes that the force is to the *right*, in agreement with experiment.

This procedure is perfectly general and applies to any direction of current and any orientation of the wire and magnetic field. In some cases, however, the applied magnetic field is not exactly perpendicular to the wire and so cannot be made to line up exactly parallel to the field produced by it. In this situation, the applied magnetic field may be split up into two components: one parallel to the wire (which produces no force on the wire) and one perpendicular to the wire (which produces the force according to the above convention). The following examples should clarify all the above points.

a.   The right-hand figure shows the side view of the situation, i.e. as seen by looking along the wire. The application of the above convention shows that the force on the wire will be towards the observer for the left-hand figure.

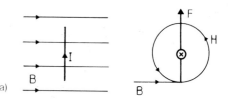

a)

b.   In this case the circular lines of force are clockwise since the electrons are travelling *towards* the eye. The application of the convention shows that the force on the wire will be away from the observer as applied to the left-hand figure. Notice that this is in the opposite sense to example (a), as would be expected from property b in (13.2).

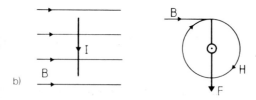

b)

c.   In this case the two sets of lines of force cannot be made to be parallel, so that there is no force. This agrees with property c(iv) in (13.2), so that there is no force on the wire when the directions of the current and the applied magnetic field are parallel, since sin $0 = 0$.

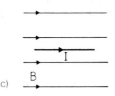

c)

d.   In this situation we must first split the magnetic flux density B up into two components parallel and perpendicular to the wire as shown in the illustration by B_0 and B_{90}. The above example has shown that B_0 will have no effect on the wire and can therefore be ignored. Application of the convention then shows that the force on the wire is in the upward direction, as shown for example (a) above.

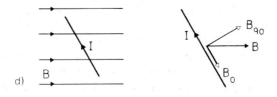

d)

Exercise 13.1

   a. What is the direction of the force on the wire in Figure 13.1?

   b. Determine the direction of force on the wire for the following:

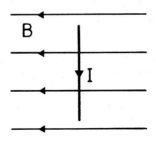

13.3 INTERACTION OF TWO ELECTROMAGNETIC FIELDS

We have seen that a force exists on a current-carrying conductor when in the presence of a magnetic field and that this is known as the Motor Principle. It is immaterial whether the magnetic field interacting with that of the conductor is produced by a permanent magnet or whether it is itself produced electromagnetically. If the latter, then the two current-carrying conductors each produce a magnetic field which interact so as to produce mutual forces between the conductors. A simple example of two electromagnetic fields interacting is given by two solenoids placed close together. When a current flows each solenoid behaves like a bar magnet, with a north and a south pole at either end (12.4). They therefore attract or repel each other depending upon the directions of the currents. Two further examples are given below.

13.3.1 Two infinite parallel wires

Figure 13.3 shows two 'infinite' parallel wires C and D which carry currents I_C, I_D respectively. Figure 13.3(a) shows the plan view of the wires, while Figure 13.3(b) is the view obtained by looking along the wires towards C and D, where the electron flow is into the paper for both wires. Now, since the direction of the magnetic field is anti-clockwise around a moving electron (12.2), the magnetic flux density at wire D due to wire C (B_C) is 'upwards', while that at C due to D (B_D) is 'downwards' as shown in Figure 13.3(b). We now use the convention (outlined in 13.2.1) to determine the direction of the forces on each wire. Considering wire D first, the point at which the magnetic lines of force due to wire D and wire C are parallel and in contact is given by P in Figure 13.3(b). Drawing an imaginary line from P through wire D, in accordance with our convention, shows that the force on the wire is to the left, i.e. towards the other wire C. A similar argument may be used to show that the force on wire C is towards D, so that there is a mutual force of attraction between the wires.

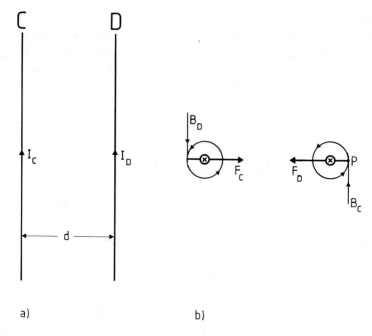

Fig. 13.3 The mutual forces between two infinite parallel wires carrying an electric current. This is used to define the unit of current (ampere).

Exercise 13.2

In what direction are the forces if (a) the current in one wire is reversed and (b) the current in both wires is reversed?

Insight

The magnetic flux density from an infinite length of wire is given by $B = \mu_0 I / 2\pi d$ (Table 12.1), and the force per *unit* length on wire is $F = BI \sin \theta$ (Equation 13.1, where $l = 1$). In Figure 13.3, $\theta = 90°$, so that $\sin \theta = 1$. Thus the force per unit length on wire D due to the current in C is

$$F_D = \frac{\mu_0 I_A I_B}{2\pi d}$$

and the force per unit length on wire C due to the current in D is

$$F_C = \frac{\mu_0 I_B I_A}{2\pi d}$$

Hence, $F_C = F_D$ so that there is an *equal* and *opposite* force on the two wires, as would be expected from Newton's Third Law of Motion (7.4).

The above formula may be used to define the SI unit of electrical current of 1 ampere by substituting unity for d, I_A and I_B, whereupon

$$F_D = F_C = \frac{\mu_0}{2\pi} \, \text{N m}^{-1}$$

Definition

A current of 1 ampere flows in one infinite straight wire if an equal current in a similar wire placed 1 metre away in vacuum produces a mutual force of $\mu_0/2\pi$ newton per metre of length (i.e. 2×10^{-7} newton per metre, since $\mu_0 = 4\pi \times 10^{-7}$ H m^{-1}). See also Appendix VII.

13.3.2 Magnetic deflection of an electron beam

Figure 13.4 shows an electron beam travelling in a vacuum and passing through a magnetic field produced by (say) a 'magnetic deflection coil' as used in a cathode ray tube (CRT) or television tube.

The path taken by the electron beam is circular when it passes through the magnetic field, since the direction of the force is always at right-angles to the direction of travel of the electron beam, and this direction changes as the beam

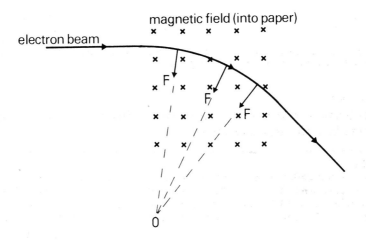

Fig. 13.4 Magnetic deflection of an electron beam. The electrons enter the magnetic field from the left and are deflected in a circular path. The direction of force on the electrons changes as they are deflected.

is deflected. After leaving the magnetic field the beam travels in a straight line.

The angle of deflection of the electron beam increases as the magnetic flux density (B) increases, so that a means of controlling the direction of the beam is possible by varying B. This leads to the concept of 'scanning' the electron beam as in a vidicon television camera tube or television monitor tube by applying a varying magnetic field in each of the X and Y directions. Further consideration of such systems is beyond the scope of this book.

Insight

The force on an electron charge e travelling at velocity v at an angle θ with respect to a magnetic flux density B is given by

$$F = Bev \sin \theta \qquad\qquad \text{Equation 13.2}$$

This is effectively the same fomula as Equation 13.1 (i.e. $F = BIl \sin \theta$) since $v = l/t$ (distance in unit time) so that $ev = (e/t) \cdot l = Il$, since the electric current I, which each moving electron represents is e/t (i.e. charge per unit time).

13.4 THE MOTOR PRINCIPLE IN RADIOGRAPHY

The Motor Principle is relevant to radiography whenever electrical energy is transformed to mechanical energy via magnetic energy. Obviously, this includes the use of motors (e.g. to drive a rotating anode) as well as meters. However, there is another phenomenon which must be considered before explaining the action of such devices, and that is 'electromagnetic induction', which is the topic of the next chapter. We shall return to the subjects of motors and meters in chapters 14 and 17 respectively.

Exercise 13.3

a.   What is meant by the Motor Principle (Effect)? Give a simple example and describe the convention you use to determine the direction of the force on the current-carrying conductor. Upon what factors do the direction and magnitude of this force depend?

b.   Verify that the direction of the deflection of the electron beam shown in Figure 13.4 is correct. In what direction would the deflection be if (i) the direction of electron flow were reversed and (ii) protons were used instead of electrons?

c.   Make a list of as many examples as you can of the use of the Motor Principle in radiography (include image intensification).

SUMMARY

1.   The Motor Principle (Effect): A current-carrying conductor experiences a force when placed in a magnetic field. This means that electrical energy may be transformed into mechanical energy via the interaction of magnetic fields, as in an electric motor.

2.   Force on a current-carrying wire subjected to a magnetic flux density of B is: $F = BIl \sin \theta$, so that:

a. F is maximum when $\theta = 90°$ and zero when $\theta = 0$

b. $F \propto B$, I and l.

3. Sign convention for determining *direction* of force on current-carrying conductors:

a. arrange lines of force from the two sources to be parallel and in contact (point P).

b. draw an imaginary line from P through the conductor — this gives the direction of force on the conductor.

(*Note:* Fleming's Left and Right Hand Rules are described in Appendix I.)

4. Two electromagnetic fields may interact, producing an equal and opposite force on each conductor, e.g. two 'infinite' parallel wires may either repel or attract each other when passing current. This leads to the definition of an ampere (Appendix VII).

14. Electromagnetic induction

It is important to appreciate the difference between 'electromagnetic induction' and 'electromagnetism' since one is just the reverse of the other. They may be described as follows:

Electromagnetism: the production of a magnetic field by electricity (Chapter 12).
Electromagnetic Induction: the production of electricity by a changing magnetic field (also known as the generator effect).

This chapter on electromagnetic induction is therefore concerned with the generation of electricity from magnetism.

14.1 CONDITIONS NECESSARY FOR ELECTROMAGNETIC INDUCTION

As an illustration of electromagnetic induction, consider the simple experiment as depicted in Figure 14.1. A solenoid L is joined to a meter which can measure both the magnitude and direction of any electric current flowing through the solenoid.

The following effects are observed experimentally when the magnet, M, is moved relative to the solenoid:

  a. No current is induced in L if the magnet is stationary with respect to the solenoid (Fig. 14.1(a) and (c)).
  b. A current is induced in L whenever the magnet is moved towards or away from the solenoid (Fig. 14.1(b) and (d)).
  c. The magnitude of the induced current is greater if the magnet is moved *faster.*
  d. Reversing the movement of the magnet reverses the direction of the induced current, as does reversing the pole nearest the solenoid also.

From this simple experiment, therefore, we may conclude that *only a changing magnetic field* is able to induce electricity in a conductor, and that the electricity induced is in some way dependent upon how fast the magnetic field changes. These concepts are discussed more fully in the following sections.

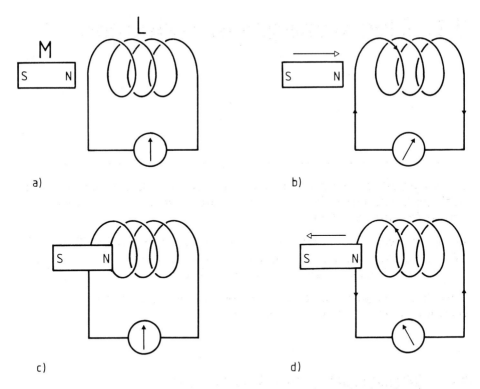

Fig. 14.1 An example of electromagnetic induction. A current flows only when there is relative movement between the bar magnet and the solenoid.

14.2 FARADAY'S LAWS

The laws of electromagnetic induction due to Faraday may be defined as follows:

1. A change of the magnetic flux linked with a conductor induces an EMF in the conductor.
2. The magnitude of the induced EMF is proportional to the *rate* of change of magnetic flux linkage.

Law 1 may be described as *qualitative* in the sense that it describes under what conditions an EMF is induced. Law 2 is *quantitative*, since it states the magnitude of the EMF obtained.

In order to understand Faraday's Laws, a clear idea of the concepts of 'EMF' and 'magnetic flux linkage' must be established. EMF (i.e. 'Electromagnetic Force', 10.3) is the 'driving force' capable of causing an electron flow in a circuit, and measures the difference in electrical potential energy across a source of electricity (in volts). Electrons 'fall down' a potential difference in the same way that water falls down a waterfall created by two levels of water.

It is important to note that Faraday's Laws do not specify whether the conductor needs to be completely isolated from or connected to an 'external' circuit — for in either case the induced EMF depends only upon the 'rate of change of magnetic flux linkage' and is independent of any other considerations. An analogy would be a 12 volt car battery, which has an EMF of 12 volts whether it is connected to a car bulb (an external circuit) or not — although here the source of the EMF is chemical rather than electromagnetic.

In (11.4) and (12.4) magnetic flux and magnetic flux density are discussed. The magnetic flux through a volume V may be visualised as being proportional to the number of lines of force passing through that volume, as shown in Figure 14.2. If a magnetic flux of 10 weber (11.4) passes through V, then the *magnetic flux linkage* with V is said to be 10 weber also.

In summary, moving the magnet relative to the solenoid (Fig. 14.1) changes the lines of flux which pass through the solenoid and so an EMF is induced according to Faraday's First Law. A rapid movement of the magnet increases the rate at which such 'flux linkage' with the solenoid alters, thus inducing a larger EMF by Faraday's Second Law.

Insight

Mathematically, Faraday's Laws give

$$E = - \frac{dN}{dt},$$

where E is the induced EMF in volts and N is the flux linkage in weber. (The negative sign is due to Lenz's Law — 14.3.) Thus, if a flux linkage change of *1 weber/second* is associated with a conductor, then an EMF of *1 volt* is induced across the conductor.

Now, a changing magnetic flux linkage associated with a particular conductor may be accomplished by either of two methods:

a. by relative movement between the conductor and the magnetic flux
b. by varying the magnitude of the magnetic flux while the conductor is stationary.

A dynamo, or AC generator (14.8), uses the first method to induce an EMF, while an AC transformer (Ch. 16) uses the second method.

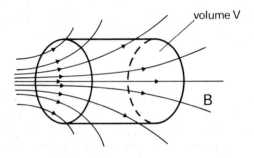

Fig. 14.2 The 'magnetic flux linkage' associated with a volume V.

14.3 LENZ'S LAW

Lenz's Law is concerned with the *direction* of the induced current which results if the conductor is connected to an external circuit, i.e. it concerns 'closed' rather than 'open' circuits. Faraday's Laws apply equally well to both open and closed circuits, as mentioned above.

Lenz's Law

The *direction* of the induced current in a conductor caused by a changing magnetic flux is such that its own magnetic field *opposes* the changing magnetic flux.

This law is a consequence of the Law of Conservation of Energy (7.2), since if the direction of the current was such that it *helped* whatever agency was causing it, then it would be possible to have perpetual motion and obtain 'something for nothing', in defiance of the Conservation Law.

For example, when the north pole of a bar magnet is moved towards a solenoid, as in Figure 14.1(b), a current will flow in the solenoid in such a direction that it produces a north pole at the end closest to the magnet, and a south pole at the other. This has the effect of producing a force of repulsion between the bar magnet and the solenoid, so that *work* must be done against this force in order to keep the magnet moving towards the solenoid. Thus mechanical energy is transformed into electrical energy. (If the current in the solenoid were to flow in such a direction as to attract the north pole of the magnet, then the magnet could be released and it would gather speed and increase the current it induced. Thus, energy would be produced for nothing, and the Conservation of Energy would be violated.) Other examples of Lenz's Law are given in this book, e.g. in motors and generators (14.7 and 14.8), transformer cores (16.1.1) and moving coil meters (17.5.3). However, a general method of determining the direction of the induced current is required, as was the case for the forces due to the Motor Principle — (13.2.1), and this is the subject of the following convention.

14.4 SIGN CONVENTION FOR INDUCED CURRENT

The method for finding the direction of the induced current (electron flow) is very similar to that described in (13.2.1) for the Motor Principle. Again, in an attempt to avoid confusion, Fleming's Hand Rules are not used, but may be seen in Appendix I.

Convention

Draw an arrow from the conductor in the direction of its movement and intersect this at point P with another arrow representing the direction of the magnetic flux. The induced current is then in such a direction that one of its resulting magnetic lines of force passing through P is in the same direction as that of the magnetic flux.

The following two examples should clarify the use of this convention.

Example 1

A wire is viewed 'end-on' in Figure 14.3, and is moved to the right. Applying the convention above results in the two arrows meeting at point P in the right-hand figure. The current induced in the wire must therefore flow in such a direction as to produce clockwise lines of force, i.e. the electron flow is towards the eye of the observer.

We may verify Lenz's Law for this example in the following manner: an induced current flowing towards the observer will itself produce a magnetic field which will interact with the existing magnetic field. We may thus use the convention for the Motor Principle to ascertain that the direction of the force on the wire is to the left, i.e. in the *opposite* direction to the original movement. Hence, the direction of the induced current is 'such as to oppose the original motion', i.e. Lenz's Law. Thus, if the wire is released, it will quickly come to rest under the restraining action of the force in the opposite direction to the original motion. This applies to any direction of the original motion of the wire except that parallel to the magnetic flux, B, since no magnetic flux change occurs and so no EMF and current are induced.

Example 2 — Rotation of aluminium frame

If a non-ferrous metal (e.g. aluminium) frame is supported so that it may rotate freely when spun (Fig. 14.4), it is found that the presence of a magnetic field causes it to stop very rapidly (e.g. if a bar magnet is suddenly moved close to it), irrespective of its direction of rotation.

This occurs because the presence of a magnetic field will induce a current in the frame so as to 'oppose its motion' (i.e. Lenz's Law) relative to the magnetic field — i.e. a force will be produced in the opposite direction to its rotation, thus slowing it down. Note that the opposing force exists only while the aluminium frame is *moving* — once it stops the force is also zero, since the

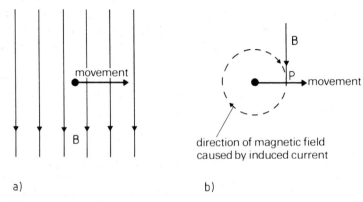

a)   b)

Fig. 14.3 An example of the use of the convention described in the text for establishing the direction of the induced current (Lenz's Law).

EMF (and hence current) are only induced by a *changing* magnetic flux, by Faraday's Laws. Thus, the frame will *not* start to rotate in the opposite direction!

We may verify these findings with the use of the sign convention above, as follows: suppose the frame rotates clockwise when viewed from above and the magnetic field is from left to right (Fig. 14.4(b)).

The above convention applied to the left-hand vertical part of the frame is shown in the figure, and results in an induced electric current flowing away from the eye of the observer. The current is induced in the opposite direction in the right-hand vertical part of the frame, however, so that electrons are able to flow around the whole frame (up on side and down the other).

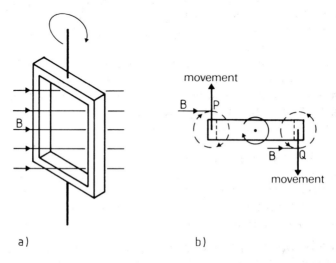

a)   b)

Fig. 14.4 A further example of Lenz's Law. The rotating aluminium frame rapidly comes to rest in the presence of a magnetic field. This is the way the moving-coil meter is 'damped'— see Chapter 17.

Each of the magnetic fields produced by the induced current will interact with B, because of the Motor Principle. The force produced on the conductor will be from P through the left side, and Q through the right side of the frame respectively (by the convention in Ch. 12), i.e. in *opposition to the movement of the frame.*

This is a particularly important example of Lenz's Law, as it applies to the 'damping' of a moving coil meter, the coils of which are wound on an aluminium frame (17.5).

Insight

The way in which EMF is induced, leading to Faraday's Laws, is discussed here for the example (a) above, i.e. moving a wire at right-angles to a magnetic field. Consider a straight wire of length *l* which is in a uniform magnetic flux density *B* directed into the paper. The wire is moved at constant velocity *v* to EF, over a distance *d*, as shown in the figure.

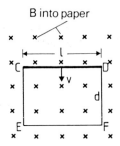

B into paper

Each electron within the wire is therefore moving relative to a magnetic field in the same direction as v so that a force will exist on it due to the Motor Principle.

The sign convention shows that the force on each electron is from D to C (left as an exercise for the student), so that C becomes negatively charged and D becomes positively charged (since electrons have flowed away from D) — thus a difference of electrical potential (i.e. an EMF) exists across CD. A steady EMF is established such that the force on an electron acting along DC due to the Motor Principle is exactly balanced by the force acting along CD (i.e. in the opposite direction) due to the electrostatic force of repulsion from C and attraction from D.

Equation 13.2, in (13.3.2) gave the equation $F = Bev \sin \theta$ for the force acting on an electron moving at velocity v through a magnetic flux density of B. In this particular example, $\sin \theta = 1$, so that the force F_1 due to the Monitor Principle is $F_1 = Bev$ to the left. The electrostatic force on an electron is just the electric field strength, E, times the charge on the electron, e (9.4). Now, $lE = $ EMF $=$ the work done in moving a unit charge from C to D (9.6).

$$\therefore \quad E = \text{EMF}/l$$

and the electrostatic force F_2 to the right is

$$F_2 = eE = \frac{e}{l} . \text{EMF}$$

Now, $F_1 = F_2$ so that

$$\frac{e}{l} . \text{EMF} = Bev.$$

$$\therefore \quad \text{EMF} = Bvl \qquad\qquad \text{Equation 1}$$

Thus we have an expression relating the induced EMF to B, v and l, which can now be expressed in terms of the 'rate of change of magnetic flux linkage'.

The total magnetic flux which has been linked with the wire is that passing through the area CDEF, i.e. $B \times d \times l$, since B is the magnetic flux per unit area. The *rate of change* of magnetic flux linkage is therefore Bdl/t, where t is the time taken to move the wire from CD to EF. But $v = d/t$, so that rate of change of flux linkage $= Bvl$. Thus, by comparison with Equation 1 we have finally:

induced EMF = rate of change of flux linkage

Exercise 14.1

a. In which direction may the wire be moved in the figure in order to induce (i) the maximum and (ii) zero EMF?

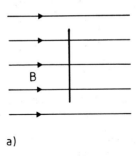

a)

b. The bar magnet having its north pole pointing downwards is dropped through a horizontal loop of wire. What is the direction of the induced current in the wire when the magnet is (i) above and (ii) below the wire?

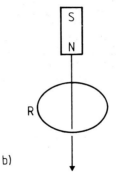

b)

14.5 MUTUAL INDUCTION

If the changing magnetic field from one current-carrying conductor is placed near a second conductor, then an EMF and current will be induced in the second conductor, by Faraday's and Lenz's Laws. However, the changing current thus induced will produce its own magnetic field which will induce an EMF and current in the first conductor. Thus, each condutor induces electricity in the other and the effect is therefore known as 'mutual induction'. For example, the coil P in Figure 14.5 is connected to a battery via a switch SW and placed close to the coil S, which is connected to a sensitive meter M to measure any current induced in S. When SW is closed an electron flow rapidly builds up to a steady level around P. During this short time, a *changing* magnetic flux is linked with the coil S so that an EMF and current are induced in it, but acting in opposition ot the changing flux, by Lenz's Law, and the

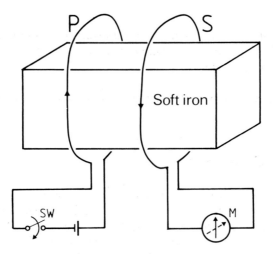

Fig. 14.5 Mutual induction. A changing current in coil *P* (the 'primary') induces a current in coil *S* (the 'secondary'), and vice versa. The soft iron magnifies the effect by improving the magnetic flux linkage between the coils.

pointer in meter M is deflected transiently in one direction. The effect of S on P is to slow down the rate of growth of current in P, again by Lenz's Law. After a short time the current in P is constant and that in S is zero (by Faraday's First Law) since the magnetic flux linkage is constant. When SW is opened, a changing (collapsing) magnetic flux is produced in P which again induces an EMF and current in S. However, this time the direction of the induced current is in such a direction to oppose the *reduction* in magnetic flux (in contrast to when SW is closed), so that the current flows through S in the opposite direction, and the pointer of the meter M is deflected transiently to the other side. The current in S may be greatly enhanced if a bar of soft iron is put through one or both coils, as in the figure. This is because the magnetic flux linkage between P and S is greatly improved owing to the magnetisation of the soft iron bar. Hence, the *change* of flux linkage is also increased, leading to higher values of induced EMF and current, by Faraday's Laws.

The EMF, E_s, induced in any nearby conductor (the 'secondary') may be shown by experiment to be:

a.   proportional to the rate of change of current in P (the 'primary')

b.   dependent upon the detailed design of the two conductors and the flux linkage between them. This is called the *mutual inductance* (*M*).

Thus,

$E_s = M \times$ rate of change of primary current   Equation 14.1

The greater the mutual inductance, *M*, the greater the mutual effect between two conductors. *M* is measured in *henry*, and may be defined as:

Definition

A mutual inductance of 1 *henry* exists between two conductors if one volt is induced in one conductor when there is a current change of 1 ampere/second in the other.

An AC transformer operates on the principle of mutual induction, as explained in Chapter 16.

14.6 SELF-INDUCTION

Consider the solenoid in Figure 14.6(a). If SW is closed, a current starts to build up in the solenoid. Now as this current increases, *each* turn of the solenoid produces a changing magnetic flux which is linked with the *other* turns of the solenoid (the flux from one turn is shown in the figure). Thus from Faraday's and Lenz's Laws, a so-called 'back EMF' will be induced in the solenoid, i.e. in opposition to the 'forward EMF' from the battery. This effect is known as 'self-induction' and means that the current in the solenoid may take an appreciable time to reach its maximum value if the 'self-induction' is large. The 'self-induction' of an electrical system is defined in a very similar manner to mutual induction above, i.e.

$E_B = L \times$ rate of change of current   Equation 14.2

Here, E_B is the 'back EMF' and L is the 'self-inductance' measured in henry.

Definition

A conductor has a self-inductance of 1 henry if a back EMF of 1 volt is induced when the current flowing through it changes by 1 ampere/second.

A graph of the current flowing through the solenoid is shown in Figure 14.6(b). As can be seen, the induced 'back EMF' slows down the growth of the current. However, it eventually reaches its maximum value given by Ohm's

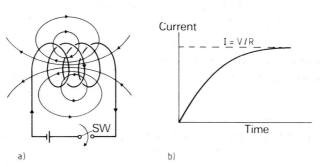

a)   b)

Fig. 14.6 Self-induction. The change of magnetic flux linked with all the turns induces a 'back-EMF' which slows down the growth of current in the coil.

Law (10.5). If the wire of the solenoid were unwound to become straight, then there would be no flux linkage, no back EMF, and so the current would rise to its maximum value very quickly.

As in the case of mutual induction, self-induction is enhanced if a soft iron bar is placed in the solenoid, as the magnetic flux linkage between the coils is increased.

An autotransformer operates on the principle of self-induction, as explained in Chapter 16.

Insight — Units of permeability

In (11.2) it was stated that the SI unit of permeability was 'henry/metre' — this is discussed here, and, although rather involved, the relationships between the units may prove to be helpful to the reader.

Biot and Savart's Law (12.4) gives

$$B = \frac{\mu}{4\pi} \cdot \frac{Il\sin\theta}{r^2}$$

so that, by cross-multiplication, the units of μ are:

$$\frac{\text{tesla} \times \text{m}^2}{A \times \text{m}} = \frac{\text{Wb m}^{-2} \times \text{m}^2}{A \times \text{m}} \quad \text{(since 1 tesla} = \text{Wb/m}^2\text{)}$$

i.e. $\text{Wb}A^{-1}\,\text{m}^{-1}$ Equation 1

Faraday's Law is $E = -dN/dt$ where N is the flux linkage in weber. Also, for a conductor of self-induction L henry, $E = -L(dI/dt)$, so that (combining these two expressions) $L = dN/dI$. Thus, the units of L (and M) are

$$\frac{\text{magnetic flux}}{\text{ampere}}$$

(i.e. $\text{Wb}\,A^{-1}$) so that 1 henry $= 1\ \text{Wb}\,A^{-1}$, or 1 henry/metre $= 1\ \text{Wb}\,A^{-1}\,\text{m}^{-1}$, i.e. the same as Equation 1 above, so that the units of μ are $H\,\text{m}^{-1}$.

14.7 THE ELECTRIC MOTOR

Although the electric motor is, of course, the prime example of the Motor Principle in that it converts electrical energy into mechanical energy, it cannot be properly understood without considering also the effects of electromagnetic induction. A simplified DC electric motor is shown in Figure 14.7 where a battery is connected to a single coil of wire KLMN via 'brushes' B and 'commutator' C. The coil of wire is in the magnetic field of a permanent magnet, the direction of whose magnetic field is from left to right in the figure.

When the current is first switched on, the electron flow is in the direction as indicated on the diagram, and the coil suffers a clockwise force due to the Motor Principle (i.e. an upward force on KL and a downward force on MN, as may be verified by the use of the convention in 13.2.1). The commutator C also turns with the coil KLMN so that the current always flows in the same direction relative to the permanent magnet. Hence the coil always experiences a

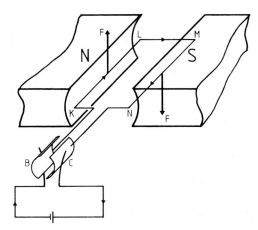

Fig. 14.7 The DC electric motor.

clockwise force and keeps rotating. Without the commutator, KLMN would eventually stop at right-angles to the magnetic field.

Thus, we have a conductor which is moving relative to a magnetic field — i.e. undergoing a change of magnetic flux linkage — so that an EMF and current must be induced according to Faraday's and Lenz's Laws of electromagnetic induction (14.2 and 14.3). The faster the coil rotates, the greater is the induced EMF and current because the rate of change of flux linkage increases (Faraday's Second Law). The direction of the induced EMF is in the opposite direction to that applied, so as to produce an induced current which will oppose (Lenz's Law) the motion of electrons along KLMN. This induced EMF is therefore known as a 'back EMF' since it acts in opposition to the 'driving' EMF from the electrical supply (battery). Thus the faster the coil rotates, the smaller is the *net* current which flows in it until, for a free-moving frictionless motor, the rotational speed becomes such that no current flows at all because the 'forward' and 'back' EMFs cancel each other out. It is for this reason that an electric motor does not rotate more and more quickly: it achieves a steady speed owing to the 'back EMF' induced in the windings by electromagnetic induction.

When the motor is 'under load' (i.e. performing mechanical work) then the rotation speed reduces so that a net current may flow and the electrical work then performed is transformed into mechanical work (and heat, etc.).

14.8 THE ELECTRIC GENERATOR

In contrast to the electric motor, the generator is designed to transform mechanical energy into electrical energy, i.e. the reverse of the motor. This is why electromagnetic induction is also called the 'generator effect'. However, an electric motor may be operated as a generator, and vice versa.

A DC generator (or 'dynamo') is shown in Figure 14.8(a) — note the similarity to the motor depicted in Figure 14.7(a). The coil KLMN is forced to

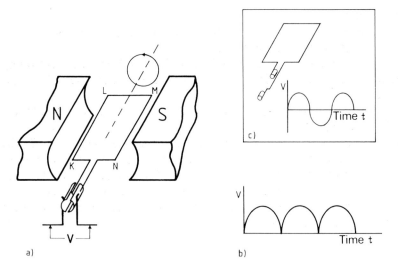

Fig. 14.8 (a) a DC generator, or 'dynamo', producing a waveform as in (b). Inset shows an AC generator, or 'alternator', with corresponding waveform (sinusoidal).

rotate, thus inducing an EMF (V in the figure) due to the laws of electromagnetic induction. The function of the commutator is to produce a 'rectified' voltage and current (Ch. 20) as shown in Figure 14.8(b).

If the two ends, K and N, of the coil are brought to separate commutators (inset in Fig. 14.8) then an *alternating* EMF is induced. This arrangement is called an AC generator or 'alternator'. Another design whereby the magnets move around a stationary coil is called a 'magneto'.

In all cases, if there is no external electrical circuit connected, then no current is able to flow and only sufficient work to overcome frictional resistance is necessary to keep the rotational movement at the same speed. As soon as an external circuit is connected, however (i.e. an 'electrical load'), then a current is able to flow both in the winding and in the circuit. It should now come as no surprise to discover that this current will flow in such a direction so as to *oppose* the motion of the coil, i.e. Lenz's Law. This means that *mechanical* work must be performed to overcome this resisting force, so that mechanical energy is transformed into electrical energy.

The effect of suddenly increasing the 'electrical load' of the generator (i.e. suddenly drawing more current from it, as in an X-ray exposure, for example) is to increase the opposing force on the coil due to the Motor Principle. As in all other examples, the 'Motor Effect' and the 'Generator Effect' act in opposition. Hence the generator slows down momentarily and the induced EMF (which is dependent upon the speed of rotation) is slightly reduced. Thus, an increased current load produces a lower available potential difference, as is the case for other electrical supplies (e.g. a battery).

The diagram of the voltage waveform of the alternator (as shown in inset) is known as a 'sinusoidal' variation (1.9.1) and is the most common form of alternating current (AC). The use of such alternating voltages and currents is described more fully in the following chapter.

Exercise 14.2

a. Explain what is meant by the term 'electromagnetic induction'. How does it differ from electromagnetism?

b. State and explain Faraday's and Lenz's Laws of electromagnetic induction. Hence list the factors upon which the magnitude of the induced EMF depends.

c. In what circumstances is it possible to have an induced EMF without an induced current?

d. What is meant by the terms 'mutual' and 'self' induction. Define the unit (henry) in which each is measured. Discuss the application of mutual and self-induction in the production of a stable kV_p for an X-ray tube (see Ch. 16).

e. What is the effect on an alternator of suddenly increasing the load (current) drawn from it? Explain why this results in a lower potential difference (voltage) from the alternator.

SUMMARY

1. Electromagnetic induction (also the 'generator effect'): the production of electricity by a changing magnetic field linked with a conductor. This is the opposite of electromagnetism.
2. The 'magnetic flux linkage' of a conductor is the number of magnetic lines of force which pass through the conductor — measured in weber.
3. Faraday's Laws:

   1. A *changing* magnetic flux linked with a conductor induces an EMF in the conductor.
   2. The EMF is proportional to the *rate* of change of magnetic flux.

An EMF is induced whether the circuit is *open* (no current) or *closed* (current) with an external circuit.
4. Lenz's Law: The *direction* of the induced current in a closed circuit is such as to oppose the change producing it. This means that the original magnetic flux and the induced magnetic flux act in opposition, and is a consequence of the law of conservation of energy.
5. Mutual Induction: A mutual induction of 1 henry exists between two conductors if an EMF of 1 volt is induced in one when the current changes by 1 ampere per second in the other.
6. Self-Induction: A conductor possesses a self-inductance of 1 henry if a 'back EMF' of 1 volt is induced when the current in it changes by 1 ampere per second.

15. Electricity (AC)

Direct current (DC) electricity (Ch. 10) is a flow of electrons in one direction only. This chapter concerns alternating current (AC) which is an alternating flow of electrons, i.e. they flow first one way and then the other.

The most common type of AC is *sinusoidal*, where the magnitude of current (or voltage) varies as a sine-wave with time (1.9.1). The next section considers this and other types of AC and DC. The generation of AC is described briefly in (14.8).

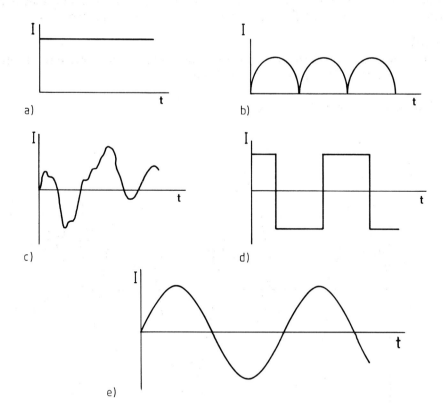

Fig. 15.1 Types of DC and AC: (a) constant DC, (b) 'pulsatile' DC, (c) irregular AC, (d) square waveform AC, (e) sinusoidal AC.

15.1 TYPES OF DC AND AC

Figure 15.1 shows some common types of DC and AC in graphical form. Figure 15.1(a) is the case considered in Chapter 10 — i.e. steady DC — where the number of electrons passing a point per second in the circuit is constant, resulting in a horizontal straight-line graph as shown. Figure 15.1(b) is a case of 'pulsatile' DC, where the electrons always move in the same direction, but do so in a series of 'jerks' or 'pulses'. An irregular AC waveform is shown in Figure 15.1(c) where there is no discernible pattern to the electron flow, although it flows in alternate directions, since it goes alternately positive and negative. ('Positive' and 'negative' directions are purely arbitrary.) A regular AC waveform is shown in Figure 15.1(d), where the electron flow jumps abruptly from one direction to an equal but opposite value in the opposite direction for an equal time. This is known as a 'square wave-form'. Lastly, a *sinusoidal* AC waveform is shown in Figure 15.1(e).

15.2 SINUSODIAL AC

Figure 15.2 illustrates the sinusoidal AC waveform in more detail, together with some of the quantities used to measure it. These are defined below.

1 Cycle
  One complete waveform, starting from any point. Usually measured from zero (i.e. ABCDE) or a peak (e.g. BCDEF).
Period (T)
  The time for one cycle — in seconds.

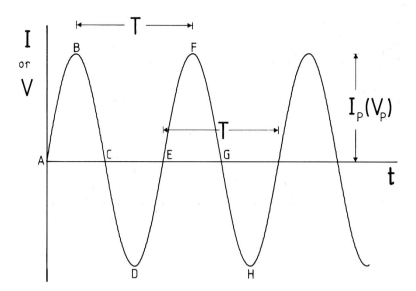

Fig. 15.2 A sinusoidal waveform.

Frequency (f)

The number of cycles which occur in one second — in cycles per second or hertz (Hz).

Amplitude

The maximum value of positive or negative current (or voltage) on the waveform.

There is a simple relationship between period (T) and frequency (f). Suppose that we have a waveform of frequency 10 Hz, i.e. 10 cycles occur every second. Since the waveform is regular, each cycle must therefore occur in 0·1 second, in order that 10 cycles may occur in one second. Generally, then:

$$f = \frac{1}{T} \hspace{6cm} \text{Equation 15.1}$$

The equation for a sinusoidal current is —

$$I_t = I_p \sin 2\pi ft$$

where I_t is the current at time t and I_p is the amplitude of the current. The corresponding formula for a sinusoidal voltage is —

$$V_t = V_p \sin 2\pi ft$$

The remainder of this chapter discusses further quantities used to measure sinusoidal AC and its use in different types of simple electrical circuits.

15.2.1 Peak current (or voltage)

The peak current, I_p, is the same as the amplitude, i.e. the maximum positive or negative value of current. Similarly, the peak voltage, V_p, is the maximum absolute value of voltage. In radiography, the peak voltage across the X-ray tube in the forward direction (i.e. the anode positive with respect to cathode) is usually quoted. For example, an X-ray unit operating at 75 kV$_p$ has a peak voltage of 75 kV across it.

15.2.2 Average current (or voltage)

The average current flowing in one cycle of a sinusoidal waveform is just *zero*, since there is no net electron flow, i.e. the electrons finish at the same point from which they start. The same conclusion applies to any numbers of cycles, so that:

$$
\begin{aligned}
I_{AV} &= 0 \\
V_{AV} &= 0 \\
&\text{for a sinusoidal waveform}
\end{aligned}
\hspace{3cm} \text{Equation 15.2}
$$

However, if the AC waveform is *rectified* (Ch. 20) then a value for the average current is obtained. 'Half-wave' rectification (20.1) produces a waveform

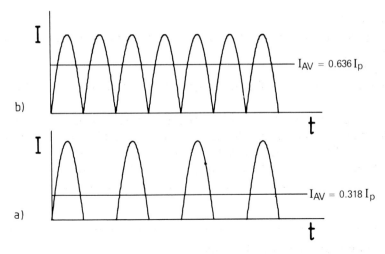

Fig. 15.3 (a) Half-wave rectification and (b) full-wave rectification of sinusoidal AC.

where alternate half-cycles are missing, as shown in Figure 15.3(a). This produces a form of 'pulsatile DC' (15.1) which results in a net electron flow and therefore a value for the average current. A 'full-wave rectified' current is shown in Figure 15.3(b) on the same scale. Again, a 'pulsatile DC' is produced where the average value is just twice that of the 'half-wave' rectified current, because there are twice as many peaks over the same time. It may be shown mathematically (see Insight below) that:

$$I_{AV} = 0\cdot318I_p$$
$$V_{AV} = 0\cdot318V_p$$

for half-wave rectification

Equation 15.3

and that,

$$I_{AV} = 0\cdot636I_p$$
$$V_{AV} = 0\cdot636V_p$$

for full-wave rectification.

Equation 15.4

Insight

The average current is defined as that steady current which is required to flow over a given time to produce the same total charge as the waveform being considered.

i.e. average current, $I_{AV} = \dfrac{\text{total charge}}{t} = \dfrac{1}{t}\displaystyle\int_0^t I_t \, dt$

For half-wave rectification; I_{AV} must be taken over one complete cycle (i.e. $t = 1/f$) and is therefore given by —

$$I_{AV} = \frac{\displaystyle\int_0^{1/2f} I_p \sin 2\pi ft + 0}{1/f}$$

$$= I_p . f . \left[-\frac{\cos 2\pi ft}{2\pi f} \right]_0^{1/2f}$$

$$= \frac{I_p . f}{2\pi f} . [(-\cos \pi) - (-\cos 0)] = \frac{2I_p}{2\pi} = \frac{I_p}{\pi}$$

Now, $\dfrac{1}{\pi} = \dfrac{1}{3 \cdot 14159} = 0 \cdot 318$

so that $I_{AV} = 0 \cdot 318 I_p$

and $V_{AV} = 0 \cdot 318 V_p$ $\Bigg\}$ for half-wave rectification

For full-wave rectification, we need only integrate over a half-cycle, so that

$$I_{AV} = \frac{I_p . 2f}{2\pi f} \left[(-\cos \pi) - (-\cos 0) \right]_0^{1/2f}$$

$$= \frac{2I_p}{\pi}$$

i.e. twice the value obtained above.

i.e. $I_{AV} = 0 \cdot 636 I_p$

$V_{AV} = 0 \cdot 636 V_p$ $\Bigg\}$ for half-wave rectification

---

15.2.3 Effective (RMS) current (or voltage)

If an AC supply is connected across a resistor, then electrons will flow first one way and then the other, producing no *net* movement of electons within the re-sistor. Under these circumstances the average current is zero, as discussed above. This does not mean, however, that the net *heating* effect will be zero, because work must be done on the electrons to move them in either direction. Thus we would not expect that electrons moving in one direction would heat up the resistor, while electrons moving the other way would cool it down again! The 'average current' is therefore a quantity which is not suitable for determining the *energy* or *power* expended in a circuit when connected to an AC supply. The quantity of importance is the so-called 'effective' current, and may be defined as:

Definition

The *effective current* is that value of constant current which, flowing for the same time, would produce the same expenditure of electrical energy in a circuit as the alternating current.

The effective current is also known as the 'Root Mean Square' (RMS) current, as shown below. The effective or RMS *voltage* is defined in a very similar manner, i.e.

Definition

The *effective voltage* is that value of constant voltage which, being present for the same time, would produce the same expenditure of electrical energy in a circuit as the alternating voltage.

In (10.6.2) it was shown that the general equation for DC electrical power is $W = VI$ where W is expressed in watts, V in volts and I in amperes. In an AC circuit, both V and I are continually changing so that it is the effective values of each which must be used.

i.e. $W = V_{eff} \times I_{eff}$ Equation 15.5

Here, W is the *average* power generated in the circuit, taking into account at least one half-cycle of AC.

Similarly, if we consider an alternating current flowing through a resistor R, then, by analogy to (10.6.3), we have

$$W = I_{eff}^2 R$$

Equation 15.6

$$W = \frac{V_{eff}^2}{R}$$

Note

Ohm's Law for DC is $V = IR$ (see 10.5).

For *AC*, the same equation may be used *provided* that the same type of units are used, i.e. if V is in effective units, so must be I, and so on.

The effective values of current and voltage are related to the peak values by the following relationships:

$$I_{eff} = 0 \cdot 707 I_p$$

Equation 15.7

$$I_{eff} = 0 \cdot 707 V_p$$

Thus, for a sinusoidal waveform, the effective or RMS value is slightly over 70% of the peak value of current or voltage. This relationship is derived in the Insight below.

Insight

Consider the case of an alternating current flowing through a resistor, If the instantaneous value of the current is I_t at time t, then the instantaneous power generated in the resistor at that moment is $I_t^2 R$ watt. The average power is therefore $(I_t^2)_{AV}. R$ watt. Also, the average power is $I_{eff}^2 R$ watt from the above definition of an effective current.

$$\therefore I_{eff}^2 = (I_t^2)_{AV} = \text{mean} (I_t^2) \qquad \text{('mean' is the same as 'average')}$$
i.e. $I_{eff} = \sqrt{[\text{mean}(I_t^2)]}$

Thus, the effective current is the 'Root Mean Square' of the AC current, i.e. the square root of the mean (i.e. average) square of the current. This is illustrated in Figure 15.4.

Mathematically therefore,

$$I_{eff}^2 = \frac{\displaystyle\int_0^{1/2f} I_t^2 dt}{1/2f}$$

Using the relationships $I_t = I_p \sin 2\pi f t$ and $\cos 4\pi f t = 1 - 2 \sin^2 2\pi f t$

we obtain

$$I_{eff}^2 = fI_p^2 \int_0^{1/2f} (1 - \cos 4\pi f t)\, dt$$

which, when integrated and simplified, produces

$$I_{eff}^2 = \frac{I_p^2}{2}$$

By taking the square root of both sides, we obtain finally:

$$I_{eff} = \frac{I_p}{\sqrt{2}} = 0.707\, I_p$$

since $1/\sqrt{2} = 0.707$.

This is an agreement with Equation 15.7

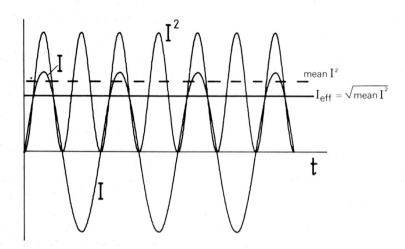

Fig. 15.4   Graphical representation of an 'effective' (RMS) value of current.

15.3 AC AND THE X-RAY TUBE

An X-ray tube requires a high potential difference (voltage) across it and a current flowing through it in order to produce X-rays. The mains voltage is far too small to use directly across an X-ray tube, so that a means of increasing it to tens of thousands of volts is required. This is relatively easily accomplished using a 'step-up transformer' which requires AC in order to operate (16.1). However, the mains voltage is too high to use directly across the filament, the latter supplying the electrons forming the mA through the X-ray tube, In this case, a 'step-down transformer' is used (Ch. 16) to provide the low voltage and high current necessary for the heating of the filament. Thus, an AC supply may be either increased or decreased relatively easily using transformers.

In AC circuits the voltages or currents are usually expressed in terms of their effective values, unless otherwise stated. However, the following convention applies when considering the voltages and currents applied to an X-ray tube:

a.   the voltage across the tube (kV) is expressed in terms of the *peak* voltage, i.e. kV_p.

b.   the current flowing through the tube (mA) is expressed in terms of the *average* current.

c.   the mains voltage and currents are expressed in terms of effective (or RMS) values.

15.3.1 Voltage across tube (kV_p)

The advantages of expressing the potential difference across the X-ray tube in terms of the kV_p value are:

(i)   the maximum energy of X-ray photon emitted from the anode is the same value in keV (6.4.1 and 28.2)

(ii)   the voltage rating of the high tension (HT) cables may be directly compared to the kV_p to see whether they will be able to withstand the maximum voltage applied to them.

If an X-ray unit provides a 'constant potential' supply to the X-ray tube (Ch. 20), the peak and average values of the voltage are the same, as the supply is effectively DC (in practice, a voltage 'ripple' (20.4) produces a small difference between the peak and average voltages across the tube).

15.3.2 Current through the tube (mA)

The mA meter measures the *average* current flowing through the X-ray tube. This is proportional to the average intensity of the X-ray beam during the exposure and has the additional advantage of giving a true reading of milli-coulomb when multiplied by the exposure time in seconds (i.e. mAs). Thus, mA × s = mAs, which represents the total charge which has flowed through the X-ray tube during the exposure.

15.3.3 Mains voltage (current)

The electrical mains is a source of *power* and is therefore most often expressed in terms which make calculations of power most convenient, i.e. effective of RMS values. Thus, if the electrical mains is 115 volts in the USA, this represents the effective value, and the corresponding peak value is $115/0.707 = 163$ volts, from Equation 15.7. The RMS mains voltage in the UK is a nominal 240 volts which gives a peak value of $240/0.707 = 339$ volts.

Exercise 15.1

a. What is meant by 'sinusoidal' alternating current? Illustrate your answer with a graph of current against time.

b. Explain what is meant by 'peak', 'average' and 'effective' (or 'RMS') values of sinusoidal current. What are the relationships between these quantities, assuming that the current has been fully rectified?

c. A 10 volt RMS supply is connected across a 100Ω resistor. What is:

(i) the RMS current
(ii) the peak current
(iii) the average current
(iv) the average power produced in the resistor?

(*Hint:* you may use Ohm's Law, if the same type of unit is considered for both current and voltage.)

d. What is meant by an 'effective' (or 'RMS') alternating current? Use your answer to determine the value of DC current which would produce the same power in the 100Ω resistor in question (c) above.

15.4 BASICS OF AC CIRCUITS

15.4.1 Phase difference

Hitherto we have considered only the case where the peak voltage occurs at the same time as the peak current. The current and voltage are then said to be 'in phase'. This is not necessarily so for AC circuits, however, and a 'phase difference' is then said to exist between the voltage and current waveforms. This is illustrated in Figure 15.5(a), where I 'lags' behind V, and in Figure 15.5(b) where I 'leads' V, where I and V are the current and voltage waveforms respectively. A waveform displaced to the right occurs later than, and therefore 'lags', the waveform to which it is compared. The angle between the two waveforms is the 'phase angle' where 360° is equivalent to 1 cycle (1.9.1). This is shown in Figure 15.6, where the 'phase angle' θ exists between the current I and voltage V. Figure 15.6 is known as a *vector diagram*, and OC is the 'current vector' and OA is the 'voltage vector', both of which rotate completely anti-clockwise at a rate of f revolutions per second, where f is the frequency of the AC supply. The example in the figure is that of the voltage vector leading the current vector by θ. The magnitude of the current and voltage at any time is

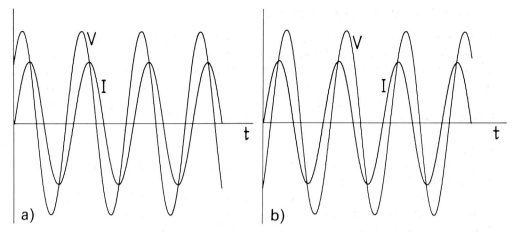

Fig. 15.5 Phase difference between current and voltage waveforms: (a) **I** 'lags' **V**, (b) **I** 'leads' **V**.

given by the 'vertical' distance of the tip of each vector, e.g. the length OB for voltage vector OA, as shown in the figure. The angle θ is of course maintained between the two vectors throughout the rotation of both.

15.4.2 Reactance and impedance

There are two measures of the 'AC resistance' of a circuit: the *reactance* and the *impedance*. Both are measured in ohms (as in DC resistance), but measure different quantities as explained below.

Referring to Figure 15.6, a phase difference of θ exists between the voltage across and the current flowing through a particular AC circuit. The *reactance*, X, is defined as the ratio OB/OC where OB is measured in volts and OC is in amperes. The important point to note is that the voltage OB and the current

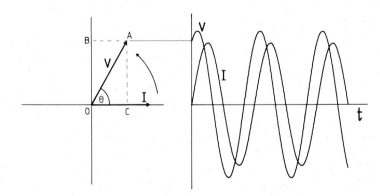

Fig. 15.6 A vector diagram. The two vectors **V** and **I** rotate anticlockwise and the 'vertical' height of each gives the instantaneous values of the voltage and current. The angle θ is maintained throughout the rotation. **V** lead **I** (or **I** lags **V**) in this diagram.

OC are at right-angles. As shown later (15.5.2 and 15.5.3), reactance is produced by capacitors and inductors, but not by resistors.

The *impedance*, Z, is defined as the ratio OA/OC where OA is measured in volts and OC is measured in amperes, as before.

To summarise: Resistance, reactance, and impedance are all measured in ohms and are expressed by the ratio of 'volts to amps'. However, the direction of the voltage vector is different in each case, being 'in phase' with the current for resistance, at right-angles to the current for reactance and at a particular angle to the current (the phase angle) for impedance. Impedance is thus the general term for 'resistance of flow' of which reactance and resistance are particular cases. The examples shown in Section 15.5 should make these concepts clear.

15.4.3 Power, power factor, wattless component and kVA

If an instantaneous current I flows in a circuit due to an instantaneous voltage V, then the power W at the instant is just $W = VI$ (10.6.2). However, in most cases we are not concerned with the variation of power over one cycle, but with the average power over one or more cycles. In this case, the effective or RMS values of current and voltage are required (15.2.3) such that:

$$W = V_{\text{eff}} \times I_{\text{eff}}$$

However, this formula only holds in the case when there is no phase difference between V and I, i.e. $\theta = 0$ in Figure 15.6. It will be shown (15.5) that reactance does not contribute to the average power drawn from a supply — hence only the power produced in the *resistances* in the AC circuit need be considered. The latter is obtained simply by resolving V along I (i.e. $V \cos \theta$), so that the final expression for AC power is:

$$W = V_{\text{eff}} \times I_{\text{eff}} \times \cos \theta \qquad \text{Equation 15.6}$$

The *power factor* is the value of $\cos \theta$, which is unity for a circuit containing only resistors, and may be less than unity for other circuits, in which case a phase difference occurs between V and I.

The *wattless component* of the voltage V is $V \sin \theta$ and represents the component of V which produces no average power, because it is in phase with the reactance. Likewise, the current flowing through a reactance is termed a "wattless current'.

The power rating of transformers is often quoted in units of 'kVA', i.e. kilovolts times amperes. This specifies the maximum value of the output of the transformer when running continuously into a *resistive* load, i.e. V and I are in phase ($\theta = 0$ in Fig. 15.6). The RMS values of 'kV' and 'A' are used to obtain the values of kVA.

Example

If the maximum output of a transformer is 20 kVA, and it is connected to an X-ray tube running at an RMS voltage of 50 kV, what is the maximum current permitted for continuous exposure? From the definition of kVA,

$$20 = 50 \times I$$
$$\therefore \quad I = 0.4 \text{ A} = 400 \text{ mA}.$$

A particular X-ray tube, however, may have a much lower rating than this (Ch.22) but 400 mA is the maximum current that the *transformer* may safely deliver at 50 kV.

15.5 SIMPLE AC CIRCUITS

Section 15.4 gave a general account of phase, reactance, impedance etc. and how they apply in general to AC circuits. In this section these concepts are applied to individual circuit components and a simple LRC circuit in order to show their practical application.

15.5.1 Resistor

Figure 15.7 shows the connection of an AC supply across a resistor. In this case there is no phase difference between the voltage and the current, i.e. they are 'in phase', so that the vector diagram shows the current and voltage vectors pointing in the same direction. They both rotate together, giving sinusoidal voltage and current waveforms which peak at the same times and cross the axis at the same times.

The average power generated in the resistor is just given by:

$$W = V_{\text{RMS}} \times I_{\text{RMS}}$$

as explained in (15.2.3).

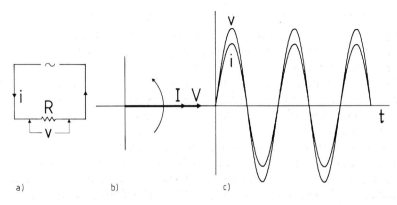

Fig. 15.7 (a) Circuit, (b) vector diagram, and (c) waveforms for a resistor. **V** and **I** are 'in-phase'.

15.5.2 Capacitor

It is evident from a comparison of Figures 15.8 and 15.7 that an AC supply connected across a capacitor introduces a phase difference between the voltage and the current.

The vector diagrams indicates that the voltage across the capacitor lags behind the current flowing in and out of the plates by 90°, giving sinusoidal current and voltage waveforms as shown. Thus, a perfect capacitor possesses reactance (V/I in the figure) and no resistance.

It may be shown (see Insight below) that the value of the reactance is given by

$$X_c = \frac{1}{2\pi fC} \qquad\qquad \text{Equation 15.7}$$

where f is the frequency of the AC supply (in Hz) and C is the value of the capacity in farads. Thus, the reactance is inversely proportional to both the capacity and frequency of supply.

The average power generated in a capacitor is *zero* as, over each half-cycle, the capacitor gives back to the circuit the same power that it receives. There is thus no net expenditure of power, agreeing with Equation 15.6, since cos 90° is zero.

Exercise 15.2
Draw a graph of one cycle of sinusoidal AC current. On the same graph draw the voltage waveform as shown in Figure 15.8, i.e. V lagging I by 90°. For 10° intervals, calculate and superimpose a graph of V times I and show that this gives a waveform of twice the frequency of I with an average value of zero over one cycle. Repeat the same procedure for a resistor (Fig. 15.7) and hence show that the power generated in a resistor over one cycle is not zero.

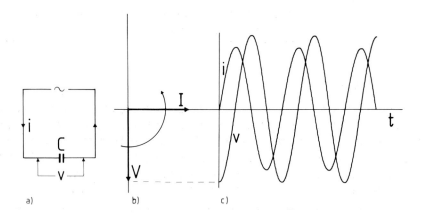

Fig. 15.8 (a) Circuit, (b) vector diagram, and (c) waveforms for a capacitor. **V** lags **I** by 90°

Insight

For a capacitor, the charge (q) and the voltage (v) are in phase, as is seen by the simple relationship $C = q/v$. However, electric *current* is the *rate of flow* of charge and it is this which has a 90° phase difference with respect to the voltage.

Mathematically, therefore, $i = dq/dt$ and since q varies as a sine wave (being 'in-step' with v), i will vary as $d(\sin 2\pi ft)/dt$, i.e. $2\pi f \cos 2\pi ft$. A cosine waveform is shifted 90° 'to the left' compared to a sine waveform, so that i leads v by 90° (Fig. 15.8).

In order to derive an expression for the reactance of the capacitor, we need to use the following relationships:

$X_c = V/I$; where V and I are peak values
$C = q/v$; $i = dq/dt$ (as discussed above)
$v = V \sin 2\pi ft$

Combining these relationships, we obtain

$$i = \frac{dq}{dt} = C\frac{dv}{dt} = C\frac{d(V \sin 2\pi ft)}{dt}$$

$$\therefore \quad i = (CV \cos 2\pi ft) . 2\pi f$$
$$= 2\pi fC . V \cos 2\pi ft.$$

Thus, the peak value of $i = 2\pi fCV (= I)$

$$\therefore \quad X_c = \frac{V}{I} = \frac{V}{2\pi fCV}$$

$$\therefore \quad X_c = \frac{1}{2\pi fC}, \text{ in agreement with Equation 15.7}$$

The power at any moment is $v \times i$

$$= V \sin 2\pi ft . I \cos 2\pi ft$$

$$= \frac{VI}{2} \sin 4\pi ft \text{ (since 'sin } 2\theta = 2 \sin \theta \cos \theta\text{')}$$

giving a power variation of twice the frequency of the supply (i.e. $4\pi ft$ rather than $2\pi ft$).

The average value of a sine-wave is zero, so that the net power taken by the capacitor from an AC supply is zero.

15.5.3 Inductor

The voltage across an inductor is out of phase compared to the current flowing through it. This is evident from the appropriate vector diagram and waveforms of Figure 15.9, where it is seen that the voltage *leads* the current by 90°. (This is the opposite way round to the capacitor (15.5.2).) A perfect inductor therefore possesses reactance (V/I in the figure) and no resistance.

The reactance of an inductor, X_L, may be shown to be given by:

$X_L = 2\pi fL$ Equation 15.8

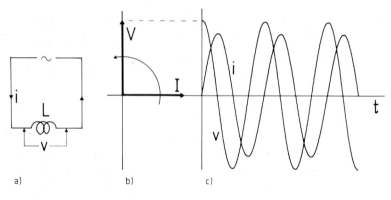

Fig. 15.9 (a) Circuit, (b) vector diagram, and (c) waveforms for an inductor, V leads I by 90°.

where f is the frequency of the AC supply and L is the value of the inductance in henry. Thus the reactance of an inductor *increases* with the frequency, f, unlike that of a capacitor (Equation 15.7). We have seen that the net power drawn from an AC supply by a capacitor is zero. The same is true of an inductor, so that we may say that a reactance consumes no power, while resistance does consume power.

Insight

The 'back EMF' induced in an inductor is proportional to the rate of change of current in the inductor (14.6). Thus, by differentiating the current with respect to time, i.e. di/dt, we obtain a quantity which is proportional to the voltage. A similar argument as put forward in the previous Insight will then suffice to show that the voltage leads the current by 90°, since the voltage contains a cosine term (the differential of a sine). Notice that this is the opposite way round to the case of a capacitor, where the current leads the voltage by 90°. This is shown by the vector diagrams in Figures 15.8 and 15.9.

We may derive an expression for the reactance of an inductor by combining the following relationships:

$X_L = V/I$; where V and I are peak values

$v = L\dfrac{di}{dt}$; where v is the voltage applied across the inductor

$i = I \sin 2\pi ft$.

Thus, $v = L\dfrac{d(I \sin 2\pi ft)}{dt} = 2fLI \cos 2\pi ft$

The maximum (peak) value of v is therefore $V = 2\pi fLI$ and the reactance is therefore

$X_L = \dfrac{V}{I} = 2\pi fL$

in agreement with Equation 15·8.

The instantaneous *power* generated in the inductor is v times i, i.e,

$2\pi fLI \cos 2\pi ft \times I \sin 2\pi ft = \pi fLI^2 \sin 4\pi ft$

This expression, like that of the previous Insight, represent a sine waveform of double the frequency of the current or voltage waveform, and whose average value is zero. Thus there is no net power generated in a pure inductor.

15.5.4 RCL in series-resonance

As an example of how the circuit components of resistor (R), capacitor (C) and inductor (L) may be used in an AC circuit, consider Figure 15.10 where the AC supply is connected across a circuit consisting of an R, C and L joined in series. The use of a vector diagram is shown to advantage in this example, as we may draw the resistance R in phase with the current, the reactance of the inductor, X_L, 90° ahead of the current, and the reactance of the capacitor 90° behind the current. The voltages across each circuit component (v_R, v_L, v_C,) are out of phase with each other, just as are the reactances, and it is the *vector sum* of the voltages which is equal to the supply voltage. Likewise, it is the vector sum of

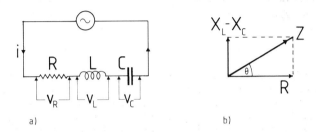

a)   b)

Fig. 15.10 A resistor, capacitor and inductor connected in series to an AC supply. The vector diagrams shows the resistance (R), the net reactance ($X_L - X_C$) and the overall impedance (Z) of the LRC circuit.

the resistance and reactances which produces the impedance Z which, in general, will have a phase difference with respect to the current (θ in Fig. 15.10(b)). Moreover, the voltage and impedance vectors (V and Z) will be coincident, so that the voltage and current will also have a phase difference of θ between them.

The calculations of these quantities is quite easy, and proceeds as follows:

a.   Since X_L and X_C are acting in opposition, they may be subtracted to form a resultant reactance of ($X_L - X_C$) acting along the direction of X_L.

b.   ($X_L - X_C$) and R may be combined together using Pythagorus' theorem (Fig. 15.10(b)) to form the impedance, Z, where: $Z^2 = R^2 + (X_L - X_C)^2$

i.e. $Z = \sqrt{[R^2 + (X_L - X_C)^2]}$

c.   The phase angle θ is obtained by taking the tangent of θ (1.9.1), i.e. $\tan \theta = (X_L - X_C)/R$

i.e. $\theta = \tan^{-1}\left(\dfrac{X_L - X_C}{R}\right)$

d. The value of the peak current is obtained from the definition of impedance (15.4.2)

i.e. $Z = V/I$

$$\therefore \quad I = \frac{V}{\sqrt{[R^2 + (X_L - X_C)^2]}}$$

Equation 15.9

If V is expressed in terms of peak voltage, I will be in peak current; if V is in RMS units, so will be I.

Example: $R = 26\Omega$; $L = 100\text{mH}$; $C = 50\mu\text{F}$; $f = 100\text{Hz}$.
Therefore, $X_L = 2\pi f L = 2\pi \cdot 100 \cdot 10^{-1} = 20\pi = 62\cdot8\Omega$
and $\qquad X_C = 1/2\pi f C = 10^6/2\pi \, 100 \cdot 50 = 36\cdot8\Omega$
(N.B. all units must be in henry, farad, etc.)
Thus, the net reactance $(X_L - X_C) = 62\cdot8 - 36\cdot8 = 26\cdot0\Omega$, and the impedance, Z is

$$\sqrt{[R^2 + (X_L - X_C)^2]} = \sqrt{(676 + 676)} = 36\cdot8\Omega$$

The phase angle, θ, is given by $\tan \theta = 26/26 = 1$, so that $\theta = 45°$.

Resonance

In Figure 15.10(b), Z is always greater than R because it is the hypotenuse of a triangle. The current becomes smaller as Z increases ($I = V/Z$) or greater as Z decreases. The smallest value of Z which it is possible to have is that when $X_L = X_C$, so that $\theta = 0$ and the impedance is composed solely of the resistance R. The current is then at a maximum for the circuit. This effect is called *resonance* and depends upon the values of L, C and f as shown below.

Now, $X_L = 2\pi f L$; $X_C = 1/2\pi f C$, so that resonance will occur when $2\pi f L = 1/2\pi f C$, i.e.,

$$f^2 = \frac{1}{4\pi^2 LC} \text{ (by cross-multiplication)}$$

i.e. $f = \dfrac{1}{2\pi \sqrt{LC}}$ 　　　　　　　　　　　　　　Equation 15.10

For given values of L and C, the value of f obtained from this equation is that frequency at which the maximum current occurs, i.e. 'resonance'. Higher or lower frequencies than this 'resonant frequency' produce lower currents, so that a resonance curve similar to that shown in Figure 15.11 is obtained. The principles of resonance in AC circuits is put to good use in radio receivers for example, where a variable capacitor is used in series with an inductor to produce a resonant frequency of the same value as the broadcast frequency of the radio station. The circuit then resonates and is insensitive to other frequencies so that only one 'station' is heard.

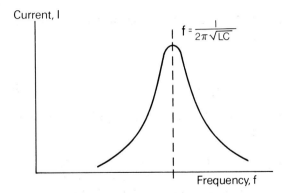

Fig. 15.11 Resonance in a LRC circuit. The current is at a maximum at the 'resonant frequency', and is said to 'resonate'.

15.6 THREE-PHASE AC

Devices which use electricity have a wide range of power requirements, from electronic circuits consuming less than a milliwatt, to electric kettles working at kilowatts, to very powerful transformers using megawatts of power. Any national electrical supply system for general use must therefore be able to cope with this wide variation in requirements for electrical power, and it does this by making available one or more 'phases' of AC. This is made possible by the winding geometries of the AC generators. In a three phase supply, there are basically three sets of windings placed symmetrically around the rotor, which may be shown diagrammatically by the windings W_1, W_2 and W_3 in Figure 15.12.

Each set of windings of the generator has a sinusoidal AC voltage induced in it (14.8), but they are displaced from each other because of the different times at which they encounter the regions of strongest magnetic field within the generator.

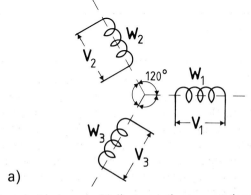

Fig. 15.12 Three-phase electrical supply: (a) diagrammatic representation of three sets of windings in the AC generator.

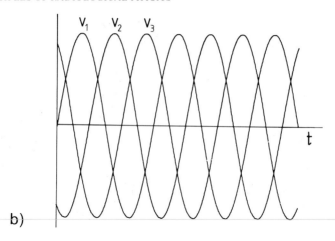

b)

Fig. 15.12 Three-phase electrical supply: (b) the 120° separation between the three 'phases'.

The voltages V_1, V_2 and V_3 from windings W_1, W_2 and W_3 are known as *phase voltages*, and are separated by 120° from each other, as shown in Figure 15.12(b) (i.e V_2 lags 120° behind V_1; V_3 lags 120° behind V_2, etc.); thus a phase difference of 120° exists between each phase. (*Note:* As an aid to drawing Fig. 15.12(b), it is useful to check that the intersection of two curves is always opposite the peak of the third curve.) These phase voltages must be 'stepped-up' to a very high value (132 000 volts) in order to transmit the electrical power efficiently over long distances (10.7), then 'stepped-down' again and taken to houses, hospitals, etc. This is accomplished using 'star' and 'delta' connections of the phase voltages as outlined below.

15.6.1 Star and delta connections

The two methods of connecting the phase voltages together are the 'star' and 'delta' connections as shown in Figure 15.13. If we assume that an RMS PD of 240 volts is induced in each winding of the generator (i.e. the same as the mains voltage), then the voltages available from the delta connections are three in number, and correspond to the original phase voltages as shown in Figure 15.12(b). However, the star connection enables the selection of six voltages: the three phase voltages, and three 'line' voltages one of which is shown across W_1 and W_3. The central connection of the star is called the *neutral* and is kept near earth potential by equalising the power outputs from the three phases as closely as possible.

The line PD is 415 volts from a star connection, not 480 volts as looks reasonable from Figure 15.13. This is because of the phase difference between the phase voltages of W_1 and W_3. It may be shown (see Insight below) that the line voltage is also sinusoidal, and has a magnitude which is a factor of $\sqrt{3}$ greater than the phase voltage. The four wires L_1, L_2, L_3 and N are distributed to domestic, hospital and industrial users, and the appropriate voltages ('phase' or 'line') are available, i.e. phase voltages for domestic use, and both

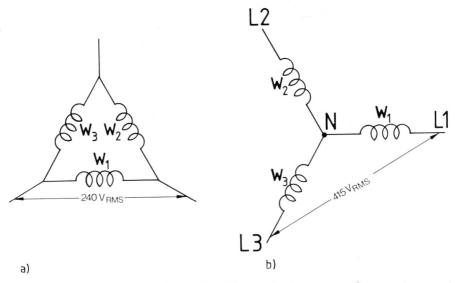

Fig. 15.13 Three-phase connections: (a) delta, (b) star.

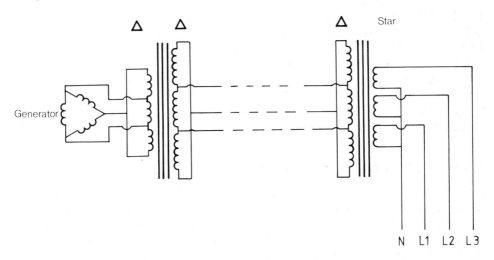

Fig. 15.14 Generation and distribution of three-phase supplies. The consumer has a choice of three 'phase' voltages (e.g L1 − N) or three 'line' voltages (e.g. L1 − L2).

phase and line voltages for hospital and industrial use. The star connection has been termed the 'three-phase four-wire supply' for obvious reasons.

The transfer of power from a generator to a city (for example) is shown diagrammatically in Figure 15.14.

Insight

The voltage across L_1 and L_3 in Figure 15.13 is the *difference* between the voltages across $L_1 - N$ and $L_3 - N$. For example, if the potential at N is zero, and $L_1 - N$ is 10 volts and $L_3 - N$ is 4 volts, then the voltage (i.e. the potential difference) across $L_1 - L_3$ is $10 - 4 = 6$

volts. Thus, we may use the vector diagram shown in the figure to calculate the line voltage across $L_1 - L_3$.

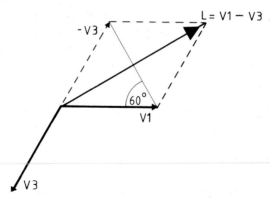

Now, $\sin 60° = \sqrt{(3)}/2 = \dfrac{L/2}{V_1}$ from the figure.

Thus, $L = \sqrt{(3)}V_1$, i.e. the line voltage is $\sqrt{3}$ times the phase voltage. In the UK the voltage is therefore 415 volts.

15.6.2 Three-phase X-ray circuits

Three-phase supplies are used in radiography for two main purposes: (i) the generation of X-rays at high power and at constant potential, and (ii) in the induction motor circuit used to rotate the anode. The induction motor is discussed in (21.2.2) and the three-phase HT rectification circuit is explained in (20.4.3).

Exercise 15.3
    a.   Why is kV measured in peak units, mA in average units and mains voltage in RMS units when considering X-ray circuits?
    b.   What is meant by the statement that the current and voltage are 'in-phase' in a particular AC circuit? Illustrate your answer with a suitable graph.
    c.   What is meant by 'phase difference' in AC circuits? Show how this may be illustrated by a 'vector diagram' and on a graph of voltage and current against time, assuming that the voltage leads the current by 45° in a particular circuit.
    d.   Define electrical resistance, reactance and impedance. In what units is each measured? What is the reactance of (i) a capacitor of C farad (ii) and inductor of L henry when connected to an alternating supply of frequency f hertz?
    e.   Explain the terms 'power factor', 'wattless component' when applied to an AC circuit. Why is the average power generated in a pure reactance zero?
    f.   What is meant by 'resonance' is an AC circuit? Illustrate your answer by considering a resistor, capacitor, and inductor connected in series and joined to an alternating electrical supply.

SUMMARY

1.   Sinusoidal AC is described mathematically by the formula $I = I_p \sin 2\pi ft$ and $V = V_p \sin 2\pi ft$ where I_p, V_p are the peak current and voltage and f is the frequency of the AC supply in cycles/second, or hertz.

2.   One *cycle* is one complete waveform; the *period* is the time for one *cycle;* the *frequency* is the number of cycles per second, and the *amplitude* is the maximum value of current or voltage.

3.   Frequency, $f = 1/T$ where T is the period.

4.   Average current (voltage) = 0 for sinusoidal waveform.

Average current (voltage) = 0·318 × peak current (voltage)
    for half-wave rectified AC.

Average current (voltage) = 0·636 × peak current (voltage)
    for full-wave rectified AC.

5.   Effective (or RMS) current: 'that value of constant current which, acting over the same time, would produce the same expenditure of electrical energy in a circuit as the alternating current'.

6. $I_{RMS} = 0·707I_p$; $V_{RMS} = 0·707V_p$. All AC voltages and currents are normally RMS values unless otherwise stated. $(0·707 = 1/\sqrt{2})$

Voltage across X-ray tube expressed in peak, i.e. kV_p. Current through X-ray tube expressed in average, i.e. mA. Mains voltage is expressed in RMS values.

7.   AC circuits involving the use of capacitors and/or inductors produce a *phase difference* between the current and voltage waveforms. These may be represented by rotating vectors.

8.   Resistance, reactance and impedance are all measured in ohm, and are the ratio of volts to amperes (both peak or RMS) at (a) 0°, (b) 90°, and (c) θ, to the current respectively. θ is the phase difference between the current and voltage waveforms.

9.   Inductors have reactance of $2\pi fL$ which *leads* the current by 90°. Capacitors have reactance of $1/2\pi fC$ which *lags* the current by 90°.

10.   Reactance consumes no net power from an AC supply.

11.   The power used in a circuit is given by

$$W = V_{RMS} \times I_{RMS} \times \cos \theta,$$

$\cos \theta$ is the 'power factor', $V \sin \theta$ is the "wattless voltage' and $I \sin \theta$ is the 'wattless current'.

12.   Resonance occurs in an AC circuit when the current is greatest (at a particular frequency). For a series RCL circuits the resonant frequency, $f = 1/2\pi\sqrt{LC}$, and the current is $I = V/R$.

13.   Three-phase AC consists of three sinusoidal waveforms 120° apart. These may be connected in a 'star' or 'delta' configuration.

14.   The phase voltage is that across the individual windings; the line voltage is that obtained across each of the three connections to the star and delta connections. For a delta connector, the line and phase voltages are equal; for a star connection, the line voltage is $\sqrt{3}$ × the phase voltage.

16. The AC transformer

The AC transformer has an electrical input and an electrical output. The electrical output potential difference (voltage) may be considerably greater or smaller than the input voltage. The transformer is then called a 'step-up' or a 'step-down' transformer respectively. A transformer is thus a device for changing *alternating* voltages and currents from one level to another. It has the great advantage of simplicity of construction and efficiency, and hence is used in a very wide range of applications.

In radiography, for example, the mains voltage is too great to be connected directly across the filament of an X-ray tube (the resulting high current would rapidly destroy the filament) and too small to be connected directly across the X-ray tube. In the latter case of course, many thousands of volts are required in order to produce an X-ray beam of sufficient intensity and energy. Thus a 'step-down' transformer may be used to reduce the voltage applied to the filament (the 'filament transformer') and a 'step-up' transformer to supply the necessary high voltage (or 'high tension') across the X-ray tube (the 'high tension transformer').

Two other types of transformer are encountered in radiography: the autotransformer and the 'saturated' or 'constant voltage' transformer. These will be considered later in this chapter (16.4 and 16.5).

16.1 THE PERFECT (OR IDEAL) TRANSFORMER

Definition

A perfect, or ideal, transformer is one whose output electrical power is equal to its input electrical power, i.e. no power is 'lost' in the transformer itself.

There is, of course, no such thing as a perfect transformer, although efficiencies (16.2) of 98% and more in real transformers are not uncommon. Thus, the concept of an ideal transformer is not very far from practical reality, and its advantage lies in the simplification of the mathematics used to describe the behaviour of transformers.

Consider such an ideal transformer shown in Figure 16.1, where two isolated coils of wire (or 'windings') share a common soft-iron core. Other shapes and configurations of windings exist, but the one shown in the figure is the simplest and is similar to the construction of the high tension transformer. The input, or

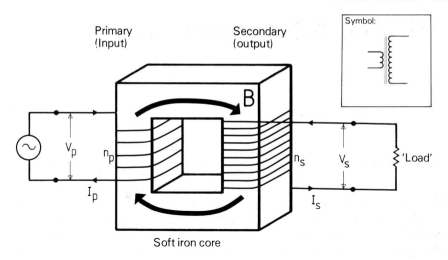

Fig. 16.1 An 'ideal' transformer. The electric currents flowing in the primary and secondary windings and the magnetic flux within the core alternate in direction — the situation at one particular moment is shown. In practice, the core is laminated, as in Fig. 16.2. Also shown is the symbol for this 'step-up' transformer.

'primary' side of the transformer has an alternating voltage V_p across it, and there are n_p turns wound around the core. Corresponding values V_s, n_s exist on the output, or 'secondary', side of the transformer. It will be evident from the study of Chapter 14 that the principle of operation of the transformer is that of *mutual induction* (14.5), because of the following sequence of events:

a.   The alternating current, I_p, produces a *changing* magnetic flux density (B) within the soft iron core.

b.   The *changing* magnetic flux is linked with the secondary coil, so that an EMF is induced according to Faraday's and Lenz's Laws of electromagnetic induction (14.2 and 14.3).

Note than an alternating supply is *essential* for the operation of the transformer since no EMF will be induced in the secondary if the magnetic flux linkage is constant (Faraday's Laws). The alternating supply ensures that the magnetic flux linkage to both windings is continuously changing, thus inducing an EMF in each winding.

The purpose of the soft iron is to contain all the magnetic flux within it so that the flux linkage between the primary and secondary windings is as near perfect as possible. It is able to do this because of its strong induced magnetism, resulting from a high permeability (11.2).

The mathematics of the transformer are very simple if we start by considering the effect of the changing magnetic flux on a single turn placed anywhere around the soft iron core. Here we assume that no magnetic flux is lost from the core, so that the rate of change of flux does not depend upon the location of the single turn of wire. Hence the EMF induced (which depends only upon the rate of change of magnetic flux) *is independent* of the *position* of the turn or, to put it another way, the *EMF induced in any single turn of wire is the same*. This is simply because, by Faraday's second law, the EMF is proportional to the rate of change of flux linkage, the latter being the same for each single turn.

If we call v the voltage* induced per turn, then the primary voltage V_p, is given by the number of primary turns multiplied by v:

i.e. $V_p = n_p \times v$ or $\dfrac{V_p}{n_p} = v$

and the secondary voltage is V_s, is obtained in the same manner

i.e. $V_s = n_s \times v$ or $\dfrac{V_s}{n_s} = v$

Thus, $\dfrac{V_p}{n_p} = \dfrac{V_s}{n_s}$ (since both are equal to v)

By cross-multiplication, we obtain the useful formula:

$$\frac{V_s}{V_p} = \frac{n_s}{n_s}$$

Equation 16.1

This equation is true for both peak and effective (RMS) values of voltage, provided that V_s and V_p are both expressed in the same units.

The ratio V_s/V_p is known as the 'voltage gain' of the transformer, which is greater than unity for a step-up transformer and less than unity for a step-down transformer.

The quantity n_s/n_p is known as the 'turns ratio' of the transformer. Thus, if the turns ratio of a particular transformer is 200 (sometimes expressed as 200 : 1), then we know from Equation 16.1 that (a) there are 200 times as many turns on the secondary as on the primary, and (b) the voltage across the secondary is 200 times that of the primary.

The *current* flowing in the secondary may be calculated from a consideration of the electrical power of both primary and secondary. Now, the input power $= V_p \times I_p$ watts (assuming RMS values), and the output power $= V_s \times I_s$ watts (15.2.3). As defined above for a perfect transformer these two quantities are equal, since no power is expended in the transformer, so that

$V_p \times I_p = V_s \times I_s$

i.e. $\dfrac{I_s}{I_p} = \dfrac{V_p}{V_s}$

By comparison to Equation 16.1, it may be seen that

$\dfrac{V_p}{V_s} = \dfrac{n_p}{n_s}$

---

*In this chapter, following common usage, the terms 'voltage' and 'EMF' are used interchangeably — see 10.3 for the definitions of both.

so that the above equation may be written as:

$$\frac{I_s}{I_p} = \frac{n_p}{n_s} \qquad \text{Equation 16.2}$$

for a perfect transformer.

An inspection of Equations 16.1 and 16.2 shows that if the voltage is *increased* by a factor n_s/n_p, then the current is *reduced* by the same factor. Obviously, if both the voltage and current were increased, the output power would be greater than the input power, so disobeying the law of energy conservation (7.2). Thus, the voltage can only be increased at the expense of the current, and vice versa.

16.1.1 Faraday's and Lenz's Laws applied to transformers

The formal statements of Faraday's and Lenz's Laws of electromagnetic induction have been discussed previously (14.2). We may summarise here by stating that the induced EMF in a conductor is proportional to the rate of change of the magnetic flux linkage with the conductor and the induced current acts in opposition to the changing magnetic flux.

The application of Faraday's Law to the transformer is straightforward, since the changing magnetic flux (caused by the alternating supply connected to the primary winding) is linked to both primary and secondary windings so inducing an EMF in each. In fact an equal EMF is induced in each turn, as discussed in the previous section.

Lenz's Law may be used to determine the direction of the induced current in the secondary — i.e. it always acts so as to oppose the changing magnetic flux in the core. It is therefore 180° 'out of phase' (15.4.1) with the primary current, since the latter causes the magnetic flux. The same argument applies to the direction of induced eddy currents within the core (16.3.2), i.e. 'out of phase' compared to the primary current.

Insight

Many students find it surprising to learn that it is current drawn from the secondary of a transformer which determines the primary current, feeling that 'cause' and 'effect' have been interchanged.

However, if we consider a transformer whose secondary winding is 'open-circuit' (i.e. not connected to anything), then no current can flow in it, although an EMF is induced in it. What current flows through the primary? The answer, for a perfect transformer, is *zero* since the changing magnetic flux passing through the primary winding induces a 'back-EMF' (by self-induction — 14.6) exactly equal to the EMF of the electrical supply. These two EMFs act in opposition and so cancel each other, so that no current flows. (In a practical transformer, a small current would flow in order to overcome the transformer 'losses' — see below). Thus, we may say that the primary current is zero if the secondary current is zero.

If now the secondary winding is connected across an external circuit (e.g. a light bulb), then the EMF induced in the winding will cause a current to flow (so that the bulb lights), but in such a direction as to act against the changing magnetic flux within the core. The flux is thus reduced which means that the back-EMF in the primary is reduced (due to a reduced rate of change of flux linkage with it) and a *primary* current therefore flows, since the EMF of the supply is now greater than that of the back-EMF. Thus, a current in the secondary has caused a current to flow in the primary, the relative magnitudes of each being given by Equation 16.2.

16.2 PRACTICAL TRANSFORMERS

It is not possible to construct an ideal transformer in practice because there are always 'power losses' within the transformer itself. This means that the power from the transformer secondary is always less than the power applied to the primary by an amount equal to these power losses. The efficiency of a practical transformer may be defined as follows:

Definition
   The *efficiency* of a transformer is the ratio of its output power to its input power.

Obviously, the efficiency is always less than unity, or less than 100% if expressed as a percentage. For example, if 100 watt of electrical power is supplied to the primary of a transformer, and 95 watt is produced in the secondary, then the efficiency is 0·95 or 95%. In this case 5% of the power is 'wasted' in the transformer windings and core, i.e. it is not available as useful electrical power.

Equation 16.1 gives a reasonably good estimate of the voltage gain for practical transformers, i.e. the voltage gain is equal to the turns ratio. However, Equation 16.2 no longer applies because of the power losses in practical transformers as illustrated by the following example.

Example
A transformer has a turns ratio of 100 : 1 and an efficiency of 95%. If a current of 0·5 A RMS flows in the primary when a voltage of 5 V RMS is applied across it, what is (a) the output RMS voltage (b) the output RMS current?
   We know that the voltage gain is equal to the turns ratio (Equation 16.1).

$$\therefore \quad \frac{V_s}{5} = \frac{100}{1}$$

   i.e. $V_s = 500$ volts RMS on the secondary.

We also know that the efficiency is the output power: input power, so that

$$\frac{V_s \times I_s}{V_p \times I_p} = \text{efficiency}$$

i.e. $500I_s = 0.95 \times 5 \times 0.5$ (by cross-multiplication).

$$\therefore \quad I_s = \frac{0.95 \times 5 \times 0.5}{500} = 4.75 \text{ mA RMS flowing}$$
in the secondary

Note that an ideal transformer would have produced the same output voltage, but a secondary current of 5 mA.

16.3 TRANSFORMER LOSSES

A more detailed analysis of the sources of the power losses in transformers is considered in this section. These are shown summarised in Table 16.1, and discussed in turn below.

Table 16.1 A summary of the losses associated with a practical transformer.

Transformer loss	Comments
'Copper' losses	Caused by resistance of copper windings. Also known as 'I^2R' losses.
'Iron' losses	Losses produced in soft iron core
a) Imperfect magnetic flux linkage	Very small effect
b) eddy currents	Caused by electromagnetic induction within core of transformer — reduced by 'laminations'
c) hysteresis	Caused by work done in moving the magnetic domains — reduced by appropriate choice of core material (e.g. 'stalloy')
Regulation (a consequence of transformer loss)	Output voltage decreases with increasing current load because of resistance of secondary winding

16.3.1 Copper losses

The term 'copper' refers to the copper windings, of course, which have a small but finite resistance. An RMS current I_{RMS} flowing through a resistance R produces a power within the resistor of $I_{RMS}^2 R$ watt (see 15.2.3). Hence this type of power loss is often referred to as an $I^2 R$ loss, the result being to warm the copper windings on both the primary and secondary.

One general point regarding the secondary winding of a step-up transformer: it is made of many hundreds of turns of *thin* wire because

a.   the low current produced in the secondary does not require thick wire (a high current in thin wire would over-heat and may even melt the wire)

b.   thin wire is required in order to be able to fit all the turns into the space available.

There is a common misconception concerning the use of thin wire on the secondary of a step-up transformer which is that thin wire is necessary in order to limit the current in the secondary because it has a high resistance! This is quite untrue; the current has a value determined by the laws of electromagnetic induction, and the effect of the resistance of the windings has only a small ef-fect in practice.

The low secondary current in a step-up transformer reduces I^2R losses even though the resistance of the secondary may be slightly higher than that of the primary. This is because of the strong dependence of these losses on the I^2 term. For a fuller treatment of this concept, see 'Power loss in cables' (10.7).

16.3.2 Iron losses

'Iron' losses refer to power losses in the soft iron core of the transformer. This takes three forms, as outlined below.

Magnetic flux loss
If the magnetic flux is not fully contained within the soft iron core, then the flux passing through the secondary winding will be less than that produced by the primary. The EMF induced in the secondary and the output electrical power will therefore be lower than if the flux linkage were perfect. However, this effect is very small and may be neglected for most practical purposes.

Eddy currents
From Faraday's and Lenz's Laws (14.2, 14.3) we know that a changing flux linked with a closed conductor induces an EMF and current in the conductor. Furthermore, the induced current opposes the effect of the changing flux linkage. Now, soft iron is an *electrical conductor* in addition to being a strongly magnetic material. This means that the varying flux passing through the soft iron core of a transformer will induce electric currents within the core itself, and in such a direction as to oppose the changing magnetic flux within the core. Figure 16.2(a) illustrates this point, where it is assumed that the direction of increasing electron flow in the primary of the transformer is anti-clockwise at a particular moment. Thus, by Lenz's Law, the currents induced in the core of the transformer will be clockwise, such that the magnetic flux produced by the two directions of current will act in opposition. When the current in the

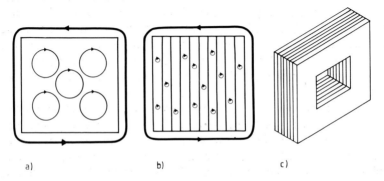

a)   b)   c)

Fig. 16.2 Eddy currents within a transformer core oppose the magnetic flux within the core. They are reduced by the use of laminations, as shown in (b) and (c).

primary is travelling clockwise during the next half-cycle of the alternating current, the induced currents in the core will be circulating in an anti-clockwise direction. These induced currents within the soft iron core are known as *eddy currents*, and are a source of power loss in the transformer, for their effect is to:

a. heat up the transformer core, due to the electrical resistance of the soft iron

b. reduce the magnetic flux in the core

The latter means that the magnetic flux linkage with both the primary and secondary windings is reduced. This reduces the 'back-EMF' in the primary (14.6), and an increased primary current therefore flows to increase the magnetic flux within the core to the value it would have had if no eddy currents were present. However, the increased current in the primary constitutes a power loss, since it is required to overcome the loss of power due to the eddy currents, and it does not contribute to the electrical power in the secondary winding.

Eddy currents may be reduced, but not entirely eliminated, by the use of a *laminated* core, as shown in Figure 16.2(b) and (c). Thin sheets, or laminations, of soft iron are riveted together so as to make the required square cross-section. Each lamination is electrically insulated from its neighbours by a very thin layer of insulation (e.g. 'shellac' varnish). The eddy currents induced in such a core are therfore confined within the small cross-sectional area of each lamination, which increases the overall electrical resistance of the core ($R \propto 1/\text{area}$ — see 10.4.1). Thus, a laminated core produces a much lower power loss within the transformer than a single-piece core, but does not reduce this loss to zero. Heat is still produced in the core and may therefore require cooling, as in the example of an oil-immersed high-tension transformer for X-ray units. The oil convects heat from the transformer which is produced in the windings ($I^2 R$) and the core (eddy currents and hysteresis).

Hysteresis

The reader is referred to (11.7) for a fuller explanation of the causes of hysteresis than is appropriate here.

Hysteresis is the 'lagging behind' of the induced magnetism in a ferromagnetic material when the applied magnetic field changes, producing a 'hysteresis loop' as shown in Figure 11.8 (p. 172). A transformer is usually designed to operate around a partial hysteresis loop, so that the magnetic flux within the core increases as the primary current increases, so enabling the secondary current to increase in proportion (but see 16.5 for 'constant voltage' transformers).

The greater the area within the hysteresis loop, the greater is the work which is performed on the magnetic domains in the core in changing their directions. The 'rate of work' is the definition of power (6.3.7), so that power is expended within the core in rotating the domains, so leaving less power available for the secondary winding of the transformer. The power loss due to hysteresis in the core increases the kinetic energy of the atoms of the core and so manifests itself in the form of heat.

Hysteresis is reduced by the choice of an appropriate material, such as 'stalloy' or 'permalloy'.

16.3.3 Regulation

Regulation in a transformer is a consequence of the resistance in the windings. If the electrical 'load' to the transformer in *increased* (i.e. a higher current is made to flow from the secondary), it is found that the potential difference across the secondary winding is *decreased* — this is known as 'regulation'.

Regulation occurs in any source of electricity which contains an internal resistance. In the case of a transformer, the internal resistance is the resistance of the secondary winding. Figure 16.3 illustrates the regulation of a transformer in graphical form. The output current is zero when the secondary winding is disconnected from the external circuit — this is the 'open circuit' condition, and the corresponding voltage is known as the 'open circuit' voltage (V_0 in the figure). When the transformer is put 'on load' so that a current may flow in the secondary and in the external circuit (e.g. X-ray tube), the output voltage falls linearly with secondary current. The regulation therefore varies with the transformer load, or to express it differently, the potential difference supplied by a transformer reduces as the current from it increases.

Definition

The *percentage regulation* is given by:

$$100 \times \left(\frac{\text{Open circuit voltage } - \text{ on load voltage}}{\text{Open circuit voltage}} \right)$$

at a given current (or 'load').

In Figure 16.3. this is simply the quantity $\dfrac{v}{V_0} \times 100\%$.

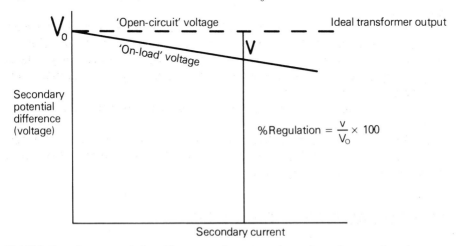

Fig. 16.3 Transformer regulation. The greater the current drawn from the secondary the smaller becomes the potential difference across it. This effect is caused by the resistance of the windings (see text).

Transformers possess 'good' regulation, i.e. the on-load voltage is close to the open-circuit voltage, so that v is small. However, the regulation present in a High Tension Transformer (HTT) for an X-ray unit, though relatively small, must be corrected or the mA and kV_p will not be independent, i.e. increasing the mA will decrease the kV_p from its intended value. Such correction (or 'compensation') circuits are beyond the scope of this book, except for the simple case of the use of an autotransformer for 'mains compensation' (16.4.2).

Insight

The primary winding of a transformer usually has such a low resistance that its effect on regulation may be ignored. If an EMF of V_0 is induced in the secondary and the resistance of the secondary is r, then a current I will produce a 'voltage drop' of Ir (Ohm's Law) across the internal resistance r. This means that the potential difference which is available to the external circuit has been reduced by an amount Ir.

i.e. $V = V_0 - Ir$

This formula explains why the regulation is linear with current, as shown in Figure 16.3. Note that $V = V_0$ if (a) $I = 0$ or (b) $r = 0$, so that there is no regulation for the open-circuit condition, or if the resistance of the secondary winding is zero.

Exercise 16.1

a.   What is meant by an 'ideal' or 'perfect' transformer? Explain its action by means of the laws of electromagnetic induction.

b.   If 110 volts is applied to the primary of an ideal transformer, and the turns ratio is 500 : 1, what is the voltage supplied by the secondary? If this is an RMS voltage, what is the value of the peak voltage?

c.   What is meant by the term 'transformer losses'? List and explain the causes of such losses and describe how these are minimised in practical transformers.

d.   Define the 'efficiency' of a practical transformer. What is the efficiency of an ideal transformer? If 240 volts is applied to the primary of a transformer which has 500 turns on the primary and 50 000 turns on the secondary, what is the primary current if 1·9 mA flows in the secondary, assuming that the transformer has a 95% efficiency?

What would the primary current have been if the transformer had been perfect?

e.   Explain why the potential difference across the secondary of a high tension transformer varies when the electrical current drawn from it is increased. Hence define 'regulation'.

16.4 THE AUTOTRANSFORMER

The autotransformer is a very useful device for selecting a range of output voltages whose values are not very different from the input voltage (usually within a factor of 2). It is constructed so that it is possible to select the number of primary and secondary turns across which the primary and secondary voltages occur. This has important consequences in radiography as a means of compensating for mains voltage fluctuations, as described below. Figure 16.4 shows a simplified drawing of an autotransformer, consisting of a laminated soft iron core (which may be in the form of a ring) and a *single* winding which is connected to switch S_1 on the primary side, and S_2 on the secondary side. Adjustment of S_1 and S_2 selects the number of primary turns, n_p, and secondary turns, n_s, respectively.

The principle of operation of the autotransformer is therefore that of *self induction* (14.6) since only one winding is present.

Mathematically, we may proceed as before in Section 16.1 and argue that the same changing magnetic flux is linked with each winding, so that the *induced EMF per turn is constant* (as for the transformer) from Faraday's Laws (14.2). If the EMF per turn is v, then the primary voltage V_p, is given by $V_p = n_p v$, and the secondary EMF is $V_s = n_s v$.

Thus,

$$\frac{V_s}{V_p} = \frac{n_s}{n_p} \qquad\qquad \text{Equation 16.3}$$

Assuming no power loss within the transformer, it may be shown (16.1) that:

$$\frac{I_s}{I_p} = \frac{n_p}{n_s} \qquad\qquad \text{Equation 16.4}$$

Thus, the same formulae which apply to an ideal transformer also apply to an ideal autotransformer, the only difference being that the primary and secondary turns are selected from the same winding. The restricted selection of

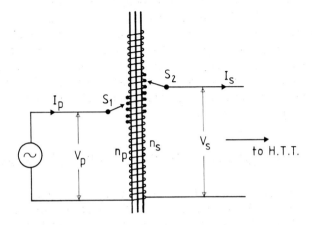

Fig. 16.4 An autotransformer. The principle of operation is self-induction within the single winding. The numbers of primary and secondary turns are selected by S1 and S2, so giving a variable voltage gain.

the number of turns on primary and secondary windings means that the ratio n_s/n_p in Equation 16.3 can only change over a limited range of values, so that the voltage gain of the autotransformer has a correspondingly small range. As stated above, this is usually between 0·5 and 2·0.

16.4.1 Losses and regulation

All the sources of power losses discussed in Section 16.3 apply to an autotransformer. However, the less severe design constraints required for an autotransformer (i.e. voltage gain of around unity) make it possible to use a thick winding of copper wire with a consequent reduction in the winding resistance (particularly of the secondary winding) when compared to a transformer ($R \propto 1/A$ — see 10.4.1). Thus, the 'copper losses' are lower in an autotransformer and the regulation of an autotransformer is better than that of a transformer, since both of these sources of losses are dependent upon the resistance of the windings.

16.4.2. Mains compensation

The autotransformer is positioned between the electrical mains input and the input to the high tension transformer. If fulfills three functions: to select the kV_p value, to correct for long-term mains voltage variations and for mA compensation. Only the first two functions are discussed here.

In Figure 16.4, the electrical mains is connected to the primary across n_p turns, selectable by switch S_1. The secondary voltage is connected across the primary of the high tension transformer (HTT) which has a *fixed* voltage gain. The kV_p across the X-ray tube is therefore adjusted by the selection of the voltage applied to the primary of the HTT, and this is accomplished by means of switch S_2 — the 'kV_p control'. A more detailed circuit is shown in Figure 17.11 (p. 261).

If the mains voltage varies, as it must owing to regulation (16.3.3) of the electrical supply as the 'load' varies during the day, then the secondary voltage from the autotransformer and the kV_p will also vary in sympathy, leading to under- or over-exposed radiographs (X-ray intensity $\propto kV_p^2$ — 4.7). However, if S_1 is adjusted manually so that the *voltage per turn* is kept constant as determined by the 'mains compensation meter' (M_1 in Fig. 17.11) then the voltage applied to the HTT is constant for a given setting of S_2. A numerical example of such mains compensation is given in (17.7.1).

16.5 THE 'CONSTANT VOLTAGE' TRANSFORMER

Some X-ray units use a 'constant voltage' transformer in the filament circuit so as to ensure a well-stabilised supply to the filament. The output of the X-ray tube (i.e. the X-ray intensity) is very sensitive to the temperature of the filament which in turn means that the electrical supply to the filament must be very stable.

The 'constant-voltage', or 'saturated core', transformer uses magnetic saturation in the core of the secondary winding to limit the maximum magnetic flux linkage with the secondary, and hence the maximum secondary voltage. The output voltage of such a device is therefore 'constant' in the sense that it has an upper limit as is its normal working value. Any increase in primary voltage cannot then increase the secondary voltage or current, although a significant *reduction* in primary voltage may be sufficient to bring the secondary core out of magnetic saturation and hence reduce the secondary voltage.

The construction of the constant-voltage transformer is shown in Figure 16.5. The magnetic flux produced in the primary core A passes through two other 'magnetic circuits': the much thinner secondary core B, and a central 'high magnetic resistance' (called 'reluctance') path in core C. The thinner core B ensures that the magnetic flux passing through it is sufficient to bring it to saturation (11.7) and the core C is used as a path for the excess magnetic flux. This path, being of high 'reluctance', ensures that the majority of magnetic flux passes through B.

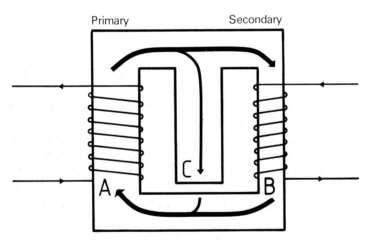

Fig. 16.5 A 'constant-voltage' or 'saturated-core' transformer.

16.6 TRANSFORMER RATING

The term 'rating' means the maximum combination of factors which a system can withstand without damage. A transformer is designed only to operate up to a given maximum set of conditions which, if exceeded, may cause damage to the electrical insulation of the winding by overheating or electrical breakdown. Chapter 22 describes the rating of X-ray tubes.

There are basically two types of exposures in radiography: screening at low power, and short higher-power exposures. Each of these produces heat within the high tension transformer (with which we are primarily concerned) owing to the 'losses' within it (16.3).

In particular, a long exposure must be undertaken at a relatively low current, or the heat generated within the transformer will not be convected away sufficiently quickly by the oil surrounding the HTT to keep the temperature within safe limits. However, short exposures may use higher values of current since the *total* energy deposited in the windings, given by 'power × time' (6.3.7), may still be low enough to cause no damage.

The detailed specification of the rating of any one transformer may be very complicated, dealing with every conceivable combination of exposure factors. However, we may reduce these to just three basic considerations:

a. The maximum kV_p which the secondary winding may produce (typically 125 kV_p)

b. the maximum *continuous* current the transformer can supply (e.g. as in screening)

c. the maximum current supplied for *short* exposures.

Exercise 16.2

a. What is the principle of operation of an autotransformer? Compare the action of an autotransformer to a transformer, noting any similarities and differences.

b. Describe two purposes of an autotransformer in an X-ray circuit, showing a simple circuit diagram.

c. Why does an autotransformer show 'better' regulation than a transformer?

d. Why cannot the secondary of an autotransformer be used to produce the potential difference required by an X-ray tube?

e. If a 10 volt battery is connected to the primary of a transformer whose turns ratio is 50, what is the secondary voltage? (Be careful!)

f. Why is an alternating supply (AC) used in X-ray circuits? Illustrate your answer with reference to the 'filament' circuit and 'high-tension' circuit of an X-ray tube. (Hint: Assume 6 volts is required by the filament supply, 50 kV_p for the X-ray tube, and the mains is 240 volts).

g. What do you understand by the term 'transformer rating'? Explain two ways in which damage may occur to the transformer if the rating is exceeded. Hence explain why the high tension transformer of an X-ray unit is contained within an oil bath.

SUMMARY

1. A transformer works by mutual induction, and an autotransformer by self-induction.

2. An alternating supply (AC) must be used, since a *changing* magnetic flux is required to induce an EMF.

3. A perfect (or ideal) transformer has an equal input and output power i.e. no power is 'lost' within the transformer.

$$\frac{V_s}{V_p} = \frac{n_s}{n_p},$$

where $\dfrac{V_s}{V_p}$ is the 'voltage gain' and $\dfrac{n_s}{n_p}$ is the 'turns ratio'.

This formula is only approximately true for a practical transformer.

5.   For no power loss, input power = output power and $\dfrac{I_s}{I_p} = \dfrac{n_p}{n_s}$.

Thus, the voltage gain is at the expense of the current, and *vice versa*.

6.   Practical transformers consume power, so that less is available for output. Efficiency is output power/input power.

7.   Transformer losses (see Table 16.1):

    a.   Copper losses — 'I^2R' in windings
    b.   Iron losses — magnetic flux losses
                eddy currents
                hysteresis.

8.   Eddy currents are reduced by a laminated core, and hysteresis losses by the use of a suitable core material, e.g. stalloy.

9.   % Regulation is: $\dfrac{\text{open circuit voltage} - \text{on load voltage}}{\text{open circuit voltage}} \times 100$

at a particular value of current. It is caused by the resistance of the windings, especially the secondary winding of a step-up transformer. Transformers have good regulation.

10.   The autotransformer has a better regulation than a transformer because the winding may be made much thicker. It is only used for small voltage changes between output and input compared to a transformer.

11.   A 'constant voltage' transformer uses a saturated core to limit the EMF induced in the secondary.

12.   The 'rating' of a transformer is a statement of what maximum combination of factors it is able to withstand without damage (e.g. max. kV_p, continuous current, and current for short exposures).

17. Meters

17.1 THE METER AS A MEASURING INSTRUMENT

Whenever a measurement of any quantity is made, there is a very important underlying assumption concerning the way the measurement is performed, and that is that the *act of measurement of a quantity must have no significant effect on the quantity itself*. For example, a thermometer must not affect the temperature of a body it is measuring by extracting too much heat energy from that body and thus reducing its temperature. In a similar manner, the measurement of an electrical quantity (such as current or potential difference) by the use of a meter must not alter it significantly from the value it would have had if the meter were not connected in the circuit.

Meters are used to measure the basic electrical units of current, potential difference, frequency, power and phase. Of these, only the measurements of current and potential difference are considered in this book since they are most relevant to radiography.

The way in which a meter is connected in an electrical circuit depends upon whether current or potential difference is to be measured. However, the meters all have one or more scales over which a pointer moves, and there is usually a statement of the current (or voltage) required to produce a full-scale deflection (f.s.d.) of the pointer printed somewhere on the scale. These points are discussed further in the remainder of this chapter.

Note

'Digital' meters (i.e. meters which have a numerical display) are not considered in this book.

17.2 THE MEASUREMENT OF CURRENT

Since an electric current is a flow of electrons (10.1), we may measure a particular current by causing the electrons to flow through the meter as well as the circuit. Thus a meter for measuring current is connected *in series* with the circuit, as illustrated in Figure 17.1. It may be connected *anywhere* within the simple circuit shown and will read the same value of current in any position. However, because of the construction of the meter (17.4 and 17.5) it has its own electrical resistance (r_m in Fig. 17.1(b)) and so adds to the overall resistance in the circuit which, by Ohm's Law (10.5), inevitably results in a

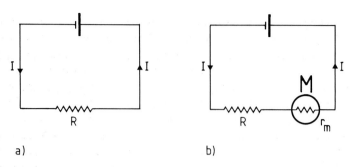

Fig. 17.1 The principle of using a meter to measure an electric current. The meter M is placed in series in the circuit so that the current being measured flows through the meter. An accurate reading is obtained if the internal resistance of the meter (r_m) is small.

reduced current. Hence, the meter alters what it is trying to measure and so cannot produce an exact reading of current. However, provided that the internal resistance of the meter is very low compared to the other resistances (R in the figure) then the difference between the true and the indicated current is so small as to be negligible.

To take a specific example, suppose that a 6V battery is connected across a 60 Ω resistor (producing a current of 0·1 A, from Ohm's Law), and a meter of 60Ω internal resistance is connected into the circuit. The total resistance is then 120 Ω and the current flow is 0·05 A — exactly one half of the value before the meter was connected! However, if the internal resistance of the meter had been 0·6 Ω, then the total resistance would have been 60·6 Ω and the current 0·099 A, which would have been sufficiently close to the true value of 0.1 A for all but the most precise work. Thus, although it is inevitable that the use of a meter will reduce the current which it is measuring, the use of a *low internal resistance* minimises this effect to an acceptable level, resulting in accurate measurements of current.

A current-measuring meter is often referred to as an 'ammeter', a 'milliammeter', or a 'microammeter' depending upon whether it is suitable for the measurement of amperes, milliamperes or microamperes respectively. For example, a milliammeter may have a full-scale deflection (f.s.d.) or 1 mA, 10 mA etc., but not 1 μA or 1 A. It is often necessary to use a meter to measure a current which would normally be far too large for it, e.g. to use a milliammeter to measure a current of an ampere or more. Obviously, such a meter cannot be connected directly into a circuit such as Figure 17.1(b), or damage to the meter might well occur. In this situation, the measuring range of the meter must be extended to higher currents, and such 'range-changing' is accomplished by the use of electrical 'shunts' as described below.

17.2.1 Shunts

Suppose we wish to measure a current of maximum value 1 A (i.e. 1000 mA) with a meter of f.s.d. 1 mA. We must 'by-pass' 999 mA around the meter and permit only 1 mA to flow through the meter in order to prevent damage to it.

The 1 mA flowing through the meter will produce a full-scale deflection on the scale. This 'by-pass' is called a *shunt* and is shown in Figure 17.2. by the resistance R_s connected across the meter. The electron flow therefore splits at point A such that only 1 mA flows through the meter when the total current is 1 A. Similarly if only 0·5 A total flows then the currents through the meter and the shunt are halved also, i.e. 499·5 mA flows around the shunt and 0·5 mA flows through the meter so that the pointer is deflected only half-way across the scale. If the pointer on the meter indicated a current of 0·2 mA (say), then we would know that this meant that there was a current of 0·2 A flowing in the main circuit. We may therefore either multiply the indicated reading on the scale by a known factor, or we may replace the previous scale which read up to 1 mA by one which reads up to 1 A. Many meters have a large number of scales of different f.s.d. values, and the operator must be sure which is the correct scale for any particular measurement.

Obviously, the meter current and the shunt current join together again at B (Fig. 17.2) so that no current is 'lost' from the main electrical circuit. The mathematics required for the calculation of the value of the shunt resistor R_s is straightforward and is just an exercise in Ohm's Law (10.5). However, we need the following definition before proceeding:

Definition

The *multiplying factor* for a current-measuring meter is the ratio of the currents required to produce a given deflection of the pointer when the shunt is connected to when it is disconnected.

In the above example, where a meter of 1 mA f.s.d. was desired to measure up to 1 A, the multiplying factor was just 1000 mA / 1 mA = 1000. Note that the multiplying factor is always greater than unity.

The potential difference V shown in Figure 17.3 exists across both the meter of resistance R_m and the shunt resistance R_s. A current i flows through the meter, and I through the external circuit, so that $(I - i)$ flows through the shunt. The multiplying factor is just I/i: the current flowing through the circuit divided by the current flowing through the meter, it being assumed that these

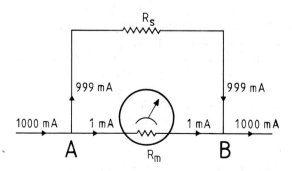

Fig. 17.2 The use of a 'shunt' to enable a meter to measure a higher current. A 1mA meter is illustrated with a shunt (R_s) enabling the meter to measure up to 1 A (1000 mA).

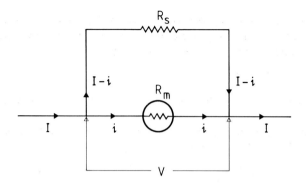

Fig. 17.3 The use of Ohm;s Law to calculate the value of shunt resistance for a given 'multiplication factor'.

would both produce the same meter reading when the shunt is connected across the meter for the larger value of current, I.

We may apply Ohm's Law to each resistor as follows:

$$V = iR_m;\ V = (I - i)R_s$$
$$\text{Thus,}\quad (I - i)R_s = iR_m$$

or $\left(\dfrac{I - i}{i}\right)R_s = R_m$ by cross-multiplication.

Simplifying this expression, we have:

$$\left(\frac{I}{i} - 1\right)R_s = R_m$$

i.e. $R_s = \dfrac{R_m}{\dfrac{I}{i} - 1}$

However, I/i is just the 'multiplying factor', as described above, so that we may express this equation in words as follows:

---

shunt resistance = $\dfrac{\text{meter resistance}}{\text{multiplying factor} - 1}$ Equation 17.1

This is a general equation relating the meter resistance, shunt resistance and multiplying factor. However, most examples of the calculation of shunt resistances are so simple that it is very quick and just as easy to use Ohm's Law directly, as shown in the following examples.

Examples

a.   A meter has a resistance of 2Ω and has a full-scale deflection of 10 mA. What shunt resistance must be used in order that the meter may measure up to 100 mA?

In the solution to this problem we assume that 100 mA is flowing in the circuit, 10 mA through the meter and therefore 90 mA through the shunt. Applying Ohm's Law ($V = IR$) to the meter:

$$V = 10 \times 2 = 20 \text{ mV}$$

Applying Ohm's Law to the shunt: $V = 90 \times R_s$ mV, where R_s is the shunt resistance.

Since the potential difference across the meter and the shunt are the same (see Fig. 17.2), we have

$$20 = 90 R_s$$

i.e. $R_s = \dfrac{2}{9} \, \Omega$

Thus the shunt resistance is 1/9 of the meter resistance, so that the current is split up in the ratio 1 : 9. Note that the equation 7.1 would have given the same result, since the 'multiplying factor -1' is 9 in this example.

b. A meter has an f.s.d. of 10 μA and a resistance of 0·1 Ω. What shunt resistance is required if the meter is to measure up to 5 mA? Proceeding as in the above example,

Ohm's law for the meter: $V = 10 \times 0{\cdot}1 = 1\mu V$
Ohm's law for the shunt: $V = 4999 \times R_s \, \mu V$
(since 4999 μA flows through the shunt).

(*Note*: both currents are expressed in μA — the choice is arbitrary providing they are the same.)

Thus, $1 = 4999 R_s$, so that $R_s = \dfrac{1}{4999}$

or (almost exactly) $R_s = \dfrac{1}{5000} = 0{\cdot}0002 \, \Omega$

Both these examples show that the resistance of the shunt is considerably *less* than the meter resistance. This is because a greater current must flow through the shunt than through the meter, and this can only be so if the shunt has a lower resistance to electron flow than the meter itself.

Exercise 7.1

a. Why is the resistance of a current-measuring meter made as small as possible?

b. What is meant by the terms: internal resistance of a meter, full-scale deflection (f.s.d.), shunt and multiplying factor?

c. A meter has a resistance of 2Ω and an f.s.d. of 1 mA. What shunt resistances are required in order that the meter may be able to measure up to:

(i) 5 mA   (ii) 10 mA   (iii) 200 mA   (iv) 1 A?

(Approximate values for shunt resistance for large multiplying factors are acceptable.)

d. How would you connect all the shunt resistances calculated in the previous example in one circuit so that the appropriate shunt resistor may be selected by a switch?

17.3 THE MEASUREMENT OF POTENTIAL DIFFERENCE

Suppose that we have the circuit shown in Figure 17.4 in which we wish to measure the potential difference (voltage) across the resistor $R1$. Potential difference is a measure of the electrical potential energy between two points (9.6), and does not 'flow', unlike current. It can therefore only be measured by connecting the 'voltmeter' *across* the two points in question. An ideal voltmeter would be able to measure the potential difference across two points without drawing any current away from the main circuit. In this way the meter would not be altering the potential difference it was measuring (17.1), for, to take an extreme example, if the resistance of the voltmeter was zero then it would 'short-out' $R1$ so that a potential difference no longer existed! From this example, it may be seen that an accurate voltmeter must have a *high resistance*. This is the opposite situation to the current-measuring meter, where a low resistance is necessary. However, the reason in both cases is the same, namely that the use of any measuring device must not alter significantly the quantity it is trying to measure (17.1).

Now in practice a meter to measure voltage is just the same as one to measure current, but with the exception that a high resistance is placed *in series* with it, as shown in Figure 17.5. The potential difference across the two points A and B is to be measured by the meter of resistance R_m. The meter is connected to a high resistance R — this limits the maximum current, i, flowing the meter to a small value.

Applying Ohm's Law twice:

a. to the meter: $v = iR_m$, where v is the PD across the meter
b. to the series resistor: $V - v = iR$

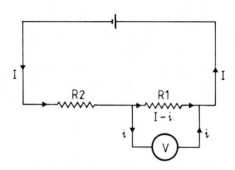

Fig. 17.4 The use of a meter to measure a potential difference. The meter is connected across the two points (i.e. in 'parallel').

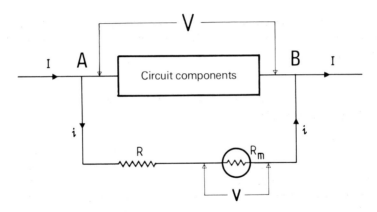

Fig. 17.5 A high resistance is placed in series with a meter to enable it to measure potential difference — it becomes a 'voltmeter'.

In this case the current through the meter, i, is the same as that through the series resistor R so that

$$\frac{v}{R_m} = \frac{V - v}{R}$$

$$\text{i.e.} \quad R = R_m\left(\frac{V}{v} - 1\right)$$

Now the term V/v is similar to I/i in the discussion on shunts (17.2.1) and is also called the 'multiplying factor':

Definition

The *multiplying factor* for a meter measuring potential difference is the ratio of the potential differences required to produce a given reading when a series resistance is in position to when no series resistance is present.

The above equation may be expressed in words, as follows:

Series resistance = meter resistance × (multiplying factor − 1)   Equation 17.2

This equation differs from Equation 17.1 in that the term (multiplying factor − 1) is on the numerator rather than the denominator.

As in the case for the calculation of shunt resistors (17.2.1), the value of the series resistance is easily performed in practice by the repeated application of Ohm's Law (i.e. is not necessary to memorise Equation 17.2), as the following examples show:

Examples:

a. A meter produces a full-scale-deflection when 1 mV is connected across it. How can it be made to measure up to 500 mV? The internal resistance of the meter is 10 Ω

Connecting a series resistance, R, to the meter will produce a current i in both the resistance and the meter when connected to 500 mV (see Fig. 17.5).

Ohm's Law for the meter gives:

$$1 = i . 10 \quad \text{i.e.} \quad i = 1/10 \text{ mA}$$

Ohm's Law for R gives $499 = iR$

$$\therefore \quad R = \frac{499}{i} = \frac{499}{1/10} = 4990 \, \Omega$$

b   A meter has an f.s.d. of 0·2 mA and an internal resistance of 0·5 Ω. What series resistance is required so that it may measure up to 10 V?

If we assume that the maximum value of current which the meter can withstand (i.e. 0·2 mA) is flowing both through the meter and the series resistance, we need only apply Ohm's Law to the resistor + meter:

$$10 = 0·2 \times 10^{-3} \times (R + 0·5)$$

$$\therefore \quad R + 0·5 = \frac{10}{0·2 \times 10^{-3}} = 50 \times 10^3$$

$$\therefore \quad R = 50 \text{ k}\Omega \text{ (approximately)}$$

Note that the resistances used in series with the meter are large, unlike those used for shunts, which are very small. The large series resistors are required in order to reduce the current flowing through the meter to a value which will not damage it, and also to take as little current as possible away from the circuit being measured (17.1).

Exercise 17.2

a.   A meter gives a full-scale deflection if 5 mV is connected across it. What resistance must be placed in series with it if it is desired to use the meter to measure up to 100 mV? The internal resistance of the meter is 0·5 Ω.

b.   If the pointer of the meter in the above question reads 4 mV on the original scale, what is the potential difference being measured?

c.   A meter has an f.s.d. of 5 mA, and this occurs when 10 mV is connected across it. What is the resistance of the meter? What shunt resistance is required so that the meter can measure up to 20 mA, and what series resistance is required so that the meter can measure up to 1 V?

17.4 THE MOVING IRON METER

In the previous sections the general principles of the measurement of voltage and current were outlined. These principles apply whatever the details of the construction of a particular meter. Two types of meter are now considered: the moving iron meter in this section, and the moving coil meter in section 17.5.

The moving iron meter has a wide variation in design. Basically, however, it works on one of two mechanisms: the repulsion or attraction of soft iron, as described below in simplified form.

17.4.1 Repulsion

Figure 17.6(a) shows the basic construction of this type of meter. Two lengths of soft iron A and B are placed within the current-carrying solenoid S. A is fixed to the inside of the solenoid, but B is free to move and is attached to a central spindle C which rotates in sympathy with the movements of B. When no current flows through the solenoid, the spring D keeps the spindle and pointer rotated fully anti-clockwise so that the pointer reads zero and the soft iron pieces are close together. When a current flows, however, a magnetic field is set up within the solenoid (12.4) which magnetises both A and B in *the same direction*, i.e. adjacent ends become magnetic north or south poles. Since 'like poles repel' (11.2) a mutual force of repulsion is set up between A and B, which increases as the current through the solenoid increases. B is able to move and therefore is pushed away from A and, in so doing, moves the pointer P on the scale G which has been previously calibrated in units of current or voltage. The pointer comes to rest when the clockwise force of repulsion between A and B is exactly balanced by the anti-clockwise force due to the spring. However, the *damper F* is necessary in order to reduce the oscillations of the pointer so that a reading may be taken reasonably quickly. This is difficult if the needle is swinging wildly backwards and forwards! Thus the function of the damper is to quickly reduce the oscillations of the needle but without affecting the final reading, and this is accomplished by the plate H travelling through a restricted space in F, so that the air may only flow between H and the inside of F with some difficulty. This arrangement is known as an 'air damper' or 'dashpot'.

One main disadvantage of the moving iron meter (both types) is the *non-linear* scale, where the graduated marks are at different spacings along the scale. This is because the force between the soft iron pieces A and B depends upon their *separation* as well as on the current in the solenoid. Thus, a disproportionate increase of current is needed to deflect the needle at the larger values of deflection. This leads to difficulties in reading the non-linear scale, particularly where the scale markings are close together.

17.4.2 Attraction

As its name implies, this type of moving iron meter works by attraction rather than repulsion. The details of spring, spindle, pointer and air-damper are the same as for the repulsive type (17.4.1); the difference being that there is only one soft iron piece (B in Fig. 17.6b) and the solenoid S is arranged so that B, when deflected, may pass within it.

A current flowing in S magnetises B and pulls it towards S in a clockwise direction against the action of the spring D — the final reading on the scale being the deflection of the pointer when the clockwise force on B is exactly balanced by the anti-clockwise force due to the spring. The function of the damper is to achieve a quicker reading as described in the previous section.

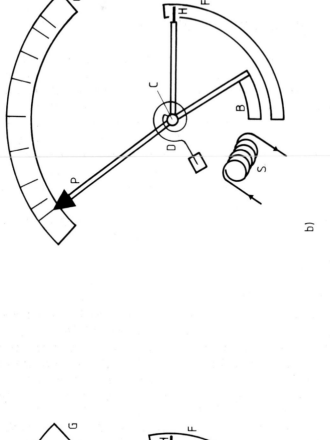

Fig. 17.6 Moving iron meters: (a) repulsion (b) attraction types. Note the non-linear scales and the air-dampers. Key: S — Solenoid; A and B — soft iron; C — spindle; P — pointer; D — spring; G — scale; F — air damper; H — piston.

Again, the scale is non-linear owing to the attractive force on B depending upon the distance between S and B as well as on the current.

17.5 THE MOVING COIL METER

The moving coil meter has several advantages over the moving iron meter. These include accuracy, increased sensitivity (enabling smaller currents to be measured) and a linear scale. It is for these reasons that the moving coil meter is more often used than the moving iron meter in X-ray equipment wherever an accurate measurement of current or voltage is required. However, the moving iron meter may measure *alternating* currents and voltages directly, whereas the moving coil meter must be supplied with 'rectified' AC (17.6). In practice, it is convenient to use a moving iron meter for the mains compensation meter (17.7.1) and the pre-reading kV meter (17.7.2), and a moving coil meter for the mA meter (17.7.3) and mAs meter (17.7.4). However, individual X-ray units may vary from this pattern, and may not have (say) a pre-reading kV meter at all, if the unit has a high degree of automatic compensation.

17.5.1 Construction and operation

The basic construction of the moving coil meter is shown in Figure 17.7. An electric current flowing in the turns of copper wire (via the two springs) causes a rotating force on the turns, due to the presence of the permanent magnetic pole pieces (i.e. the Motor Principle — Chapter 13). Since the copper wire turns are attached to an aluminium frame, both the wire and the frame and spindle assembly rotate against the restoring action of the springs until the rotating force due to the Motor Principle is exactly balanced by the opposing rotating force due to the springs (i.e. an 'equilibrium' is established). In this situation the pointer, which is connected to (and therefore rotates with) the upper spindle, indicates the value of the current by means of a calibrated linear scale. An increase in the current will then result in a new equilibrium between the force due to the Motor Principle and the force due to the springs at a greater deflection of the pointer. Switching the current off enables the springs to restore the pointer to its 'zero' position.

Exercise 17.3
   a. What would happen if the permanent magnet were removed and a current then passed through the copper turns?
   b. What would happen if springs were not used?
   c. Why is the frame aluminium rather than steel?

More detailed descriptions of the functions of the components of the moving coil meter are given below.

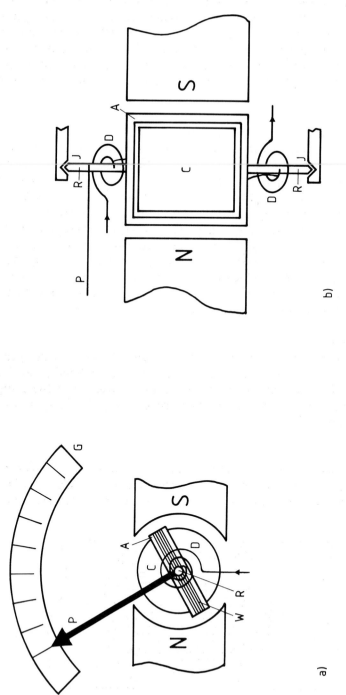

Fig. 17.7 The moving coil meter: (a) plan, (b) side view. Note the linear scale. Key:
A — aluminium frame; W — copper windings; R — spindle; D — spring; C — fixed iron core;
P — pointer; G — scale; J — jewelled bearings; N–S pole-pieces of permanent magnet.

a. Permanent magnet

This is of the 'horse-shoe' type and is made of a substance of high coercivity (11.7) in order to retain its magnetism at a constant value over a long time (i.e. steel). It has curved pole-pieces so that there is a small, constant gap between the surfaces of the poles and the copper turns. This arrangement ensures that the magnetic field strength (11.3) experienced by the copper turns is constant, irrespective of the angle of the windings and aluminium frame with respect to the magnet.

b. Fixed iron core

As would be expected from its name, the fixed iron core does not rotate at all. Its function is to ensure that the direction of the lines of force of the magnetic field (11.3) in the air gap are directed toward (or away from) the *centre* of the core. These are called *radial* lines of force and are illustrated in Figure 17.8. Such a design means that the magnetic lines of force are always directed along the *plane* of the frame. As shown later, this is a necessary condition for the production of a linear scale. In addition, the soft iron core results in an increased magnetic flux (11.4) passing through the copper turns, so making the meter more sensitive by increasing the rotating force due to the Motor Principle for a given current. Also the soft iron core acts as a "keeper" for the permanent magnet, helping it to retain its magnetism.

c. Jewelled bearings

The frame and spindle assembly rotate on jewelled bearings, which provide it with an almost frictionless and hard-wearing support (similar to those in clockwork wrist-watches). Significant amounts of friction at these supports would produce incorrect readings, of course, owing to the 'jerky' movements which would result.

d. Springs

The springs have two main functions: they serve to connect the current into and out of the meter, and they help to produce a linear scale (17.5.2). In addition, the springs are *counter-wound* (i.e. one is clockwise and the other is

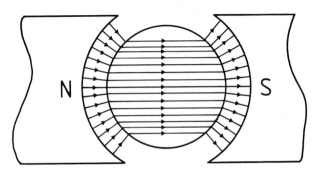

Fig. 17.8 The radial lines of magnetic field in the air-gap between the magnetic pole-pieces and the soft iron core.

anti-clockwise) with respect to each other in order to cancel the effect of temperature changes on the springs. An increase of temperature, for example, produces spring expansions which result in equal and opposite forces of rotation, so that there is no net effect due to temperature changes. Springs wound in the same sense would double the effect of the temperature changes of one spring, of course, and so would produce difficulties in maintaining both the accuracy and stability of the meter readings.

e.   Aluminium frame

The function of the aluminium frame is to produce damping of the pointer deflection, without affecting the final reading of the pointer over the scale. The damping action is produced as a result of the laws of electromagnetic induction (17.5.3).

17.5.2 The linear scale

The scale on the moving coil meter is *linear*, i.e. the graduations are spaced an equal distance apart on the scale, unlike the moving iron meters (17.4). This linearity is accomplished by a combination of factors:

a.   the use of curved pole-pieces
b.   the use of a fixed cylinder of soft iron placed symmetrically between the pole-pieces (the soft iron core is shown in Fig. 17.7)
c.   the effect of the springs when the spindle rotates.

We have already seen (Fig. 17.8) the effect of the curved pole-pieces and the soft iron cylinder on the lines of magnetic force, i.e. they become *radial* in the air gap between them. This means that the rotating force present on the copper turns when an electric current flows through them is always at *right-angles* to the plane of the turns, irrespective of the angular position of the turns, This situation is illustrated in Figure 17.9, where the same current is flowing through the copper turns for two different positions of the frame, AE and CD.

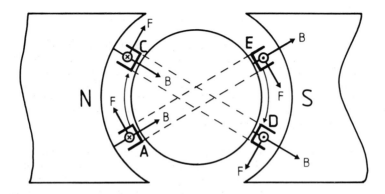

Fig. 17.9 The force (F) exerted on the copper windins is always at right-angles to the plane of the windings. This is necessary to produce a linear scale.

Since the direction of the magnetic lines of force is radial, they must always lie along the plane of the frame.

The force produced by the interaction of the two magnetic fields is, according to the Motor Principle (13.2), always at right-angles to both the direction of the magnetic lines of force and to the direction of the electric current. Since both B and I (Fig. 17.9) are fixed *relative to the frame*, then so is the force, i.e. it is always at right angles to the frame, so that the turning force on the frame does not depend upon the position of the frame. (Verification of the direction of current required to produce a clockwise turning force as shown in the figure is left as an exercise to the student using the convention in 13.2.1 or otherwise.) However, this situation is not sufficient, of itself, to produce a linear scale, since the springs are also necessary to produce a reading on the scale, for without them the pointer would just keep going!

The springs produce a restraining force which is proportional to the deflection of the pointer, and it is this property (known as Hooke's Law) which is ultimately responsible for the linear scale of the moving coil meter.

To summarise, the sequence of events is as follow:

a.   a steady current I flows in the turns of copper wire

b.   a rotating force is produced on the frame by the Motor Principle, and the whole assembly rotates

c.   the rotating force on the frame is *constant* as the frame rotates

d.   the spindles rotate against the restoring force of the springs, the restoring force increasing in proportion to the angle through which the spindle and frame have rotated

e.   a point is reached where the two forces cancel each other out, and the deflection of the pointer on the calibrated scale gives the required reading of current (or voltage).

If now the current is doubled, the rotating force is doubled and the frame will rotate until the restoring force due to the spring also doubles. This will occur at double the deflection of the pointer because of the linear behaviour of the springs. Thus the scale is also linear, since the pointer deflection is proportional to the current.

Insight

The magnitude of force on a current-carrying conductor is given by '$F = BIl \sin \theta$' (Equation 13.1). The rotating force, or couple, G, on the frame of width d is $F \times d$ so that $G = BIldn \sin \theta$ for n turns of wire. Thus, if B, l, d, n, and $\sin \theta$ are constant, $G \propto I$ only. Now l, d, n are fixed, and B and $\sin \theta$ are constant because of the curved pole-pieces and the cylinder of soft iron ($\sin \theta = 1$, i.e. $\theta = 90°$, the angle between I and B). Thus we have a rotating couple $G \propto I$.

When the pointer has reached its final value, the rotating couple, G, due to the Motor Principle is balanced exactly by the restoring couple, R, due to the springs. In addition, we know that $R \propto$ deflection of pointer, so that G is also proportional to the deflection of the pointer. Since $G \propto I$ (from above) we obtain finally that $I \propto$ pointer deflection, i.e. the angle of deflection is proportional to the current, so that a linear scale results.

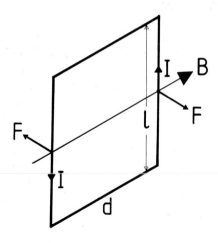

17.5.3 Damping

Without damping, the pointer would oscillate backwards and forwards on the scale for some considerable time before coming to rest and enabling an accurate reading to be taken. For the moving iron meters (17.4.1 and 17.4.2) this damping is provided by 'air dampers' (or 'dashpots'). In the case of the moving coil meter the damping is provided by the *aluminium frame*, for when it moves through the magnetic field of the permanent magnet a current is induced in the frame in such a direction as to oppose the motion. This is just an example of Lenz's Law of electromagnetic induction (14.3) which may be paraphrased here as: 'A changing magnetic flux associated with a closed conductor induces a current whose direction opposes the change producing it.'

What this means in practice is that if the current through the copper windings starts to rotate them in a clockwise direction (due to the Motor Principle), then the aluminium frame also moves and has a current induced in it in the *opposite* direction (due to Lenz's Law). There are, in consequence, two rotating forces on the frame (apart from the effect of the springs): the clockwise one due to the current in the copper turns, and the anti-clockwise one due to the opposing induced current in the frame. The net effect is to reduce the speed of rotation of the frame so that the pointer does not significantly 'over-shoot' its final reading.

One very important point is that the damping effect on the movement of the pointer caused by the induced current in the frame does *not* affect the final reading, as there is no induced current (and therefore no damping force) when the frame is stationary, since induced EMF's and currents require a *changing* magnetic flux linkage with a conductor. The example of a rotating frame in a magnetic field is also described (14.4), where the directions of the induced currents are derived from first principles.

17.6 AC AND METERS

The previous sections considered only the case where a steady direct current or voltage was being measured. We now investigate the behaviour of the meters previously described when we wish to measure sinusoidal AC (15.2).

It is fairly easy to see that a change in the *direction* of the current passing through the meters described above only affects the pointer on the moving coil meter and not those of the moving iron meters. This is because the repulsion type still repulses and the attraction type still attracts whatever the direction of the current, while the moving coil meter is deflected in the opposite direction if the current is reversed. Thus a moving iron meter will produce a deflection of its pointer in one direction if an alternating current is passed through it, while a moving coil meter will not be able to respond sufficiently quickly to the rapid changes of current direction and so will give a zero deflection. However, as we have seen in (15.1) (and shall see in Chapter 20 in more detail) alternating current may be rectified to produce 'pulsatile DC', i.e. pulses of direct current (see Fig. 15.1(b)). Figure 17.10 illustrates the behaviour of both types of meter when measuring DC and different types of alternating current or voltage. In all cases, a meter having a zero at the centre of the scale is assumed.

17.7 METERS AND X-RAY CIRCUITS

Many modern X-ray circuits use sophisticated automatic electrical and electronic control of mA, kV_p, and mains voltage. Such units may not use any meters at all. It is possible that future developments in X-ray circuits may lead to the introduction of numerical displays in preference to meters with pointers (similar to 'digital' watches). However, meters are simple, relatively cheap and have an accuracy which is adequate for most applications in X-ray circuits so that they are likely to be widely retained on the control panels of X-ray circuits for some time to come. Figure 17.11 shows a simplified circuit employing four meters whose functions are explained below.

17.7.1 Mains voltage meter (M1)

The magnitude of the mains voltage varies throughout the day and night, depending upon the electrical 'load' presented to the generating power station. The greater the demand for current (at 'peak' times during the day), the lower is the value of the mains voltage, due to the increased 'voltage drop' across the resistance of the mains cables, and also supply 'regulation' (16.3.3). The voltage presented to the primary side of the high tension transformer (HTT) would, in the absence of suitable correction (or 'compensation'), increase and decrease with the fluctuations in the mains voltage supply, thereby leading to a similar fluctuation in the kV_p across the X-ray tube. Obviously, this would result in radiographs of variable photographic density. The effect of mains voltage fluctuation on the mA is even more critical, owing to the sensitivity of thermionic emission with temperature changes (18.3.2). Thus, it is essential to

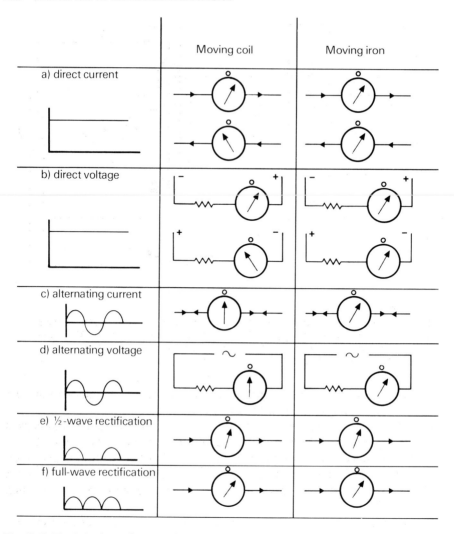

Fig. 17.10 The behaviour of the moving iron and moving coil meters to DC and AC. (*Note:* The two types of meter are not necessarily measuring the same current, although the deflections are shown as the same in the figure, for convenience.)

supply both the HTT and the filament transformer with a predictable value of voltage. This is the function of contactor S1 on the autotransformer, which is adjusted so that the 'volts per turn' (16.4.2) is always constant.

For example, for a nominal 240 V mains input, the number of primary turns on the autotransformer might be, say, 480 so that the 'volts per turn', v, is 0·5 volt. If the mains voltage now drops to a value of 220 V, then S1 is adjusted so that there are 440 turns on the primary $v = 220/440 = 0·5$ V, as before. In this way the potential difference (voltage) across a *given number of turns is kept constant*. In the above example, the voltage across 100 turns was 50 volts both before and after adjustments of S1, since the 'volts per turn' was kept constant. The secondary of the autotransformer therefore supplies a 'compensated'

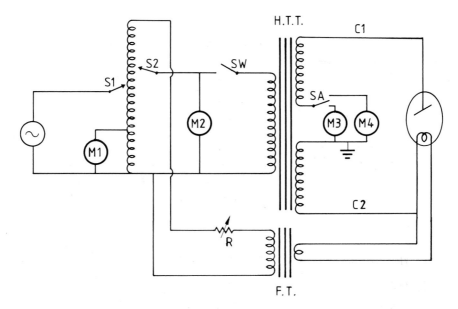

Fig. 17.11 A simplified X-ray circuit and the positions of the meters in it. M1 — mains compensation meter; M2 — pre-reading kilovoltage meter; M3 — mA meter; M4 — mAs meter. Note the earth point at the centre of the secondary winding of the high tension transformer (see text).

voltage which may be applied to both the high tension transformer and the filament to produce radiographs of predictable quality.

Meter M1 is known as the 'mains (or line) compensation meter' and is used to indicate when the 'volts per turn' is at its correct value. A typical meter for this purpose would be a moving iron meter (17.6) with a simple scale indicating the limits within which the needle should be confined. A coloured band or two closely spaced marks is all that is necessary for the scale of such a meter.

A moving iron meter in this position is the obvious choice since it measures alternating currents and voltage without any modification (unlike the moving coil meter which requires rectification), and the non-linear scale is of no significance in this situation.

The mains compensation meter may either be connected across the whole of the autotransformer or across part of it, the latter case being shown in Figure 17.11.

17.7.2 Pre-reading kV meter (M2)

When contact S2 is varied (Fig. 17.11), the number of secondary turns applied to a meter M2 is varied in proportion. When SW is closed, the voltage across these turns on the autotransformer is applied to the primary of the high tension transformer, so producing the kV required to operate the X-ray tube. S2 is therefore the 'kV control', and the purpose of meter M2 is to read the value of the kV_p which has been selected by S2 *before* taking the exposure, i.e. while switch SW is open. The meter is therefore known as the 'pre-reading kV meter' for this reason. However, it does not actually *measure* kilovoltage; it only *indicates* it. This is possible because the voltage gain (16.1) of the high tension transformer is a known constant value, being just the 'turns ratio'. For example, suppose that the turns ratio of the high tension transformer is 400. This is the same as the voltage gain of the transformer (16.1) so that 10 V on the primary produces 4 kV, and so on. Thus, if we wish to operate the X-ray tube at 80 kV$_p$, say, then we know that the required primary voltage is 1/400th of this, i.e. 200 V$_p$. The pre-reading kV meter will therefore show a deflection which, on its usual scale, would indicate 200 V$_p$. However, a rather crafty substitution of meter scales has taken place! A new scale is used whose markings are just 400 times those of the 'old' scale. No numerical calculations are therefore required. It would be somewhat time-consuming, after all, if the 'old' scale is read and each reading must then be multiplied by 400 (or some other figure) in order calculate the kV$_p$ which would actually result in practice!

Thus: 'the pre-reading kV meter *reads* voltage but *indicates* kilovoltage'.

M2 may be either a moving iron meter or a moving coil meter, but the moving coil meter would required its own rectification in order to measure the alternating voltage across the secondary windings of the autotransformer. Its linear scale is an advantage, however.

17.7.3 mA meter (M3)

Both the mA meter (M3) and the mAs meter (M4) are situated in the same place, i.e. they are both joined to the central portion of the secondary windings of the high tension transformer, and one side of each meter is 'earthed', i.e. held at zero potential. Both meters may be used at the same time if placed in series, but it is usually the case that the mA is required when 'screening' (i.e. taking a long exposure when using a fluorescent screen or image intensifier system), and the mAs is required when taking a conventional radiograph. Thus, the switch SA in Figure 17.11 is shown to indicate that either the mA or the mAs meter may be selected as appropriate.

The purpose of placing the earth point at the centre of the secondary coil of the high-tension transformer is that it produces equal (but opposite) values of kV in the two cables C1 and C2. If the earth point had been connected to one end of the secondary of the transformer, for example, then one high-tension cable would have had zero potential and the other would have had to withstand the whole of the potential difference applied across the X-ray tube. This would have meant, for example, withstanding 100 kV$_p$ rather than one cable needing to withstand only $+50$ kV$_p$ and the other -50kV$_p$. The total potential difference is still 100 kV$_p$ in the latter case, but each cable need only cope with one-half of this value.

The two meters M3 and M4 are connected to 'earth' for a very important reason: *operator safety*. This is because of the fact that they are situated on the X-ray control panel and the high-tension transformer is situated some distance away in its own oil bath (16.3.2). The high tension transformer, by its very nature, produces very high voltages which would be very dangerous if brought anywhere near a human operator. This means that the mA and the mAs meters, which are connected to the secondary of the transformer, could be a source of danger if connected to a point of high voltage on the secondary. This possibility of danger is eliminated by connecting the meters to the 'earth', as shown in Figure 17.11.

The current flowing through the X-ray tube (i.e. the mA) also flows through the secondary winding of the transformer, so that the meter M3 will indicate the mA flowing through the X-ray tube (the scale is selected to read the *average* value of mA). The filament transformer is used solely to produce a current through the filament of the X-ray tube and produce thermionic emission of electrons from it (Chapter 18) — the filament current in no way contributes to the mA — i.e. it does not pass across the tube (21.4.1)!

The mA meter is usually a moving coil meter, since the wide range of possible settings of mA requires both the accuracy of the linear scale and the sensitivity of the moving coil meter.

The circuit shown in Figure 17.11 is that of a simple self-rectified circuit, where the X-ray tube acts as its own rectifier. For a full-wave rectified circuit (20.2) the current will pass through the mA meter in both directions, so that no net deflection of the pointer will result (17.6). This problem is overcome if the meter is connected to its own rectifier, so that the current through the meter is in one direction, even though that through the secondary winding is alternating.

17.7.4 mAs meter (M4)

All the comments in the above section apply to the mAs meter: it is only the constructional details of the mAs meter which distinguish it from the mA meter.

The mAs meter is very similar to the mA meter except that it has no springs and the moving frame is somewhat heavier. Thus, if a current is passed through it for an indefinite time the pointer will keep on being deflected until it reaches the maximum value which the meter will allow (the 'end stop'). This is because there are no springs to stop the motion.

The mathematics of the mAs meter are rather too advanced for inclusion in this textbook, but the principle is fairly simple. The frame of the mAs meter is given a sudden 'kick' when the exposure is taken — this provides it with a given angular momentum. The damping effect of the frame moving within the magnetic field of the permanent magnet (Lenz's Law) then brings the frame and pointer to rest at a deflection which is proportional to the strength of the original 'kick', and this is proportional to the total electric *charge* which has flowed, i.e. the mAs (6.4.2). Thus, a deflection is produced which is proportional to the mAs, and so a suitably calibrated scale may be used to measure the mAs.

The pointer is restored to zero by passing a small negative current in the reverse direction until zero is reached on the scale. This may be done either automatically prior to the next exposure, or by the operator, after noting the mAs value which was given on the previous exposure. The ability of the mAs meter to retain its mAs reading after an exposure serves as a useful check on the exposure settings which the operator selected, or thought were selected!

Like the mA meter, the mAs requires its own rectification if a full-wave rectified high-tension circuit is used.

Insight

The scales of either of the moving iron or moving coil meters may be calibrated in peak, average or RMS units of potential difference or current, depending upon the purpose for which the meter is being used. The pre-reading kV meter described above has a scale calibrated in terms of peak units, while the mains compensation meter has an RMS scale and the mA meter has a scale indicating average current.

The simple linear relationships between all these types of units (15.2) may be used to convert one unit to another (e.g. peak to effective), or a different scale used for the meter.

Exercise 17.4

a. Describe the construction and operation of a moving iron meter. Why is the scale non-linear, and why is it necessary to 'damp' the movement of the pointer?

b. Describe the construction and operation of a moving coil meter. How is such a meter damped, and why is the scale linear?

c. Make notes on the following details of construction of a moving coil meter:

(i) permanent magnet
(ii) fixed soft iron core
(iii) spindle
(iv) aluminium frame
(v) counterwound springs
(vi) jewelled bearings
(vii) pointer
(viii) scale
(ix) copper windings

d. Draw a simplified X-ray circuit, showing where the following meters are situated:

(i) mA
(ii) pre-reading kV meter
(iii) mains compensation meter
(iv) mAs

e. How may a moving coil meter with an internal resistance of 2 Ω and an f.s.d. of 1 mA be used to measure

(i) 100 mA DC
(ii) 10 V DC
(iii) 100 mA AC (full-wave rectified)?

SUMMARY

1. Meters are connected in such a way as to alter the quantity they are trying to measure to a negligible extent. For the measurement of current, this means that the meter should have a *low* resistance, and, for voltage, a *high* resistance. Current is measured by connecting a meter in series with the circuit, and voltage by connecting a meter in parallel.

2. A meter may measure currents beyond its normal range by the use of 'shunts', which take some of the current around the meter from one side to the other. The 'multiplying factor' is the ratio of the f.s.d. with the shunt to that without it. For a useful increase in range, the shunt resistance is always less than the meter resistance — simply calculated using Ohm's Law.

3. A meter may measure a voltage by means of a high value of series resistor. This limits the current drained from the circuit being measured and enables the voltage to be read on the scale of the meter. The necessary value of the resistance in series with the meter is calculated using Ohm's Law.

4. Moving iron meters: repulsive and attractive types. Both have non-linear scales, and are damped by an air 'dash-pot'.

5. Moving coil meter: very sensitive, works on the Motor Principle, has linear scale and is damped by the movement of aluminium frame in the magnetic field of the permanent magnet (Lenz's Law). Linear scale caused by combination of curved pole-pieces, cylindrical soft-iron core and springs. Springs also carry current to copper turns.

6. Moving iron meter measures AC directly; moving coil meter requires the AC to be rectified.

7. Mains voltage meter is used to provide a constant electrical supply from the secondary of the autotransformer.

8. Pre-reading kV meter 'measures voltage but indicates kilovoltage'.

9. mA meter measures tube current and is connected to an earth point for reasons of electrical safety.

10. mAs meter is similar to mA meter except that it has no springs.

18. Thermionic emission

18.1 THERMIONIC EMITTERS

A substance which releases electrons relatively easily when heated is known as a 'thermionic emitter', and the process of the release of the electrons is called 'thermionic emission'.

The application of heat to a body increases the kinetic energy of its atoms and increases the violence of their collisions, such that some orbiting electrons may be dislodged from their weaker outer orbits. The electrons so 'released' in the centre of the body travel only a very short distance, but some of those very near the *surface* will be able to leave the body, i.e. they have been 'emitted' by the body. Obviously the higher the temperature of the body, the greater is the thermionic emission since more electrons will be given the necessary energy to be able to break free of the influence of the surface atoms of the body. Also, thermionic emission is a phenomenon which depends on the structure of the *surface* atomic layers of the body, since electrons manage to escape only from this region. The scrupulous cleanliness of the surface of the body is therefore essential to the efficiency of thermionic emission.

Thermionic emitters are compared in terms of their *work function*, expressed in units of electron volts (eV) (see 6.4.3), where the work function is the work which must be performed by an electron in escaping from the body. Substances which are good thermionic emitters (e.g. metals) have a lower work function than those which are poor thermionic emitters, since less work is required on the part of the electrons to escape.

Table 18.1 shows the work functions of three typical thermionic emitters.

Table 18.1 Good thermionic emitters

Substance	Work function	Comment
Tungsten	4·5eV	Used as filament of X-ray tube to provide electrons for mA (working temperature about 2000°C)
Thoriated tungsten	2·5eV	Used as filament/cathode in 'directly heated' thermionic vacuum diode
Oxides of alkaline earths (e.g. calcium, barium)	1·0–1·3eV	Used as cathode for an 'indirectly heated' thermionic vacuum diode

From the foregoing discussion, it is apparent that thermionic emission depends upon the temperature and material of the body. Also, it increases with the surface area of the body.

18.1.1 Space charge

Each electron which is thermionically emitted from the surface of a body leaves the body with a net positive charge, since it was electrically neutral before heat was applied. The electrons are therefore attracted back toward the body almost as fast as they are emitted. At any moment, therefore, a 'cloud' of electrons exists around the body with contains a constant number of electrons, since electrons are joining and leaving the cloud at an equal rate. At a higher temperature the electron cloud, or *space charge*, becomes greater owing to the increased electron emission from the body. If the body is left to cool, it will reduce the space charge substantially to zero by capture of the electrons forming the space charge.

If a positively charged body is placed near the space charge some of the electrons within the space charge are attracted towards that body and an electron current flows. This is the principle of the thermionic vacuum diode and the X-ray tube (among other devices), as explained in the ensuing sections of this chapter.

18.2 THERMIONIC EMISSION IN RADIOGRAPHY

The most important, and most obvious, example of thermionic emission in radiography is the filament of the X-ray tube. The filament consists of a few turns of tungsten wire which is heated by passing an electrical current through it, so releasing thermionic electrons and forming a space charge around the filament. When a positive potential is applied to the anode of the X-ray tube the space charge is strongly attracted towards it, producing X-rays when the electrons are forced to decelerate within the anode (Ch. 28).

Thermionic emission is also put to good use in the vacuum diode (18.3) where it is used to ensure that electric current will only pass in one direction, i.e. it is used as a rectifier (Ch. 20).

Exposure switching circuits and 'constant potential' circuits may also use specialised vacuum or gas-filled valves such as the triode (18.4) and thyratron (18.5), each of which uses the principle of thermionic emission to supply electrons capable of flowing within the valve.

The modern trend is towards semiconductor (or 'solid state') devices, which have some advantages when compared to the thermionic valve devices. These are discussed in more detail in Chapter 19.

18.3 THE VACUUM DIODE

The vacuum diode is a device which will pass an electric current in one direction only, and is therefore useful in X-ray rectifier circuits (Ch. 20).

18.3.1 Structure

There are two types of vacuum diode: the *directly* heated and *indirectly* heated cathode. In the former, a current is passed through a tungsten wire to increase its temperature and thus produce the thermionic liberation of electrons which are collected by a nearby plate (the 'anode'). (Note the similarity of this type of diode to the X-ray tube.) However, this type of diode has largely been superseded by the more efficient indirectly heated cathode type of diode, and it is this type which is illustrated in Figure 8.1, together with its electrical symbol.

A centrally placed tungsten *filament* is sealed inside a thin cylindrical sheath which is filled with powdered silicon, the outside surface of the cylinder being

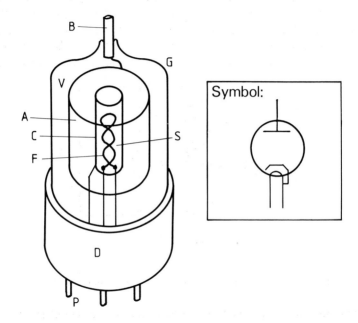

Fig. 18.1 The structure of an 'indirectly heated' thermionic vacuum diode. Key: F — tungsten filament; S — powdered silicon filling; C — cathode made of oxide coating; A — anode collecting plate; V — vacuum; B — anode connection (often has screw thread); G — glass envelope; D — base; P — pins connected to filament and cathode.

coated with a thermionically emitting substance, such as a metal oxide (Table 18.1). The oxide coating is the *cathode*, and is heated indirectly by conduction through the powdered silicon of the heat produced by the filament. The low work function of the oxide coating makes this an efficient arrangement for producing an electron space charge around the cathode. A cylindrical *anode* is placed symmetrically around the cathode assembly, and is connected to the opposite end of the valve to that for the cathode connections in the case of a diode for X-ray work, as shown in the figure. Diodes which are not used at such a high voltage may have all the connections provided through pins in the case of the valve.

The whole assembly is contained inside an evacuated glass envelope so that electron flow between the cathode and anode is unimpeded by gas molecules.

18.3.2 'Characteristic' curves

Suppose that a diode is connected as shown in Figure 18.2. Battery B1 supplies the current to the filament required to raise its temperature and so produce thermionic emission from the cathode. Battery B2 is connected across the diode such that the anode has a positive potential of V_a compared to the cathode. Under these circumstances, some of the space charge formed around the cathode manages to reach the anode, so that a current flows (i_a). The effect of the positive potential on the anode is also to detach the space charge from the immediate neighbourhood of the cathode to an area somewhere between the cathode and anode. The higher the anode potential, the closer is the main body of the space charge to the anode. Electrons thermionically emitted from the cathode have now to attempt to pass through the repelling action of the space charge. Not all of them will be able to do so, and so the current through

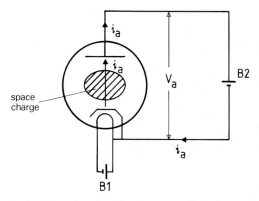

Fig. 18.2 Electric conduction through a thermionic vacuum diode (see text).

the diode is said to be *space-charge limited* due to the repelling action of the space charge.

At a particular value of anode potential, all the space charge is collected by the anode as soon as it is emitted from the cathode, and the diode is then said to be *saturated*, since the current is at a maximum under these circumstances. These points are summarised by the graph shown in Figure 18.3 — the so-called *vacuum-diode characteristic curves*.

It should be borne in mind that there are a whole family of characteristic curves for a particular vacuum diode depending upon the temperature of the cathode and therefore its rate of thermionic emission. Two such curves are shown in Figure 18.3: one of high cathode temperature (OABC) and one of lower cathode temperature (OADE). As the anode to cathode potential difference is increased from zero, an increasing number of electrons are collected by the anode from the space charge. This is the space-charge limited region OA in the figure, and is the normal working region for vacuum diodes.

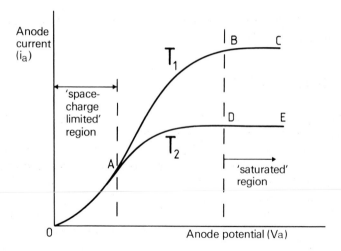

Fig. 18.3 The 'characteristic' of a thermionic vacuum diode. The upper curve has a higher temperature (T_1) than the lower curve (T_2). Diodes are operated in the 'space-charge limited' region, and X-ray tubes in the 'saturated' region (see text).

The saturated regions for the two different temperatures are BC and DE, and correspond to the situation of complete collection of the space charge so that i_a can no longer increase, no matter how large V_a is made. BC is higher than DE because of the increased thermionic emission at the higher temperature, of course. X-ray tubes are operated in the saturated region (18.6).

Diodes are operated in the space-charge limited region rather than the saturated region in order to be able to supply whatever mA value is required by the X-ray tube. They cannot do this if they already saturated and therefore cannot supply a higher current if it is needed.

Current will not flow from anode to cathode, since the anode is not capable of emitting electrons into the vacuum and so to the cathode. Hence the diode only passes current in one direction, i.e. from cathode to anode.

The 'solid state' equivalent of the vacuum diode is the $p-n$ junction diode (19.3.4).

18.3.3 Effect of gas in the diode

If gas (e.g. mercury vapour or argon) is present in the glass envelope, the electrons are impeded in their progress from the cathode to the anode by collisions with the gas atoms. If the voltage between the anode and the cathode is increased, these collisions become more energetic and result in the gas atoms being ionized, i.e. the outermost electrons are removed from orbit. Thus, more and more electrons are produced, since the newly released electrons are able to take part in subsequent ionisation. This process is called 'gas multiplication'. A high current is therefore established, which stops when the anode potential is reduced to near-cathode potential. The tube is therefore either 'off' or 'on' with no intermediate state, making it suitable for use in electronic switching circuits where a high current is required. A more useful valve is the gas-filled triode —the thyratron (18.5).

18.4 THE TRIODE

The triode valve, like the diode, operates in a vacuum and contains a thermionically emitting cathode and surrounding anode. However, the triode has a wire mesh, or *grid*, between the anode and cathode which is used to control the flow of electrons from cathode to anode by applying a potential to it. This is illustrated in Figure 18.4, together with the behaviour of the triode in graphical form, i.e. its 'characteristic'. When the grid potential is strongly negative with respect to the cathode, the electrons thermionically emitted from the latter will be unable to pass through the holes in the wire mesh of the grid due to its repelling action. Thus no current flows (point A in Fig. 18.4(b)). As the grid potential is increased in a positive direction, however, a greater number of electrons are able to penetrate the mesh and reach the anode, so that an increasing anode current is obtained (ABC in the figure) until saturation is reached (CD), when the current is at the value which a diode would pass under the same circumstances. Only one of a whole family of curves is shown in the figure.

The ability to control the current passing through the triode by altering the potential on the grid is very useful for switching the valve on and off and for signal amplification. It finds a particular application for radiography in a secondary X-ray switching circuit with a 'constant potential' correcting facility (20.4.2).

The 'solid state' equivalent of the triode is the transistor (19.4).

18.5 THE THYRATRON

The thyratron is a gas-filled (e.g. argon at low pressure) triode valve, which, like the gas-filled diode, is either 'on' or 'off', with no intermediate states. The

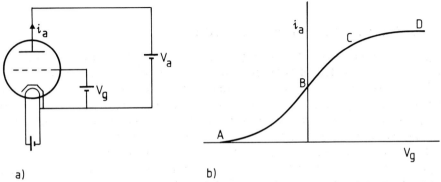

Fig. 18.4 The thermionic vacuum triode (a) shown connected in circuit, and (b) the 'triode characteristic' so measured.

potential on the grid is used to switch the thyratron 'on', but cannot then be used to switch it 'off' again, as explained below. The thyratron is switched 'off' by reducing the anode potential to nearly cathode potential so that 'gas multiplication' (18.3.3) can no longer take place.

Figure 18.5 illustrates the behaviour of the thyratron, where the dot by the anode signifies that it is a gas-filled device. Proceeding as before with the triode valve, a strongly negative grid potential compared with the cathode will prevent electron flow (point A in the graph). When B is reached, electrons which have managed to pass through the grid are able to ionise the gas and 'gas multiplication' takes place, resulting in a rapid rise in current (BC on the graph). The thyratron is said to 'strike' at a potential corresponding to B, i.e. the valve is switched into the 'on' state' (It becomes luminous when in this state owing to some electron recapture by the gas ions.) An increasing grid potential (C to D) has no further effect because the current is dominated by the gas multiplication.

If the potential is reduced from D to C, the thyratron does not switch off at C, however, but continues in its 'on' state along CE. This is due to a cloud of positive gas ions which congregate around the grid and make it effectively neutral, so that it is unable to influence the electron flow from the cathode through the valve. Thus, the thyratron can be switched 'on' by its grid potential, but cannot be switched 'off' by the same means. The only way of switching the thyratron off is to prevent gas multiplication from taking place by reducing the anode potential difference with respect to the cathode to almost zero. This ability of the thyratron to keep 'on' until its anode voltage is at, or near, zero is put to good use in X-ray switching circuits where it is desired to expose for a given number of mains half-cycles. It is beyond the scope of this book to discuss such circuits, and the reader is referred to any competent book on X-ray equipment.

The 'solid state' equivalent of the thyratron is the thyristor (19.5).

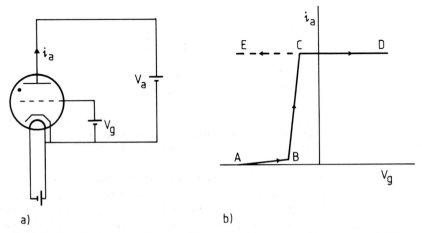

Fig. 18.5 The thermionic gas triode — the 'thyratron': (a) connected in circuit, and (b) the thyratron 'characteristic'. Note that the thyratron is either fully conducting ('on') or conducting very little ('off'), due to 'gas multiplication' (see text).

18.6 THE X-RAY TUBE AS A SATURATED DIODE

The structure of the X-ray tube (Ch. 21) conforms with all the requirements of a vacuum diode, i.e. a cathode which is a thermionic emitter placed close to a positively charged collecting plate, or anode. In fact, the X-ray tube may be used as its own rectifier in the so-called 'self-rectified' circuit (20.1.1) because of its diode action.

However, there are two fundamental differences in the mode of operation of a vacuum diode and the X-ray tube:

a.   a low 'voltage drop' is required for a diode, while a high 'voltage drop' is required for an X-ray tube (in order to produce X-rays)

b.   a diode is operated in the space charge limited region, while an X-ray tube is operated in the saturation region (Fig. 18.3).

To take the second difference first, the advantage of operating an X-ray tube in the saturation region is that mA and kV_p may be set *independently* of each other. This is because, when saturated, an increasing anode potential on the X-ray tube cannot collect any more current than is already being produced by the

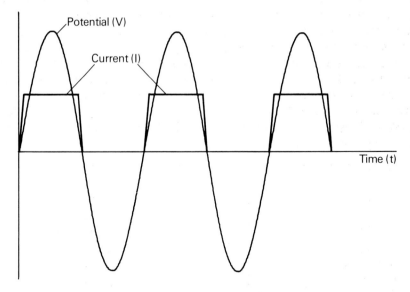

Fig. 18.6 The current and voltage waveforms of an X-ray tube operating as its own diode, or rectifier. The current waveforms are flat-topped because the X-ray tube is operated in the saturation region. This enables kV_p and mA to be adjusted independently.

filament, so that the kV_p may be adjusted without affecting the mA. (This corresponds to DE or BC in Fig. 18.3) It would be a nuisance, after all, if (say) changing the kV_p from 50 to 75 kV_p increased the mA from 20 mA to 30 mA, thus requiring the operator to manually correct for this before taking the exposure, i.e. it is desirable to be able to alter one thing at a time without affecting all the others!

Operating the X-ray tube in the saturated region and a high potential difference, or 'voltage drop', may be considered as the X-ray tube having a high effective resistance. For example, if a potential difference of 50 kV exists across the tube and a current of 200 mA is flowing through it, the effective resistance as given by Ohm's Law ($R = V/I$) is 250 kΩ. A diode, however, is operated with a copious supply of space charge, i.e. in the space charge limited region, so that its effective resistance is much lower and the voltage drop across it is low. A typical voltage drop of 500 V for the same current of 200 mA produces an effective resistance of 2·5 kΩ for the diode — very much less than for the X-ray tube. (*Note:* neither the diode nor the X-ray tube *obeys* Ohm's Law — these calculations are for illustration only.)

Figure 18.6 shows the idealised voltage and current waveforms for an X-ray tube acting as its own diode. Note that the current waveform is flat-topped owing to the saturation produced at relatively low voltages, and also that no current flows when the potential difference across the X-ray tube is negative — the so-called 'inverse voltage'.

Exercise 18.1

a. Describe the phenomenon of thermionic emission, and state the factors upon which it depends. How may thermionic emission be explained in terms of the 'work function' of a material?

b. What is the difference between vaporisation and thermionic emission? (see Ch. 8 if unclear).

c. What is meant by the 'space charge' which surrounds a thermionic emitter? Use this as a means of explaining the *characteristic* of a vacuum diode.

d. What is 'gas multiplication'? Hence explain the effect of a small amount of gas in a thermionic diode tube.

e. Discuss the similarities and differences between the operation of a triode and thyratron valve.

f. Discuss the similarities and differences between the operation of a thermionic vacuum diode and an X-ray tube. In particular, why is the X-ray tube operated in a different part of the 'vacuum diode characteristic' from the vacuum diode? Use voltage and current waveforms to illustrate your answer.

SUMMARY

1. Thermionic emission is the release of electrons from a body which occurs when the body is heated.

2. The rate of thermionic emission depends upon the type of substance, its surface area and the temperature.

3. A 'space charge' of electrons exists around a heated thermionic emitter, and may be attracted towards a positively charged plate, as in a diode.

4. A thermionic vacuum diode only passes current in one direction: from cathode to anode. Current cannot flow in the opposite direction because the anode cannot emit electrons itself (unless seriously overheated).

5. A vacuum diode is operated in the 'space charge limited region' of its 'characteristic' (Fig. 18.3), while an X-ray tube is operated in the 'saturated region' so that mA and kV_p, are independent of each other.

6. Triodes and thyratron are special-purpose valves used in exposure switching and control of kilovoltage applied across an X-ray tube.

19. Semiconductors

The use of semiconductor materials and its associated technology is becoming increasingly widespread in everyday life, particularly since it has been possible to produce many thousands of electronic circuits on a small 'chip' of silicon using so-called 'Large Scale Integration' (LSI) techniques. The most recent example of this technology is the *microprocessor*, which is an electronic device capable of being programmed to perform specific tasks. There is no doubt that the microprocessor will find many applications in control and measurement within the field of radiography and radiotherapy, since it is cheap, relatively easy to program and is able to perform an extremely wide range of functions. However, the microprocessor is a very complicated 'solid state' device and is not suitable for detailed description in this book. Other, simpler, solid state devices such as the *p–n* junction diode and thyristor have been very widely used in X-ray circuitry for a number of years — and hence are suitable for inclusion in this chapter after a general description of the properties of semiconductor materials.

19.1 INTRINSIC SEMICONDUCTORS

An *intrinsic* semiconductor is a chemically pure semiconductor (i.e. it contains

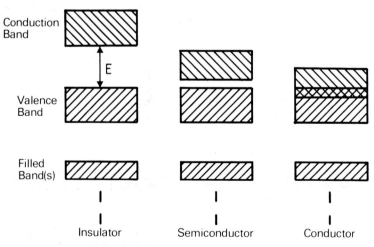

Fig. 19.1 The differences in the electron energies between insulators, semiconductors and conductors.

no impurities within it) and is assumed to have perfect regularity in its crystal structure. The concept of semiconductor materials was introduced briefly in Chapter 10 (10.1), where the properties of conductors, semiconductors and insulators were compared in terms of the 'energy band model' of the orbiting electrons of the material. The figure illustrating this (Fig. 10.2) is reproduced here as Figure 19.1. As shown in the figure, semiconductors are characterised by a small energy gap (up to a few eV) between the top of the valence band and the bottom of the conduction band. At very low temperatures all the outer electrons are contained within the valence band and are at their lowest possible energy states. Thus no electrons are able to take part in electrical conduction, since there are no 'free' electrons in the conduction band, so that the semiconductor is effectively a perfect insulator at these low temperatures. However, at normal room temperatures many electrons are able to gain sufficient energy (from the interaction of the energetic atoms) to jump up to the conduction band and so take part in electrical conduction.

19.1.1 Positive holes

Associated with each electron which has been able to reach the conduction band is a 'vacancy' left behind in the valence band; this vacancy being called a 'positive hole', or just 'hole'. A 'hole' may be filled by an electron from the *valence* band of a neighbouring atom, but in so doing the electron leaves a 'hole' in the valence band of that atom. In this way, the 'hole' may be considered to move about the crystal lattice of the semiconductor until *recombination* occurs, i.e. an electron from the *conduction* band may drop down into the vacancy, or hole, and thus 'remove' it from the valence band. At any moment all three processes are occurring: electron excitation into the conduction band (with consequent production of holes in the valence band), mobility of electrons in the conduction band and of holes in the valence band, and recombination of electrons and holes. The overall conductivity of such an intrinsic semiconductor is composed of the sum of the effects of the movements of the electrons in the conduction band and the holes in the valence band.

Insight

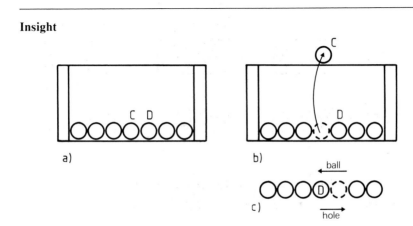

a)

b)

c)

The movement of a hole through a semiconductor may be likened to a row of ball bearings between two walls, where no sideways movement is possible because all the available space is used (as shown in the figure). Suppose that ball C has been lifted to a higher level , so that some space (i.e. a vacancy or hole) now exists between the other balls. Sideways movement is then possible: if D moves to the *left* so as to be where C was, then it leaves a space to its right, so that the hole may be considered as moving to the right, i.e. in the opposite direction to the ball D. To return to the case of semiconductors, there is no net movement possible in the valence band (because it is full — see 19.1.2) until an electron has been lifted to the conduction band. Then a neighbouring electron may move from right to the left (say) to fill this hole, only to leave a hole in its starting position, i.e. the hole moves in the opposite sense from left to right. Since the hole is associated with a positive charge (the extra charge of the nucleus over the number of electrons for that atom) the hole is referred to as a *positive* hole. Thus, if a semiconductor is passing current such that there is electron flow in the conduction band from left to right, there will also be an effective flow of positive charge associated with the movement of the positive holes in the valence band in the opposite direction.

19.1.2 Silicon

The most widely used general-purpose semiconductor material used at present is silicon, which has an atomic number of 14, and hence 14 protons in its nucleus and 14 electrons orbiting the nucleus (Ch. 25). The two inner electron shells (the 'K' and 'L' shells) are completely full and contain 2 and 8 electrons respectively. The next shell (the 'M' shell) contains 4 electrons (to make a total of 14) and this is an incomplete, or unfilled, shell in a solitary silicon atom. However, in its solid form, silicon exhibits a regular spacing and arrangement of silicon atoms (i.e. a 'crystal' structure) in which each silicon atom shares its outer electrons with those of 4 neighbouring atoms, so that each atom appears to have 8 electrons in its outermost orbit, as shown in Figure 19.2. Such electrons are termed 'valence electrons', form 'covalent bonds' and inhabit the valence band. The covalent bonds give the crystal its regularity by limiting the range of movement of any particular atom. At room temperature these bands are continuously being broken and re-formed as some of the valence electrons are given sufficient energy to reach the freedom of the conduction band (bond broken) and fall back to the valence band (bond re-formed). The 8 electron configuration per atom forms a 'closed shell' (Ch. 25) so that the valence band is effectively full until an electron from it jumps up into the conduction band. Then, as explained previously, electron flow in the conduction band and positive-hole flow in the valence band are both possible.

Intrinsic semiconductors, such as pure silicon or germanium, have very limited practical use; it is the addition of small amounts of 'impurities' to them which enable them to exhibit properties which have led directly to their exploitation in transistor radios and amplifiers, single-chip pocket calculators, microprocessors, computers etc., etc., and even to advantage in X-ray circuitry! Intrinsic semiconductors with such added impurities are known as *extrinsic* semiconductors, and are discussed in the following section.

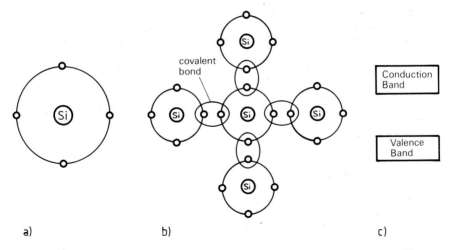

Fig. 19.2 Pure silicon as an example of an intrinsic semiconductor: (a) represents a silicon atom with 4 electrons in its outer (valence) shell; (b) demonstrates the covalent bonds formed in a pure silicon crystal by the sharing of electrons by neighbouring atoms; (c) shows the energy gap between the full valence band and the empty conduction band (at low temperatures).

19.2 EXTRINSIC SEMICONDUCTORS

The addition of controlled amounts of impurities to intrinsic semiconductors to produce extrinsic semiconductors is known as 'doping'. Doping may be 'heavy' or 'light', a typical concentration of the doping material being 1 atom for every 10 million silicon atoms (for example). The electrical conductivity of the extrinsic semiconductors so produced is very much greater than that of the intrinsic semiconductor, however, and is proportional to the concentration of the doping material (i.e. the number of impurity atoms per unit volume). The impurity atoms within the crystalline structure of the silicon are therefore the source of this greatly increased electrical conduction, and this is because the type of impurity is chosen to either enhance the electron flow in the conduction band or the positive-hole flow in the valence band. These two types of extrinsic semiconductors are known as '*N*' and '*P*-types' respectively.

19.2.1 *N*-type

The impurity added to make an intrinsic semiconductor an *N*-type ('*N*' for 'Negative') is *pentavalent*, i.e. it has 5 electrons in its outer shell. Arsenic, antimony and phosphorus are examples of pentavalent elements which are suitable for use as *N*-type impurities. Figure 19.3 illustrates the effect of introducing an atom of phosphorus, for example, into the crystalline structure of silicon. The covalent bands form as before (Fig. 19.2), but now there is an electron 'left over' in the outer orbit of each phosphorus atom, and this electron has an energy level which is only just below the bottom of the

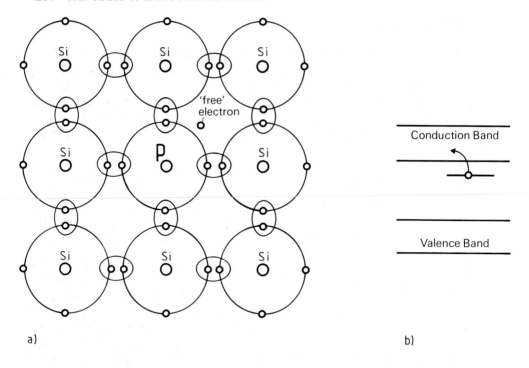

a)

b)

Fig. 19.3 Extrinsic semiconductor — *N*-type. The addition of donor impurities to an intrinsic semiconductor produces an extra 'free' electron which is able easily to reach the conduction band and take part in electrical conduction.

conduction band (Fig. 19.3(b)). At normal room temperatures it is therefore an effectively 'free' electron, since it is very easily lifted into the conduction band. It is therefore able to move through the crystal and take part in electrical conduction should a potential difference be applied across the crystal.

Since each phosphorus (or arsenic etc.) atom provides a 'spare' electron, it is an example of a so-called *donor* impurity. All suitable pentavalent atoms are also donor impurities since they 'donate' an electron to the conduction band.

However, it must also be remembered that some electrons from the *valence* band will also be able to jump up to the conduction band due to the effect of temperature, as in the case of an intrinsic semiconductor (19.1). Positive holes will therefore also be produced in the valence band and add to the conductivity. However, at normal temperatures this effect is much less than that of the extra conductivity produced by the donor electrons. Thus the so-called *majority carriers* are the electrons in the conduction band and the *minority carriers* are positive holes in the valence band in this case of an *N*-type semiconductor.

19.2.2 *P*-type

As may be inferred from the previous section, *P*-type semiconductors ('*P*' for 'Positive') enhance the conductivity of intrinsic semiconductors by increasing the flow of positive holes in the valence band. They do this simply by *increasing the number of vacancies* within the valence band, so that the electrons in that band are able to move from atom to atom, giving the appearance of positive charges moving in the opposite direction (see previous *Insight*).

Figure 19.4 illustrates the effect of using a *trivalent* impurity atom, i.e. one which has 3 electrons in its outer orbit — one less than silicon or germanium. There is a broken covalent bond between the impurity atom (aluminium in Fig. 19.4(a)) and the neighbouring silicon atoms because there are not enough electrons to form a full complement of bonds. The energy level of this broken bond is only just above the valence band, as shown in Figure 19.4(b), and so at normal room temperatures electrons from the valence band may readily jump this small gap. This means that electrons may leave the valence band of silicon and form positive holes 'behind' themselves. To put it another way, the presence of trivalent impurities results in as many vacancies, or holes, within the valence band of silicon as the number of impurity atoms. This type of impurity is known as an *acceptor impurity*, since it is able to 'accept' electrons from the surrounding silicon atoms and hence leave vacancies in the electron structure of the silicon itself.

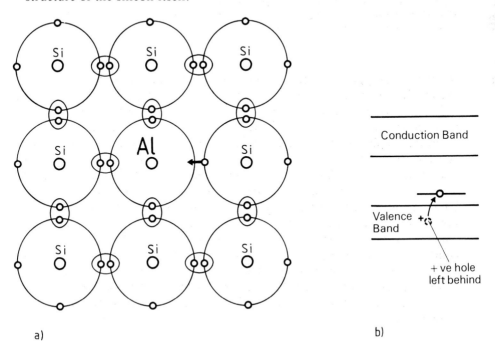

a)   b)

Fig. 19.4 Extrinsic semiconductor — *P*-type. Acceptor impurities (e.g. Al) take an electron from the valence band of the silicon [as shown in (a)] and leave a +ve hole capable of flowing through the valence band [as shown in (b)].

The *majority carriers* in this *P*-type material are positive holes in the valence band, and the *minority carriers* are electrons which find their way into the conduction band by the effect of temperature, as in a normal intrinsic semiconductor (19.1). Note that this is the opposite of *N*-type materials (19.2.1).

Table 19.1. is included here as a summary of the main points so far concerning intrinsic and the two types of extrinsic semiconductors. Note that an increase of temperature does not affect the conductivity due to the majority carriers, but only that due to the minority carriers, owing to the increased number of electrons able to reach the conduction band from the valence band as the temperature increases.

Table 19.1 Summary of properties of semiconductors

| | *Intrinsic semiconductors* | *extrinsic semiconductors* | |
		N–type	*P–type*
Typical material	Pure silicon or germanium	Silicon or germanium with added impurities	
Type of impurity	None	Pentavalent (e.g. As, P)	Trivalent (e.g. Al, Ga)
Term for impurity	—	Donor	Acceptor
Conductivity	Low	High	High
Majority carrier	(electrons and +ve holes in equal numbers)	Electrons in conduction band	+ve holes in valence band
Minority carrier		+ve holes in valence band	Electrons in conduction band
Effect of temperature	Increases numbers of both electrons and +ve holes	Increases numbers of minority carriers only	Increases numbers of minority carriers only

19.2.3 Diagrammatic representation of *N* and *P* types

In discussing the *P–N* junction (19.3) we shall need to form a mental picture of what occurs when an *N*-typed and a *P*-type semiconductor are fused together. This is made easier if a simple symbolic representation of each type is first outlined, as shown in Figure 19.5. Considering the *N*-type the 'free' donor electrons are, of course, represented by minus signs (−), while each nucleus of

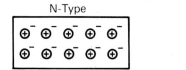
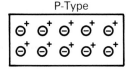

Fig. 19.5 Representation of *N* and *P*-type semiconductors. In both illustrations, the ringed charges represent immovable charges while the unringed charges represent free charges which constitute the 'majority carrier' for that material (electrons for the *N*-type and +ve holes for the *P*-type).

the donor impurity, having an excess charge because of the loss of its outer electron, is a fixed positive charge and is therefore represented by the symbol $\oplus$. In the *P*-type, it is the 'positive holes' which are 'free' and so are shown as plus signs ($+$), while the elctrons captured by the acceptor atoms give those atoms a surplus negative charge. Since the acceptor atoms themselves are fixed, the minus signs are shown ringed ($\ominus$). Thus, in either type of semiconductor the ringed charges are fixed and the 'free' charges are mobile.

There are also free positive and negative charges (not shown) in each material because of the thermal generation of electrons to the conduction band from the valence band — the 'minority' carriers.

19.3 THE *P–N* JUNCTION

Interesting effects appear when layers of *N* and *P* types are fused together to form so-called '*P–N* junctions'. Examples include the *P–N* junction diode, the transistor and the thyristor, which have one, two and three such junctions respectively.

Using the diagrammatic representation of *P*- and *N*-type semiconductors introduced in section 19.2.3. above, a *P–N* junction appears as shown in Figure 19.6. When the *P*- and *N*-types are brought together and intimate contact is

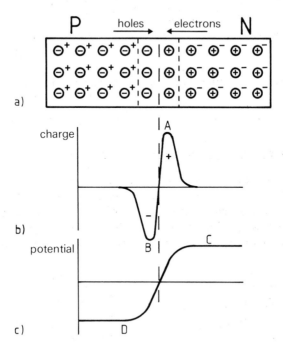

Fig. 19.6 The *P–N* junction. The diffusion of electrons across the *P–N* junction in one direction, and $+$ve holes in the other, forms a charge and potential distribution which prevents further flow. This area is known as the 'depletion layer', and the potential difference is the 'potential barrier'.

established (e.g. by 'fusing' of molten surfaces), then the free electrons of the *N*-type and the free positive holes of the *P*-type are able to penetrate across the boundary between them. This an example of *diffusion* and is due to the random movements of both types of carrier. The presence of free electrons and holes together results in recombination (19.1), i.e. the free electrons drop into the positive holes so that both charges are cancelled. Thus, for a short distance either side of the *P*–*N* junction (about 0.5×10^{-4} cm) no free carriers exist — this is therefore known as the '*depletion layer*'. However, a net charge exists on either side of the junction, as shown in Figure 19.6(b), because of the presence of the net charges on each impurity atom when its majority carrier has been cancelled. Thus, there is a negatively charged area just within the *P*-type region, and a positively charged area just within the *N*-type region. The two peaks of charge shown in Figure 19.6(b) increase in size until no further net flow of majority carriers can take place. For example, if it is imagined that a free electron of a given energy (i.e. a majority carrier of the *N*-type semiconductor) reaches A, then it will only be able to surmount the force pushing it back to the *N*-type material if its energy is greater than a certain value (because of the repulsion of the negative peak and the attraction of the positive peak when it is in the region of AB).

The charge distribution produces its own potential difference (9.6) as depicted in Figure 19.6(c) — the height of which, CD, is known as the *potential barrier* since it acts in opposition to the flow of majority carriers from either side of the barrier. For a silicon *P*–*N* junction, this potential barrier is about 0·4 volt, so that carriers of lower energy that 0·4 eV cannot surmount the barrier.

19.3.1 Minority carriers in the *P*–*N* junction

The above discussion concerned only the effect of the *P*–*N* junction on majority carriers, i.e. electrons in the *N*-type and positive holes in the *P*-type, and showed that a potential barrier was formed by diffusion which then prevented any further flow.

However, the barrier actually aids the transport of the *minority* carriers between both materials! If a free electron in the *P*-type, or a free positive hole in the *N*-type, should stray into the vicinity of the potential barrier, it is swept rapidly up (or down) the barrier into the other material. For example, an electron at D (Fig. 19.6(c)) is strongly attracted across to C, and a positive hole at D 'falls down' the potential gradient to D. At equilibrium, of course, there are equal numbers of minority carriers moving in both directions, so that there is no net flow of charge.

Now, minority carriers are thermally produced since an increased temperature increases the number of electrons which can jump up to the conduction band from the valence band. Therefore, the flow of minority carriers across the *P*–*N* junction also increases with temperature. This affects the behaviour of the *P*–*N* junction under conditions of 'reverse bias' as explained later.

19.3.2 Forward bias

If a source of potential difference (e.g. a battery) is connected to a *P–N* junction as shown in Figure 19.7(a), then a current will flow through the junction because the potential barrier is lowered (Fig. 19.7(b)). The negative side of the battery reduces the positive potential of the *N*-type and the positive side of the battery reduces the negative potential of the *P*-type, so that the original height of potential barrier is lowered and the more energetic of the electrons in the *N*-type (and positive holes in the *P*-type) are able to surmount the barrier. A steady electric current is therefore set up as long as the battery is connected. This type of connection is called 'forward bias', and produces current flow. The removal of the battery results in the full height of the potential barrier being re-established, and no further current can then flow.

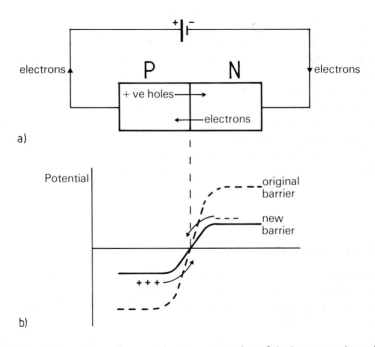

Fig. 19.7 The *P–N* junction — forward bias. The connection of the battery as shown lowers the potential barrier and allows a current to flow through the junction.

19.3.3 Reverse bias

If a battery, or other source of potential difference, is connected across a *P–N* junction in the opposite sense to that of Figure 19.7, it is known as 'reverse bias', and no current flows because the battery *increases* the potential barrier across the junction. This is shown in Figure 19.8(a) and (b), where the negative side of the battery increases the negative potential of the *P*-type, and the positive side of the battery increases the positive potential of the *N*-type so that the height of the potential barrier is increased and no current flows, since no

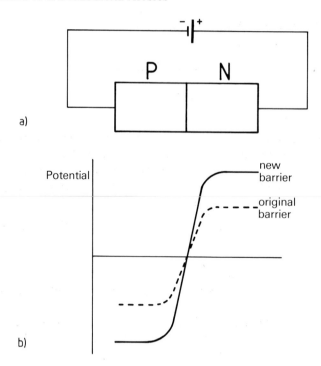

Fig. 19.8 The *P–N* junction — reverse bias. The connection of the battery in the opposite sense to Fig. 19.7 raises the potential barrier further and prevents electrical conduction.

majority carriers (electrons in the *N*-type and positive holes in the *P*-type) are able to surmount the higher barrier. However, as discussed in section 19.3.1, a small electric current due to the thermally generated minority carriers will be able to flow. The 'depletion layer' (19.3) extends further into each semiconductor on either side of the *P–N* junction under reverse bias.

19.3.4 The *P–N* junction as a diode

The previous two sections have shown that a 'forward bias' across a *P–N* junction produces a current flow, while a 'reverse bias' produces no (or very little) current. Thus, under normal circumstances:

A *P–N* junction passes electric current in one direction only.

The *P–N* junction therefore behaves in the same manner as a thermionic vacuum diode (18.3), and so is called by any of the following terms:

  a. a *P–N* junction diode
  b. a solid-state diode
or c. a semiconductor diode (or rectifier).

The symbol for the *P–N* junction diode is:

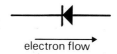

electron flow

Note that electrons may flow through the diode only *against* the direction of the arrow part of the symbol. Such solid state diodes have superior performance when compared to vacuum diodes, and so have largely superseded their use. Some of the advantages of a semiconductor diode compared to a thermionic vacuum diode include:

a.   no filament is required, leading to longer life and the expenditure of less power and heat

b.   rugged in operation

c.   smaller in size, enabling more compact X-ray units to be designed

d.   have a smaller forward 'voltage drop', therefore leaving a higher kV_p for the X-ray tube

e.   the reverse current is less than a vacuum diode owing to the small, but finite, thermionic emission from the anode of the latter.

19.3.5 *P–N* junction characteristic

If the current flowing through a *P–N* junction diode is plotted graphically against the potential difference across it, a 'characteristic' curve is produced (see also 18.3.2), as shown in Figure 19.9.

As the potential difference across the diode is increased in a forward direction, so the current through it increases, as shown by OA in the figure. No 'saturation' current exists (unlike the thermionic vacuum diode), but a current which is too high will damage the diode irreparably.

A reverse bias produces only a very low 'reverse current' (OB in the figure), all of which is due to the flow of minority carriers which have wandered close to (and been accelerated across) the potential barrier of the *P–N* junction (19.3.3). This reverse current is very sensitive to temperature, since the minority carriers are produced by thermal excitation (Table 19.1). If the reverse bias is increased, the reverse current suddenly increases dramatically (BC in the figure). This is so-called 'zener' or 'breakdown' region, and is put to good use in circuitry requiring an accurately maintained value of potential difference (the potential difference along line BC hardly changes at all, no matter what the current). The cause of the dramatic increase in the reverse current is multiplication, where the minority carriers gain so much energy in 'tumbling down' the potential barrier that they are able to ionise atoms with which they collide, resulting in more charges flowing and hence a higher current. This 'solid-state multiplication' is also referred to as the 'avalanche effect'.

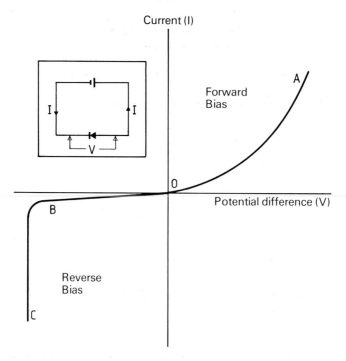

Fig. 19.9 The 'characteristic' of the *P–N* junction. Increasing the potential difference across the junction (inset) in the forward bias direction increases the current flowing through the device (OA in the figure). There is only a small current in the reverse bias direction (OB) due to minority carriers (see text). BC is the 'breakdown' or 'avalanche' or 'zener' region. The *P–N* junction thus acts as a solid-state diode, since it only allows current to flow in one direction.

19.4 THE TRANSISTOR

The transistor is a solid-state device which has largely replaced the use of valves in electronic circuits. Recently the transistor itself, as a single discrete circuit component, has been replaced in many applications by large numbers of transistors and other components on a single small silicon crystal (a 'chip'). This technique is known as Large Scale Integration (LSI), as mentioned at the beginning of this chapter, and the piece of silicon is referred to as an Integrated Circuit (IC). The transistors on such an IC are of the 'field-effect' type and are discussed in section 19.4.2. First, however, the 'junction' transistor is considered.

19.4.1 The *NPN* junction transistor

The junction transistor is composed of three alternating layers of semiconducting materials, i.e. either *NPN* or *PNP*. In both cases there are two *P–N* junctions, of course. Only the *NPN* transistor is considered here although the *PNP* transistor is very similar (the majority carriers are positive holes rather than electrons). An *NPN* transistor is shown illustrated in Figure 19.10(a),

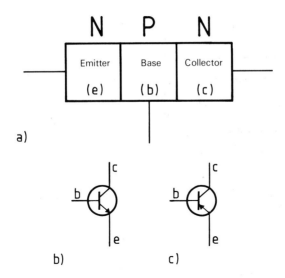

Fig. 19.10 The *NPN* junction transistor, and its symbol — (a) and (b). The symbol of the *PNP* transistor is shown in (c).

together with its electrical symbol (Fig. 19.10(b)). The central *P*-type semiconductor material is known as the 'base', as the two other types are joined to it. These form the 'emitter' and 'collector' respectively.

The factors which determine which of the two *N*-types is the emitter and which is the collector are the geometry of the device (i.e. how it is constructed) and the concentration of the impurity doping (19.2) in the two materials. Typically, the emitter contains 1000 times more 'doping' than the collector and 100 times that of the base. The emitter thus contains a ready supply of charge carriers ('extra' electrons from the *N*-type doping) which are available for flowing through the transistor as a whole. The symbols for both types of transistor are illustrated in Figure 10.10(b) and (c), where the emitter is distinguished by the arrow sign: the convention being that the direction of the arrow is in the direction in which holes would flow, i.e. opposite to the direction of electron flow. This is the same for the diode symbol (19.3.4).

Figure 19.11 shows the separation of the action of the *NPN* transistor in terms of its two *PN* junctions. In Figure 19.11(a), the base and collector are connected to a battery so that they are under 'reverse-bias' conditions (19.3.3), and only a very small current flows due to the passage of the thermally produced minority carriers across the *PN* junction, i.e. electrons from the *P*-type base, and positive holes from the *N*-type collector. Figure 19.11(b) shows the *PN* junction between the emitter and base connected in a 'forward-bias' configuration (19.3.2), when a larger current is able to flow than in Figure 19.11(a). However, if these two circuits are joined together (Fig. 19.11(c)) then it is found that almost the same current flows through both emitter and collector, while the current from the base is very small. Thus it may appear that the reverse bias across the 'base to collector' *PN* junction (as

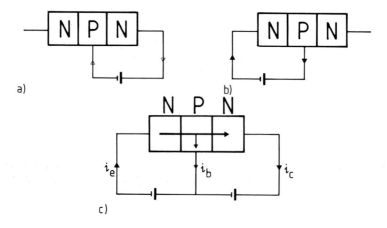

Fig. 19.11 The principle of operation of the *NPN* junction transistor. See text for details.

shown in Fig. 19.11(a)) has been destroyed since a very much larger current may now flow into the the collector than was possible before. However, it should be remembered that the reverse bias applies to the *majority* carriers (i.e. positive holes in the base). Therefore, when electrons are injected into the base from the emitter they become the *minority* carriers within the base, and as such, are readily attracted across the 'collector to base' *PN* junction. So efficient is this process that approximately 98% of all electrons injected into the base from the emitter are able to diffuse across the base and form the collector current. The remaining 2% forms the base current. The collector current is thus about 50 times the base current, the figure being constant for a particular transistor. The base current may therefore be used to control the larger collector current so that an *amplified* current (or voltage) signal may be obtained from the collector of the transistor. Amplification, however, is only one use of the transistor in electronics. Section 19.6 shows some applications of transistors in radiography.

19.4.2 The field-effect transistor

The field-effect transistor (FET) is a device which is capable of varying the current flowing through a semiconductor by means of an electric field (9.4). In this respect it is very similar in operation to the triode valve (18.4). There are several different types of FET, of which the simplest is shown in Figure 19.12, where a central rod of *N*-type material has a 'collar' of *P*-type material around it. The purpose of this collar or 'gate' is to vary the electron flow through the *N*-type material by varying the potential applied to it. One end of the transistor is the 'Source' and the other end is the 'Drain', corresponding to the direction of electron flow. If a negative potential is placed on the gate, then the *P–N* junction is under reverse bias and the electric field so produced extends the 'depletion layer' further into the *N*-type material (19.3.3). This is shown by

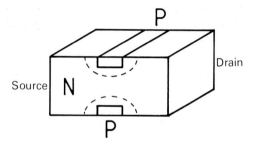

Fig. 19.12 A field-effect transistor (FET). The connection of a reverse bias between the *P*- and *N*-type semiconductors extends the depletion layer and reduces the electron flow.

the dotted lines in Figure 19.12, and is the area from which the majority carriers have been removed so reducing the overall electrical conductivity of the *N*-type. Hence, the electric current through the FET transistor decreases as the potential applied to the gate becomes more negative. At a particular 'pinch-off' potential, no current is able to flow at all. Thus, the current through both types of transistor is controlled by the application of a potential to a *P–N* junction.

The FET transistor has a high input impedance compared to a junction transistor, and means that a lower current is needed to control the device. A typical value of the input impedance (15.4.2) is $10^8 \Omega$, compared to about $10^5 \Omega$ for a junction transistor. This is an important consideration when attempting to amplify very low signals. However, an FET is more fragile than a junction transistor and is likely to be damaged by the presence of static electricity (e.g. if touched) or variations in the electrical supply.

19.5 THE THYRISTOR

The thyristor, or silicon-controlled rectifier (SCR), is the solid-state equivalent of the thyratron (18.5) and has very similar operating characteristics. It is composed of four alternating *N* and *P* semiconductor layers, as shown diagrammatically in Figure 19.13(a). A battery is shown connected so that the thyristor is in the 'forward-bias' condition. *PN* junctions *J*1 and *J*3 are forward-biased (19.3.2) but junction *J*2 is reverse-biased (19.3.3). Consequently only a small leakage current (due to minority carriers) flows through the thyristor and the external circuit. If, however, a positive pulse is applied to the *P*-type layer of junction *J*1 (as shown in the figure) then positive holes are injected into the *P*-type and flow across junction *J*1 so that the potential barrier across *J*1 is much reduced (19.3.2). Also, of course, electrons from the *N*-type flow across to the *P*-type at junction *J*1. The reduced potential difference across *J*1 means that a higher reverse potential difference than before exists across *J*2, and, if high enough, will cause breakdown to occur at *J*2 due to the avalanche effect (19.3.5). Note the similarity here to the thyratron,

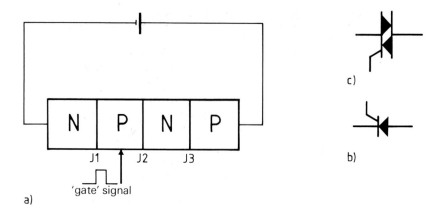

a)
b)
c)

Fig. 19.13 The thyristor. An *NPNP* thyristor is shown in (a). A 'gate' signal as shown makes the thyristor conduct until the potential difference across it is reduced to zero. (b) and (c) show the symbols for the thyristor and triac respectively.

where 'gas multiplication' takes place. The effect of the positive signal on the 'gate' is therefore to switch the thyristor hard on. However, it is usually not possible to switch the thyratron off again by putting a *negative* pulse on the gate (particularly for a thyristor designed to take a high current); it is the usual practice to switch the thyristor off by reducing the overall voltage across it to zero, when the avalanche current at *J2* can no longer be maintained. Again, note the similarity to the way the thyratron is switched off (18.5).

A *Triac* is a device which is able to switch on when both negative and positive potential differences are applied across it. It may be considered as being equivalent to two thyratrons placed in parallel but facing in opposite directions, as illustrated by the symbol of a triac as shown in Figure 19.13(c).

19.6 SEMICONDUCTOR DEVICES IN RADIOGRAPHY

Table 19.2 gives a very brief list of some uses to which semiconductor devices have been put in radiographic circuits. For example, 'wafers' of *P–N* junctions (i.e. individual thin *P–N* junction) are joined together in series to form a 'cartridge' suitable for use in high-tension rectification (Ch. 20). This is necessary in order that the solid-state rectifier so formed will be able to withstand the high reverse potential difference of the high tension supply. The mA meter is not subject to a high potential difference owing to its low resistance (17.2) and so does not require any more than single *P–N* junctions for its rectification.

Specialised electronic circuits employing semiconductor 'logic' elements are enjoying increased use in the control of X-ray tube. They replace electro-mechanical devices such as relays (12.5) and are smaller, faster in operation, more reliable and very inexpensive. Such logic circuits are made by the connection of transistors and other components into an Integrated Circuit

Table 19.2 Applications of semiconductor devices

Semiconductor device	Applications
Diode	HT rectification for X-ray tube, using cartridges of P–N junctions
	Rectification for mA and mAs meter
	Voltage-doubling circuits
	Circuit protection from electrical surges
	Power supplies (zener diodes) — to obtain constant voltage
Transistor	Electronic timing circuits
	Power supply circuits
	Safety interlock circuits to avoid exceeding the rating of the X-ray tube
Thyristor/Triac	Primary switching of HT transformer for an integral number of half-cycles
	Dimming of room lights
Logic circuits	Interlock circuits, to check system prior to exposure (e.g. anode up to speed etc.)
LSI 'chips'/ microprocessors	Sophisticated measurement and control of rating parameters (e.g. anode temperature)
	'Modelling' of complete X-ray unit for interlock circuits

package (19.4), which is sealed by a plastic or ceramic case to protect it. Unfortunately, the description of such logic devices (e.g. 'AND', 'OR' gates etc.) is beyond the scope of this book, for they form a fascinating subject in their own right.

As mentioned previously, the advent of the microprocessor is expected to make a significant impact on the automatic checking and control of X-ray units. A microprocessor is a *programmable* logic element, and may perform whatever set of operations it is programmed to do. Thus, it is a general-purpose system for the control and measurement of electronic signals. Its great advantage over ordinary logical circuitry is that it is very flexible as to the sort of operations it may perform, and may hence save a great deal of wiring, number of components and development time. A slight change of the types of operations required, or their sequences, necessitates a change in the computer program (the 'software') rather than a change to the wiring or the components (the 'hardware'). It is this adaptability, coupled to its very low cost, which is the reason for predicted impact of the microprocessor on our everyday lives, as well as a greater ranger of X-ray circuitry over which it will take control.

Exercise 19.1

    a. What is meant by the terms:

    (i) valence band
   (ii) conduction band
  (iii) free electron
  (iv) bound electron?

Illustrate your answer with diagrams where possible.

b.   What is an intrinsic semiconductor? How is the conductivity of an intrinsic semiconductor altered by adding impurities? Hence explain what is meant by:

(i) extrinsic semiconductor
(ii) P-type semiconductor
(iii) N-type semiconductor

c.   'The majority carriers in an N-type semiconductor are electrons and the minority carriers are positive holes.' Explain this statement, paying special attention to the words which are underlined. What are the majority and minority carriers for a P-type semiconductor?

d.   What is meant by the term 'P–N junction'? Show how such a junction is able to conduct an electric current when 'forward-biased', but not when 'reverse-biased'. Illustrate your answer with the 'characteristic curve' of a P-N junction.

e.   What is meant by a 'solid-state diode'? What uses does such a device have in radiography?

f.   Explain the meaning of the terms:

(i) depletion layer
(ii) potential barrier

when applied to a P–N junction. Hence show why such a junction is able to pass an electric current in one direction only.

g.   What are the advantages of a solid-state rectifier over a thermionic vacuum valve rectifier?

h.   Describe *either* the action of a transistor *or* the action of a thyristor. What purposes are *both* devices used for in X-ray circuitry?

i.   Write short notes on:

(i) electronic logic circuits
(ii) the field-effect transistor
(iii) the microprocessor.

SUMMARY

1.   A semiconductor has a conductivity between an insulator and a conductor, reflecting the small energy gap between its conduction and valence bands.
2.   An *intrinsic* semiconductor is a pure semiconductor. *Extrinsic* semiconductors have carefully measured quantities of *impurity* added to the pure intrinsic substance — this process is known as *doping*.
3.   Impurities are two types: *donor* and *acceptor*. A donor impurity is pentavalent and gives a free electron to the semiconductor, which is known as an N-*type*. An acceptor impurity is trivalent and takes an electron form the semicondutor, which is known as a P-*type*.
4.   The *majority carrier* in an *N*-type is the electron (donated by the impurity); that of the *P*-type is the *positive hole* left in the valence band.

5. An electron movement to the right in the valence band of a *P*-type is the same as a positive hole movement to the left, since the 'vacancy' moves to the original location of each electron.

6. *Minority carriers* are thermally produced and are present in all semiconductor materials at room temperature. They result from the excitation of electrons from the valence band to the conduction band (leaving positive holes behind). Minority carriers in a *P*-type are electrons in the conduction band, and minority carriers in an *N*-type are positive holes in the valence band.

7. A *P–N* junction produces a 'potential barrier' to the flow of electrons and holes which grows in height when the junction is 'reverse-biased' and diminishes when it is 'forward-biased'. Thus the *P–N* junction allows an electric current to flow in one direction only, i.e. it acts as a diode.

8. *P–N* junctions may be joined in series to produce adequate rectification for X-ray units.

9. The advantage of such solid-state rectifiers over thermionic vacuum diode rectifiers may be summarised as:

(a) smaller   (b) more rugged   (c) no filament circuitry required
(d) lower reverse current   (e) lower forward voltage drop.

10. The transistor is a 2 *P–N* junction device used in electronic control circuitry. A small 'base' current is used to control a larger 'collector' current, so that signal amplification is possible.

11. The thyristor is the solid-state equivalent of a thyratron and is composed of 3 *P–N* junctions. A 'gate' signal is used to switch the device on, after which it may only be switched off by reducing the potential difference across it to a low value. The thyristor and triac are used for primary switching of X-ray tubes for an integral number of half-cycles.

20. Rectification and exposure control

Chapters 14 to 16 have shown that it is convenient to use an alternating supply of electricity (AC) because of the ease with which it may be either 'stepped up' or 'stepped down' to levels of potential difference (PD) required by an X-ray tube. The High-tension Transformer produces a large PD (usually 50–120 kV_p) which is connected across the X-ray tube, and the filament transformer produces a low potential difference and a high current (a few amperes) to provide sufficient thermionic emission from the tungsten filament of the tube. However, as is described in more detail in Chapter 21, the X-ray tube is designed to emit X-rays when the electrons travel from the filament and strike the anode, i.e. when the anode is positive with respect to the filament and thus attracts the electrons towards itself. An alternating potential difference (PD) across the tube is therefore undesirable for two reasons:

a. the *inverse* potential difference (i.e. when the anode is negative with respect to the filament) produces no X-ray emission from the anode, since no electrons are able to strike it

b. the sinusoidally changing PD produces an X-ray beam which is continually changing in intensity, being at a maximum when the PD across the tube is also at a peak (i.e. at the kV_p), since intensity $\propto kV^2$ (28.2.2).

The inverse PD is, at best, a waste of time since only alternate half-cycles are used to generate X-rays and, at worst, may irreparably damage the X-ray tube in certain circumstances (see 20.1.1). The *ideal* situation is where a high value of steady DC voltage is applied across the X-ray tube for as long as the exposure is to last. The process whereby an alternating voltage is made to approximate to this ideal is called *rectification*. There are various types of rectification, depending upon the purposes for which a particular X-ray unit is to be used. As outlined below, the more highly powered and sophisticated an X-ray unit needs to be, the more closely does the rectification have to approach the ideal.

20.1 HALF-WAVE RECTIFICATION

As its name suggests, half-wave rectification utilises only alternate half-cycles, i.e. only one-half of the total number of half-cycles. The inverse half-cycles are therefore simply unused and the X-ray beam is alternately switched on and off for the duration of each half-cycle.

There are two basic circuits used in half-wave rectification: the 'self-rectified' and '2-diode half-wave rectified' circuits as outlined below.

20.1.1 Self-rectification

Figure 20.1 shows a simplified 'self-rectified HT circuit', i.e. a circuit which uses the X-ray tube as a diode. The tube itself therefore not only produces the X-rays, but ensures that the electrons flow only from the filament to the anode, since the X-ray tube behaves in a similar manner to a thermionic vacuum-diode (18.3.2). The voltage across the X-ray tube is an alternating sinusoidal

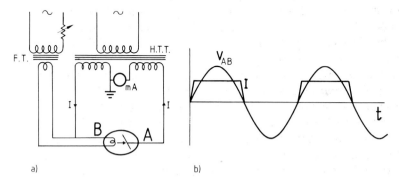

Fig. 20.1 A self-rectified circuit and its current and voltage waveforms.

waveform as shown by V_{AB} in Figure 20.1(b). However, the current waveform is flat-topped (since the X-ray tube is 'saturated' — 18.6).

General note
> The mA meter in the figures of this and other chapters is shown connected to the central point of the transformer secondary, and one side is 'earthed', i.e. connected to zero potential. See section 17.7.3 for the explanation of this arrangement.

The *advantages* of a self-rectified circuit are:

a. simplicity of circuitry
b. relatively inexpensive
c. HT transformer may be situated within the oil of the X-ray housing, making a very compact unit with no external HT leads.

The *disadvantages* of a self-rectified circuit are:

a. it is only suitable for low power work, e.g. in dentistry or for some mobile units
b. only half of the available voltage waveform is utilised
c. the inverse voltage is larger than the forward voltage owing to the effect of regulation (16.3.3) — this may, however, be corrected by additional simple circuitry

d.   the possibility of damaging the X-ray tube by exceeding the somewhat modest capability (or 'rating') of the X-ray tube when used in a self-rectified circuit.

It is the last disadvantage which imposes the most severe restrictions to the use of the self-rectified circuit. Damage to the X-ray tube will occur if a significant *reverse* current is able to flow in the X-ray tube, since this results in electron bombardment of the filament. The reverse current is able to flow if the anode becomes so hot that it starts to release electrons by *thermionic emission.* This is no surprise, since the anode, like the filament, is made of tungsten and if the filament emits electrons when its temperature is raised then so will the anode. The critical factor with the self-rectified circuit is therefore the temperature of the anode, and no exposure or series of exposures should be made which will raise this temperature to the point of significant thermionic emission. The remaining circuits of this chapter all overcome this limitation by the insertion of extra diodes.

20.1.2 Two-diode half-wave rectification

The insertion of two diodes into the secondary circuit of the high-tension transformer overcomes some of the problems associated with the self-rectified circuit described above. The circuit shown in Figure 20.2(a) shows two semiconductor diodes $D1$ and $D2$, although thermionic vacuum diodes may be

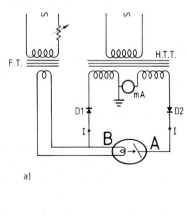

a)

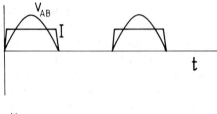

b)

Fig. 20.2 A two-diode rectifier circuit and its current and voltage waveforms. Note the absence of an 'inverse' voltage (see previous figure).

used instead. The waveforms (Fig. 202.(b)) are similar to those of the self-rectified circuit (Fig. 20.1(b)) with the important difference that there is *no inverse voltage* across the X-ray tube.

The 2-diode half-wave rectifier circuit separates the functions of rectification and X-ray production: the diodes are used to ensure that electrons cannot flow from the anode to the filament (even if the anode becomes sufficiently hot to emit electrons), and the X-ray tube is used solely to produce X-rays.

Two diodes are used so that:

    a.   the circuit is symmetrical, giving equal (but opposite) values of kV to the ends of the X-ray tube

    b.   failure of one diode does not result in damage to the X-ray tube, since the other diode will also prevent a reverse current from flowing.

For this circuit, the critical factor limiting the electrical power which may be applied to the X-ray tube is not now the temperature at which the anode becomes a thermionic emitter, but the temperature at which the surface of the tungsten anode melts (about 3000°C). The melting point of tungsten exceeds the temperature at which it becomes a significant thermionic emitter (about 1500°C) so that a higher value of mA may be used than in the self-rectified circuit before X-ray tube damage will occur. The 'working temperature' of the anode is usually limited to about 2500°C to prolong the life of the tube. For short exposures, the same X-ray tube may be used at approximately 50% more power when two diodes are connected (e.g. 1·5 times the mA for the same kV_p).

20.2 FOUR-DIODE FULL-WAVE RECTIFICATION

The two circuits described in the previous section for half-wave rectification have the serious disadvantage that only alternate half-cycles are used to produce X-rays. Thus the X-ray tube is actually switched off for one-half of the total exposure time! If every half-cycle can be used to produce X-rays, then a greater range of exposure settings may be used. In order to utilise all half-cycles, four diodes are used in the secondary circuit of the high-tension transformer (Fig. 20.3). Figures 20.3(a) and (b) are actually identical, but look somewhat different at first sight. The former is perhaps the easier to understand as it is just an extension of the 2-diode rectifier circuit (Fig. 20.2), i.e. diodes D1 and D2 are the same in both figures. Only diodes D3 and D4 have been added. D1 and D2 rectify one half-cycle (i.e. when F is negative with respect to E), D3 and D4 rectify the next half-cycle (when E is negative with respect to F) and so on. It is as if the diodes D1 and D2 were able to be quickly joined to the alternating ends of the secondary of the high-tension transformer so that D1 was always joined to the negative end, thus ensuring that the diodes would conduct and electrons would flow from the filament to the anode for each half-cycle. Obviously, such an arrangement would be extremely difficult to achieve in practice, and is quite unnecessary, as D3 and D4 may be joined as shown to cope with the inverse half-cycle. The electron flow for the two

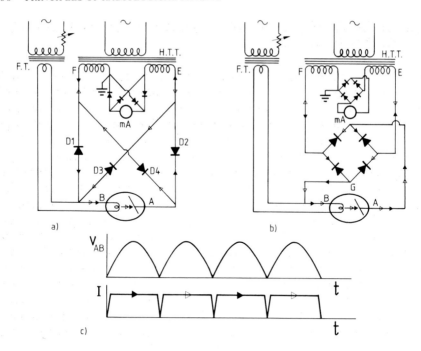

Fig. 20.3 A full-wave rectifier circuit. (a) and (b) are identical circuits, but are drawn differently. Diodes D1 and D2 conduct for one half-cycle (shown by ➤—) and D3 and D4 conduct for the next half-cycle (shown by ➔—). The voltage and current waveforms are shown in (c).

different half-cycles is shown in both Figure 20.3(a) and (b). In each case $D1$ and $D2$ conduct for one half-cycle while $D3$ and $D4$ conduct for the next.

Figure 20.3(b) is known as a *Gratz bridge circuit*, and is just a redrawing of Figure 20.3(a). A useful tip drawing the bridge circuit is to ensure that the arrows on the diode symbols all point the same way from point G, as shown in the figure.

Each of the figures shows the mA meter also fully rectified. This is because current flows both ways in the transformer secondary so that a moving coil milliammeter (17.5) would suffer rapidly alternating deflections and would not indicate the true current flowing through the X-ray tube. To do this, it must be rectified to the same extent as the X-ray tube, so that all electron flow is in one direction only. Alternatively, a moving iron meter may be used, but this is not so accurate (17.7).

Figure 20.3(c) shows the voltage and current waveforms of the full-wave rectified circuit. The voltage across transformer *secondary* is still alternating, but that across the X-ray tube (V_{AB}) has been fully rectified, i.e. the anode is always positive with respect to the filament. A current therefore flows through the tube (and X-rays are produced) for each half-cycle, as indicated by the current waveform in the figure.

20.3 COMPARISON OF HALF-WAVE AND FULL-WAVE RECTIFICATION

Figure 20.4(a) and (b) shows the current waveforms for half-wave and full-wave rectification which produce the *same value of mA*. The current waveforms for the half-wave rectifier are twice as high as those for the full-wave rectifier because the mA measures the *average* current flowing through the X-ray tube. Since every other current waveform is missing, the height of each waveform must be doubled to achieve the same average current, or, to put it another way, the *area* under each graph must be equal for each complete cycle to produce identical values of mA. This is an important consideration for short exposure times (a few cycles), since the half-wave system inevitably deposits twice the energy on the anode during its 'on' half-cycle than does the full-wave system. The anode therefore reaches a higher temperature than for the full-wave system (for the same mA). Conversely, the mA on the full-wave system may be increased by about a factor of two over the half-wave system before the same anode temperature is reached. This also allows exposure times to be reduced by one-half. For long exposure times (greater than about 5 seconds), however, the effect of individual half-cycles on anode temperature is much less important, and maximum mA and kV_p settings are very similar in both cases.

This comparison is an example of the way in which X-ray tube *rating* depends upon the type of rectification. For further discussion on rating, see Chapter 22.

20.4 CONSTANT VOLTAGE (POTENTIAL) CIRCUITS

A full-wave rectified X-ray tube is not an *ideal* system (as described at the beginning of this chapter) in that the potential difference applied across the

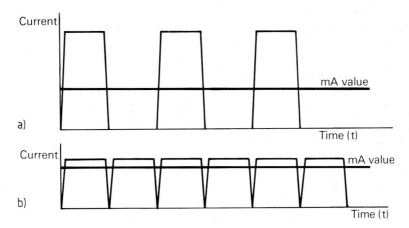

Fig. 20.4 The current and mA (average current) for (a) half-wave rectification, and (b) full-wave rectification.

tube is *pulsating*, and not constant. This has three principal disadvantages:

    a.   the anode receives rapidly varying amounts of energy
    b.   the intensity of the X-ray beam varies over each half-cycle
    c.   the quality (or effective energy — Ch. 29) of the beam varies over each
half-cycle.

The anode is better able to cope with the considerable energy being deposited on it if the energy is at a steady level over the period of exposure, so that there are no periods of higher thermal stress than others. The variation of the intensity of the beam is a serious disadvantage if very rapid sequential X-ray images are required, when some images will be darker than others depending upon which part of the half-cycle was being utilised at the time. The effect of the changing quality of the X-ray beam (see Chapter 29) is to increase the radiation dose received by the patient owing to a relatively large amount of 'soft' radiation from the smaller kV values of each half-cycle. Some of this may be removed using filters (29.1), but the best way of solving this, and the other, problems is to ensure a constant voltage (or potential) across the X-ray tube. Three methods of achieving a constant potential circuit are described briefly in the remainder of this section.

20.4.1 Capacitor-smoothed full-wave circuit

A capacitor may be used to 'smooth' the voltage applied to an X-ray tube for either half-wave or full-wave rectification circuits; the latter has been chosen here to indicate the principle. Figure 20.5 shows the inclusion of capacitors $C1$ and $C2$ to the usual full-wave rectified circuit (Fig. 20.3) to 'smooth' the voltage waveform across the X-ray tube. The capacitors are charged up quickly when the exposure starts (OC in Fig. 20.5(b)) but discharge more slowly than the usual pulsating voltage (i.e. CD rather than CF). This situation is analogous to a capacitor discharging through a resistance (see 9.10.1) — the X-ray tube acting as a 'resistance'. The voltage across the X-ray tube is therefore subject to less variation, the variation being termed the 'ripple', as shown in the figure. The voltage ripple depends upon the current flowing through the X-ray tube, since a high current means a fast loss of charge from the capacitor, and the voltage across the capacitor (V_{AB}) is proportional to the charge which remains ($V = Q/C$ — see 9.7).

    The high-tension cables also possess capacitance and therefore already smooth the voltage waveform to some extent. However, the capacity of the cables is quite small and so has a significant smoothing effect only for exposures using low mA values, e.g. in fluoroscopy.

20.4.2 Triode smoothing

The circuit shown in Figure 20.6 is an example of 'secondary switching' as well as 'constant potential'. It uses the characteristics of a vacuum triode (18.4) to switch the X-ray tube on and off as well as to correct for the residual voltage ripple present on circuits like Figure 20.5.

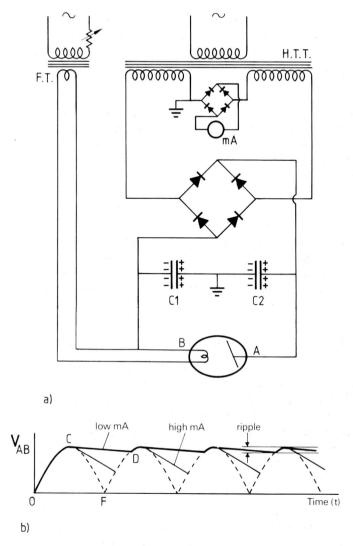

a)

b)

Fig. 20.5 A capacitor-smoothed circuit. Capacitors C1 and C2 store charge and discharge slowly through the X-ray tube, e.g. CD in (b).

Normally the X-ray tube is held in the 'off' condition by holding the grids of each triode strongly negative with respect to the cathodes. At a signal from the timer, the grid potentials are taken more positive so that each triode conducts strongly and the exposure starts. When the timer sends its next signal, the grid potentials are taken strongly negative again and the exposure is terminated. However, *during* the exposure small signals are also applied to the grids of the triodes from circuits Y1 and Y2. The higher the voltage in the ripple waveform, the more negative do these small signals become, so that the electrons are slightly more impeded in their progress through each triode at these moments. Thus the resistance to electron flow through the triodes is made to increase as

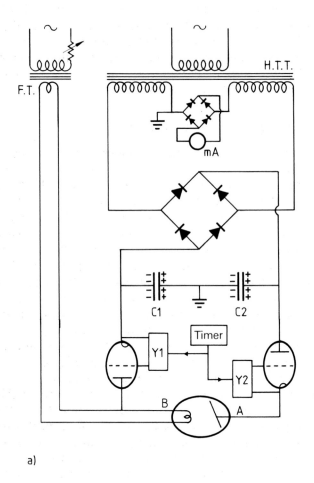

a)

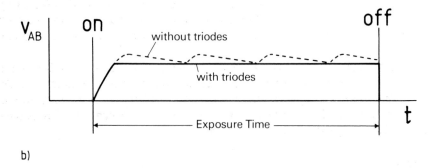

b)

Fig. 20.6 A triode-smoothed and switched secondary circuit. Control voltages from circuits Y1 and Y2 alter the 'potential drop' across each triode, and hence the potential applied to the X-ray tube, as shown in (b).

the ripple height increases so that there is a larger 'potential drop' across them. By suitable electronic design of the circuits within $Y1$ and $Y2$ the ripple across the X-ray tube may be almost completely eliminated, as shown in Figure 20.6(b). This is because the voltage corresponding to the height of the ripple is made to be dropped across the triodes, leaving the voltage to the base of the ripple applied across the X-ray tube itself.

20.4.3 Three-phase rectification

An introduction to 3-phase electrical supplies is given in section 15.6. The 3-phase rectifier circuit does not produce a precisely constant potential difference across the X-ray tube, but it does have a small voltage ripple and allows the highest X-ray beam intensities of any rectifier circuits. There are two types of 3-phase rectifier circuit: '6-pulse' and '12-pulse' per cycle. Only the former is described here, although the latter approximates even more closely to true 'constant potential'. The circuits may or may not have smoothing capacitors as described in the previous section; Figure 20.7(a) is shown without them for clarity. The explanation of the action of this circuit is rather more complicated than previously encountered owing to the rectification of three phases rather than just one. The current flow pattern through the diodes $D1$ to $D6$ changes from moment to moment, depending upon which phase has the highest voltage, so the situation for one moment of time only will be described here. This moment is shown in Figure 20.7(b) and occurs when phase 1 is at its maximum negative value and phases 2 and 3 are at half of their maximum positive values. The electron flow pattern for this situation is then shown in the figure: all the electrons flow through diode $D1$ on their way to the X-ray tube, but half flow through $D4$ and half through $D6$ on their way back to the secondary windings. A complete circuit is thus made, and no electrons are gained or lost from the system, as expected.

The effect of the rectification is to make all the negative waveforms become positive (as was the case for full-wave rectification), so that the final voltage (given by the addition of all the positive waveforms) has a total of 6 peaks per single-phase cycle, i.e. it is a '6-pulse' rectifier. The voltage ripple of such a system is small, so that an almost constant potential results across the X-ray tube.

The adoption of the 'delta' and 'star' configurations (15.6.1) for the primary and secondary windings of the high-tension transformers is because a delta connection allows a higher primary current to flow than a star connection and a star connection allows the use of an earth point as shown, ensuring equal kV stresses to either side of the X-ray tube.

Exercise 20.1

a.   Describe what is meant by the term 'rectification' when applied to an AC supply. How is this relevant to the potential difference applied across an X-ray tube?

b.   Draw a simple circuit illustrating the principle of 'self-rectification', and show how the voltage and current waveforms vary with time.

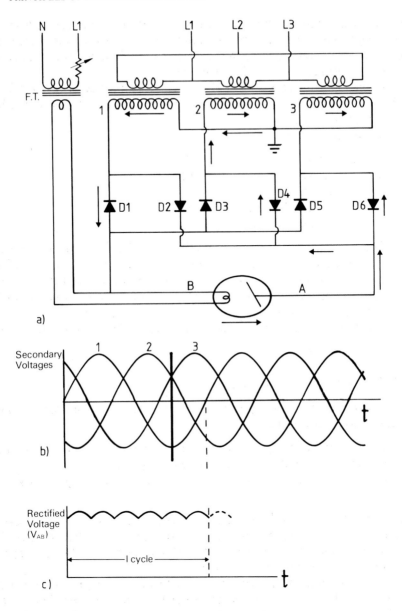

Fig. 20.7 A three-phase rectifier circuit. Electron flow through the diodes in (a) is shown for the moment of time indicated in (b). The rectified potential results in 6 pulses per cycle, as shown in (c).

c. What are the advantages and disadvantages of a self-rectified X-ray tube? Show how the '2-diode half-wave rectifier circuit' overcomes some of these disadvantages.

d. What is meant by the 'mA' passing through an X-ray tube? Why is the value of the mA different from the current passing through the tube for a half-wave rectified circuit?

e.   Draw a '4-diode full-wave rectifier circuit'. For practice, redraw this circuit using thermionic vacuum valves as the diodes. Sketch the current and voltage waveforms, and indicate the advantages which such a circuit possesses over both the self-rectified and 2-diode circuits.

f.   Using the same scales, draw the voltage and current waveforms for all the circuits in the above questions, paying special attention to the similarities and differences between them.

g.   Write short notes on:

(i) inverse voltage
(ii) thermionic emission from the anode
(iii) mA meter rectification
(iv) constant potential (voltage) rectification
(v) capacity of high-tension cables.

h.   What are the advantages of supplying an X-ray tube with a constant potential difference? Draw and describe a simple circuit diagram of any rectification circuit which provides an approximation to a constant potential.

i.   What is the effect on radiation 'quality', intensity and 'anode loading' of a constant potential compared to a full-wave rectifier circuit?

j.   What are the advantages and disadvantages of using a 3-phase rectifier circuit?

20.4.4 Primary switching

In order to deliver an X-ray exposure for an accurately-known time interval, it is necessary to do two things:

a.   heat the filament to its working temperature to produce adequate thermionic emission of electrons for the required mA

b.   supply a high voltage across the X-ray tube for the required length of time.

In addition, if the tube is of the rotating anode type, then the anode must reach its correct speed of rotation before the exposure, or it may be damaged. The sequence of events is thus to prepare ('prep') the set first, and then to apply a high voltage over a precise time interval.

A simplified circuit which uses a *contactor* to switch the high voltage on and off is shown in Figure 20.8. An X-ray contactor is a very rugged and heavy-duty electromagnetic relay (12.5) designed to have fast switching times. A timer, which may be mechanical, electro-mechanical or eletronic, energises the electromagnet S which closes the contacts C quickly by exerting a strong force of magnetic attraction. The closing of the contacts C completes the primary circuit to the high-tension transformer, so initiating the exposure. This circuit is therefore an example of *primary* switching. At the end of the exposure time as determined by the timer, the current from the timer circuit is switched off, enabling the springs in the contactor to break the contacts C and hence also the primary circuit. This removes the power to the high-tension transformer, terminates the emission of X-rays and thus the exposure.

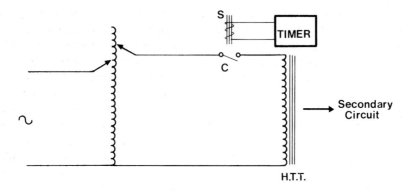

Fig. 20.8 Simplified circuit diagram of primary switching using an electromagnetic relay (contactor). The current from the timer determines how long the contact C is closed, and therefore the exposure time.

More sophisticated contactor circuits may use separate switch-on and switch-off contactors connected in series, and incorporate methods to synchronise the opening and closing of the contacts to those times when the mains voltage passes through zero during its AC waveform (Ch. 15). This prevents arcing across the contacts, leading to a longer contact life, and greatly reduces voltage 'spikes' which can otherwise be fed to the high-tension transformer leading to electrical breakdown within the X-ray tube housing. Timing the switch-on and switch-off times to the mains waveform results in exposure times which are an integral number of half-cycles, i.e. in multiples of 0·01 seconds for a mains frequency of 50Hz.

A form of primary switching which uses no moving parts is shown in Figure 20.9, where two thyristors (19.5) perform the switching. Each thyristor conducts during alternate half-cycles of the mains waveform, provided that the

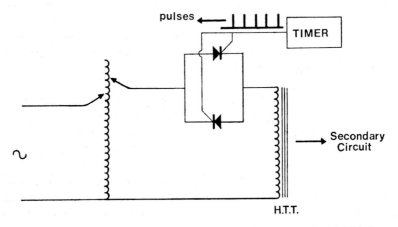

Fig. 20.9 Simplified circuit diagram of primary switching using two thyristors. The timer produces pulses for the set exposure time, so ensuring that the thyristors are switched on for alternate half-cycles (see text).

signal from the timer applied to the gates of each thyristor permits conduction to occur, e.g. the gate must be positive with respect to the source for an NPNP thyristor. A useful characteristic of the thyristor (which it has in common with the thyratron) is that conduction will continue *irrespective of the potential on the gate* until the potential across the whole of the thyratron is reduced to zero. The timer therefore need only send a train of pulses synchronised to a time slightly later than mains zero (to ensure conduction) for, once conduction has started, it will continue for that half-cycle. This circuit thus allows automatic switching of the primary circuit at times of zero mains voltage, with the advantage of 'spike' removal as outlined above. The exposure is terminated when the signals from the timer cease, leaving a potential which biases the gates of the thyratrons so that conduction is inhibited.

20.4.5 Secondary switching

An example of secondary switching is shown in Figure 20.6, where the grids of the triodes are used to switch the beam on when they are sufficiently positive with respect to the cathodes, and to switch the beam off when they are negative. It is a *secondary*, rather than a primary switching circuit, since the triodes are connected to the secondary side of the high-tension transformer.

Another form of secondary switching uses a gridded cathode arrangement within the X-ray tube, so that it becomes a specialised triode valve. It may then be switched on and off directly by the application of a positive or negative potential difference to the grid relative to the cathode.

SUMMARY

1.   An alternating electrical supply enables the easy 'stepping up' or 'stepping down' of voltages necessary for the operation of an X-ray tube.
2.   An X-ray tube produces X-rays only when the anode is positive with respect to the filament (or cathode).
3.   *Rectification* is either the elimination of the inverse half-cycles (when the anode is negative with respect to the filament) or the changing of negative half-cycles to positive half-cycles. The former is *half-wave rectification* and the latter is *full-wave rectification.*
4.   An X-ray tube may act as its own rectifier, since it is a special-purpose diode. This is a 'self-rectified circuit' which is simple and inexpensive but which may only be used at low powers owing to the possibility of reverse current arising from the thermionic emission of the anode at high temperatures.
5.   The inclusion of 2 diodes in the self-rectified circuit eliminates the possibility of reverse current flow in the X-ray tube — this is the '2-diode half-wave rectifier circuit'. This may be used at approximately 1·5 times the power of the self-rectified circuit.
6.   All half-cycles may be used if 2 more diodes are connected in the circuit — the '4-diode full-wave rectifier circuit'. The diodes act in pairs: one pair for the

positive half-cycles and the other pair for the negative half-cycles. Full-wave rectification results in more even heat loading of the anode than half-wave rectification, so higher powers may be used (approximately double that of the self-rectified circuit).

7.   Nevertheless, a 'pulsating DC' voltage across the X-ray tube has disadvantages:

   a.   anode receives rapidly varying heat loading
   b.   intensity and
   c.   quality of X-ray beam continuously changes.

These may be overcome with 'constant potential' rectification.

8.   *Constant potential* to the X-ray tube may be accomplished by:

   a.   capacitor smoothing (HT leads already have some effect)
   b.   triodes for ripple suppression
   c.   3-phase supplies.

9.   Primary switching is the technique of starting and stopping an exposure by energising and de-energising the primary side of the high-tension transformer. The time for which the primary is energised constitutes the exposure time, and this is determined by an exposure timer.

10.   Switching is accomplished when the mains voltage is at, or near, zero in order to prevent arcing across the contactor (if used), and the voltage spikes being fed to the secondary side of the high-tension transformer.

11.   Secondary switching uses electronic means to control the flow of current in the secondary side of the high-tension transformer, i.e. the mA. This may involve the use of triodes, or a special 'gated' X-ray tube.

Part C
THE CONSTRUCTION AND OPERATION OF X-RAY TUBES

21. Diagnostic X-ray tubes

The stationary anode X-ray tube is suitable for the production of X-rays at low or medium intensities, where its relative simplicity of design and construction (and therefore low cost) is a great advantage. Hence it is used for applications such as dental radiography and mobile work where no sophisticated procedures such as rapid sequential imaging are required. The higher X-ray intensities (and electrical power) needed for these applications are provided by the *rotating* anode tube since it has more efficient anode cooling. These two types of X-ray tube are discussed in turn in this chapter.

21.1 CONSTRUCTION OF STATIONARY ANODE TUBE

The X-ray tube is often referred to as the 'insert', because it is inserted (often bolted) into position inside the shield from one end. The construction of the tube, or insert, is shown diagrammatically in Figure 21.1 and discussed in the following sections.

21.1.1 Glass envelope

The glass envelope is used to enclose the vacuum within the X-ray tube and so must be strong enough to withstand the external pressure upon it. The envelope is joined to the anode stem at one end and the nickel cathode support at the other by 're-entrant' seals, so called because the glass is shaped to point

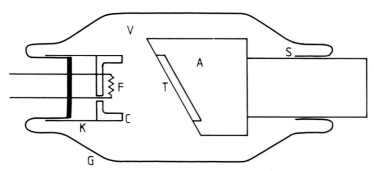

Fig. 21.1 A stationary anode X-ray tube. Key: A — copper anode; T — tungsten target; S — re-entrant seal; G — glass envelope; V — vacuum; F — tungsten filament; C — focusing cup; K — cathode support.

inwards at the area of contact. The thermal expansion (8.3) of the glass is chosen so that stresses due to thermal expansion of the two different materials are minimised.

The glass must be a good electrical insulator, or a substantial current will flow through it when a potential difference is applied between the anode and cathode. However, electrical charges are deposited on the inside of the glass during operation and must be able to 'leak' away to avoid the build up of high static charges. Thus the glass must be sufficiently conductive to allow this to happen.

A tungsten film is deposited on the inside of the glass owing to the evaporation (8.4) of tungsten from the filament. This process is unavoidable, and leads to a slight increase of the inherent filtration (29.1) of the tube. However, its main effect is to reduce the insulation afforded by the glass, and hence to increase the likelihood of electrical breakdown (i.e. sparking) after an extended operating time. The rate of growth of the tungsten film may be reduced, however, by keeping well within the rating of the X-ray tube (Ch. 22).

21.1.2 Cathode and filament(s)

The terms 'cathode' and 'filament' are often used interchangeably when discussing the operation of the X-ray tube and are, in fact, electrically connected together. However, the correct usage of the term 'cathode' implies the whole of the cathode assembly, including the filament, focusing cup, supporting wires and cathode support. Thus the filament is part of the cathode, but not *vice versa*.

The focusing cup is made of nickel or stainless steel, each of which has a high melting point and is a relatively poor thermionic emitter. It would not be desirable to produce thermionic emission from the focusing cup, since the focusing on the anode from such electrons would be poor and hence would increase the focal spot size. In addition, the thermal expansion (8.3) of these materials is close to that of the glass, so minimising the stresses to the seals during operation of the X-ray tube.

The filament is made of thin coiled tungsten (or thoriated tungsten) wire for the following reasons:

a. tungsten is a good thermionic emitter (18.2)
b. tungsten has a low vapour pressure, i.e. it does not vaporise easily (8.4) — it therefore lasts a long time
c. tungsten is rugged and able to be drawn into the thin wire required.

An X-ray tube may have two filaments of different sizes placed side-by-side, as shown in Figure 21.2. This is known as a 'dual-focus' tube. The two filaments produce two different sizes of electron foci on the anode, one for general use and the other (smaller) for 'fine-focus' applications requiring less geometric unsharpness (3.4).

One side of each filament is connected electrically to the focusing cup and the other side is insulated from it, as illustrated in Figure 21.2(c). (Obviously, the filament(s) cannot be connected to the focusing cup at *both* ends, or it

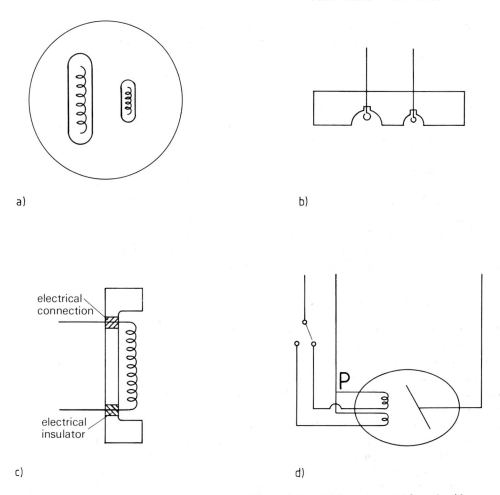

a)

b)

c)

electrical
connection

electrical
insulator

d)

P

Fig. 21.2 Details of a dual-filament assembly; (a) 'face-on' view, (b) from above, (c) from the side, (d) electrical connections.

would be 'shorted' by it!) In a dual-focus tube, therefore, one side of each fila-ment is connected together and taken to one side of the high-tension transformer (point P in Figure 21.2(d)) so that only three wires need be connected to the filament transformer and high-tension transformer, as shown. This arrangement has several advantages. In particular, it uses the minimum possible number of wires and reduces the problems of electrical insulation between the focusing cup and the filament(s). (For example, it would be possible to insulate the filament(s) from the cathode assembly and to operate them from an electrical supply which was unconnected to the high-tension transformer. However, this would require at least four wires and would produce serious problems in insulating the filament(s) from the high negative potential on the focusing cup.)

The secondary winding of the filament transformer is connected to one side of the high-tension transformer (or rectifier, if present), and it 'follows' the varying potential of the latter so reaching high potentials which could be a source of danger to the operators of the X-ray unit. It is for this reason, and for reasons of ensuring good electrical insulation and heat dissipation, that the filament transformer is contained in the same oil bath as the high-tension transformer.

Insight

All high-tension cables for X-ray units contain *three* conducting wires, even though the anode only requires one. This means that manufacturers only need to make (and X-ray departments need only stock) one type of cable. Two of the wires in the cable connected to the anode are not used.

21.1.3 Anode

(*Note:* the heat loss from the anode is described in detail in section 8.5.1.)

The anode of a stationary anode X-ray tube is constructed of the two materials copper and tungsten, and is therefore known as a 'compound' anode. The main part of the anode assembly (the block and stem) is made of copper as shown in Figure 21.3. The inclined face of the copper block has an inset of a thin (about 2–3 mm) tungsten plate, known as the 'target', on to which the electrons from the filament are focused. The target material is made of tungsten for the following reasons:

a. tungsten has a high atomic number (Z) of 74. The intensity of an X-ray beam is proportional to Z (28.1.3)

b. tungsten has a low vapour pressure, so that it does not readily vaporise (8.4) at its normal working temperature

c. tungsten has a high melting point (3387°C) so that it can withstand the heat generated during an X-ray exposure without melting

d. tungsten has a relatively good thermal conductivity (one-half that of copper — 8.2.1), thus enabling a rapid transfer of heat from the small focal area to the anode block by conduction

e. tungsten is a suitable material for machining into the shape and size required.

The face of the anode is set at an angle with respect to the axis of the X-ray beam by an amount known as the 'anode angle', as shown in Figure 21.3(a). The design of the cathode assembly described in the previous section is such that a so-called *line focus* is produced on the anode. In fact, the electrons from the filament are focused onto a thin *rectangle* (Fig. 21.3(b)) rather than a line, but the latter is a convenient term to use. If the anode angle is θ, and the true length of the line focus is r, then the 'effective' focus, a, is given by $a = r \sin \theta$ (see 3.1 for a fuller description of all these terms). The effective focus is therefore smaller than the true focus.

The advantages of using a line focus are:

a. As shown above the size of the effective focus is smaller than the real focus. The filament may thus be relatively long without giving rise to poor

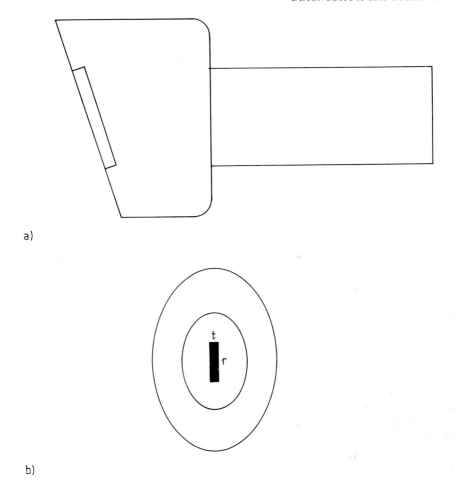

a)

b)

Fig. 21.3 The line-focus principle. (a) shows the anode viewed from the side and (b) is a view of the surface of the anode. The electrons are focused on a thin rectangle of size t times r — the 'line focus'.

geometric unsharpness. Thermionic emission from the filament is proportional to its surface area so that a long filament is able to provide the high values of mA required in many exposures.

  b.   The *area* over which the heat is deposited is the area of the real focus. The temperature rise experienced by a large area is less than that experienced by a small area for the same amount of heat, since more atoms are able to take part in the heat transfer process. The line-focus principle enables the heat to be spread over an area about three times larger than the effective focus, so enabling a reasonable compromise between the requirements of minimising the temperature rise in the target (requiring a large focal area) and minimising the size of the X-ray source (requiring a small focal area).

  The *anode heel effect* produces a reduction in X-ray intensity for those X-rays which are emitted from the anode at near-grazing angles to the face of the target. It is due to the higher absorption of those X-rays which pass through the greatest thickness of target. Hence even a new anode shows such a 'heel effect', and this is made worse by the irregularities produced in the surface of the target as a result of prolonged use of the tube. The formation of such irregularities is known as *pitting* and is caused by vaporisation of the tungsten from the target. (This forms a thin film of tungsten on the inside surface of the glass envelope of the X-ray tube (21.1), for the tungsten vapour formed during exposure condenses on the relatively cool glass surface.) The heel effect is shown diagrammatically in Figure 21.4.

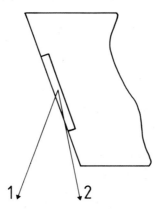

Fig. 21.4 The anode 'heel-effect'. Ray 2 is more attenuated than ray 1 owing to its longer path length within the tungsten target.

Insight
Some of the electrons which strike the anode target produce 'secondary' electrons which are emitted from the surface of the target. Many of these electrons strike the anode at points outside the original focal area, and others reach the glass and produce a static charge on it. X-rays are therefore produced at points on the target outside the area of the original electron beam. This is called 'extra-focal' radiation and contributes towards geometric unsharpness (3.4). Those electrons which reach the glass prevent further electrons from doing the same by mutual repulsion, and 'leak' away slowly between exposures owing to the small but finite electrical conductivity of the glass.

21.2 CONSTRUCTION OF ROTATING ANODE TUBE

(*Note:* the details of heat loss from a rotating tube are discussed in section 8.5.2)

The rotating anode X-ray tube forms the mainstay of the equipment used in radiographic investigations within a diagnostic department. The reason for its superiority over the stationary anode tube lies in its ability to produce higher intensities of X-ray beams than the latter. This is due to two factors: the heat deposited on the anode is spread over a much larger area, and the cooling characteristics of the rotating anode are superior (22.3.1). The construction of the rotating anode X-ray tube is shown in simplified form in Figure 21.5. The cathode has the same basic construction as described in section 21.1.2 except that it is offset from the central axis of the tube in order that electrons emitted from it strike the bevelled surface of the anode.

21.2.1 Anode assembly

The simplest anode configuration is that shown in the figure, where the anode is made of a tungsten or molybdenum disk with an accurately bevelled edge. It has a central hole through which it is connected to a molybdenum anode stem and hence to the rotor of the induction motor. The rotor, stem and anode disk are accurately balanced so that no appreciable wobbling occurs when the whole assembly rotates. The rotor moves on steel ball bearings coated in a soft metal, such as tin, which acts as a lubricant in the evacuated conditions inside the glass envelope. The positive terminal from the high-tension supply is connected to the rotor support, and there is continuous electrical connection to the anode disk itself.

The conduction of heat along the anode stem is inhibited by the poor thermal conductivity of molybdenum and by its relatively narrow diameter (8.2.1). However, some heat will inevitably reach the stator and rotor by conduction, and this could cause sufficient expansion of the ball bearings to produce seizure. The risk of this occurring is reduced by the oil surrounding the tube carrying the heat away by convection and the surface of the rotor is often painted black to increase the heat loss from the rotor by radiation (8.2.3). Many X-ray tubes also incorporate a molybdenum reflector plate behind the anode which greatly reduces the heat received by the rotor by radiation. However, damage may occur to the anode assembly by excessive

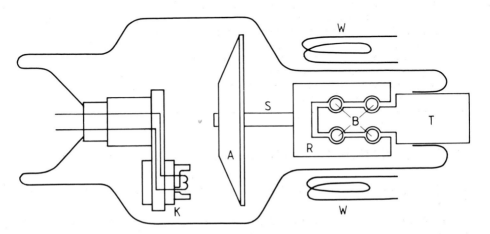

Fig. 21.5 A rotating anode X-ray tube. Key: K — cathode; A — anode disk; S — anode stem; B — ball bearings; R — anode rotor; T — rotor support; W — windings of induction motor (stator).

heat, either by the melting of the target area, or by causing the anode to 'droop' because of long exposures during fluoroscopy (for example) when the anode is not rotated.

In the more modern rotating anode tubes, the anode is made of a solid block of molybdenum with a thin coating of an alloy of tungsten and rhenium on the surface. Molybdenum has double the specific heat capacity of tungsten (8.1.2) and so produces an anode of much higher heat storage capacity in terms of Heat units (22.3.2). Rhenium has an atomic number of 75 (one higher than tungsten) and so has a good conversion of electron energy to X-rays. It also has the advantage of slowing down the ageing process on the anode surface caused by the inevitable pitting of the surface during exposures.

The effect of anode diameter and anode rotation speed on the rating of the tube is discussed in Chapter 22.

21.2.2 Induction motor

The type of motor discussed in section 14.7 would not be suitable to rotate the anode because it would be too large and it would be impossible to service (e.g. to change the commutator brushes). The type of motor used to drive the rotor is an example of an *induction motor*, and is so called because it works on the principles of electromagnetic induction, particularly Lenz's Law (14.3). The principle of this type of motor may be understood by considering the simple experiment depicted in Figure 21.6(a), where a bar magnet is moved around the rim of a supported copper disk. It is found that the copper disk *follows* the movement of the magnet, although it never manages to catch up with it. The sequence of events is as follows.

a. A moving magnetic flux from the magnet is linked with a conductor (the copper disk).

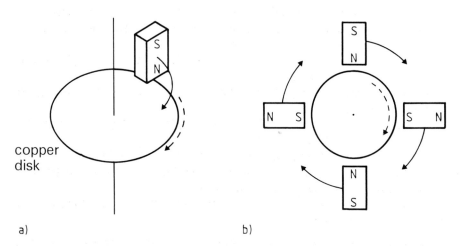

a)   b)

Fig. 21.6 An elementary explanation of an induction motor. The moving magnets in (a) and (b) cause the copper conductor to follow the movement by the induction of eddy currents within the conductor.

b.   From Faraday's Laws we know that an EMF will be induced in the disk, and from Lenz's Law the resulting current will be induced in the disk in such a way as to oppose the change producing it (14.3).

c.   The disk moves in the same direction as the magnet in order to reduce the relative motion between them. Only in this way is the 'change producing' the currents in the disk opposed, as required by Lenz's Law. In a perfect system the disk would eventually move at the same speed as the magnet, so that there would then be no relative motion and no induced currents.

A rather more efficient system is shown in Figure 21.6(b), where more magnets are used and a higher flux linkage is obtained. The copper drum follows the direction of rotation of the magnets for the same reasons as outlined above. However, it is not necessary to use permanent magnets, since current-carrying solenoids act as magnets (12.4). Hence it is necessary only to use fixed solenoids around the copper drum (the 'rotor') and to make the magnetic fields *appear* to rotate by effectively switching the solenoids on and off in rotational sequence. The magnetic field from the solenoids penetrates the glass envelope of the X-ray tube and interacts with the copper rotor on the anode assembly in the same manner as that described in Figures 21.6(a) and (b).

21.3 CONSTRUCTION OF SHIELD (HOUSING)

It would be extremely dangerous to operate an X-ray tube without some sort of suitable covering because of the presence of very high electrical potentials and the radiation hazard to the radiographer and patient alike. The tube must therefore be incorporated within a suitable container (the 'shield' or 'housing') which must be of a suitable design to satisfy the following criteria:

a.   there must be no danger of electric shock if the shield is touched

b.   no significant amounts of X-radiation should escape from the shield other than what is necessary for the taking of the radiograph

c.   the shield must give a secure support to the X-ray tube, high-tension cables and all wires connected to the tube

d.   electric discharges (arcing) must be suppressed within the housing, to avoid damage to the tube

e.   adequate heat loss from the X-ray tube to the shield and the air of the examination room must be ensured

f.   some provision should be made to be able to adjust the size of the X-ray beam, and to have some method (usually optical) of showing the position of the beam relative to the patient prior to exposure

g.   there must be adequate filtration of the beam (Ch. 29) so that harmful 'soft' radiation is removed.

It is seen that the shield must satisfy many requirements, of which only the most fundamental are listed above. A suitable design of shield is shown in schematic form in Figure 21.7, which also shows a stationary anode tube (21.1)

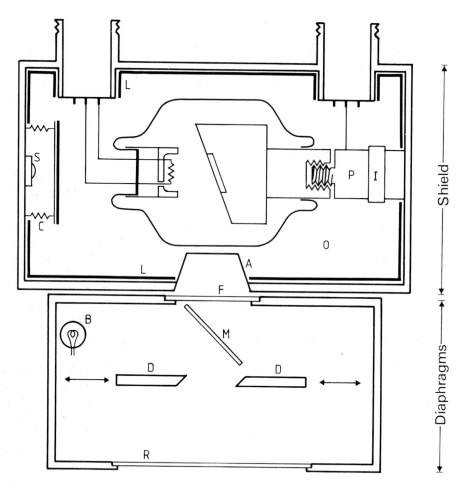

Fig. 21.7 A simplified diagram of the construction of an X-ray shield and diaphragm assembly. Key: L — lead foil; P — tube support; C — bellows; S — microswitch; I — electrical insulator; O — oil; A — shield aperture; F — aluminium filter; B — light bulb; M — mirror; D — movable diaphragms (only one set shown); R — plastic window.

in position. The insert is held in position within the shield by connecting the anode to a suitable support. This support, although joined to the metal casing, is insulated from it. The metal casing is made of steel or aluminium and is a rigid structure capable of providing a strong support for the X-ray tube, the high-tension cables and the diaphragm assembly. A lining of lead foil of about 3 mm thickness is fitted to the inside of the shield casing for radiation protection purposes (see 21.3.2) and the space between the X-ray tube and casing is filled with pure mineral oil free of air bubbles. A bellows (e.g. metal or flexible plastic) at one end of the shield is used to allow for the expansion of the hot oil, i.e. the bellows contracts when the oil is hot and expands when the oil cools down again. A micro-switch actuated by the bellows may be used to prevent further exposures if the oil is very hot — implying that the anode is near (or has even exceeded!) its maximum permissible heat loading.

The function of the oil is twofold:

a.   to suppress electrical arcing within the shield, since the oil is a good electrical insulator

b.   to carry away the heat reaching the anode stem by convection currents within the oil (for a full treatment of anode heat loss, see sections 8.5.1 and 8.5.2).

21.3.1 Electrical safety

An electric shock is, at best, always extremely unpleasant, and at worst may be fatal. High-voltage shocks are very dangerous indeed and so must be guarded against by good design and adequate servicing of equipment.

The principle of all electrical safety for the operators of electrical equipment is that it must not be possible to touch any item of equipment which will result in the operators experiencing a significant electric current passing through them. In the case of radiography, this means that the shield, and all other metal parts which it is possible to touch, must be *earthed*, i.e. connected to earth potential ('zero volts'). Human beings, being connected to earth via the soles of their feet, are already at earth potential and there is no potential *difference* (10.3) when we touch another object also at earth potential. Thus no current can flow and no shock is experienced.

The shield is held at earth potential by connecting it to the copper braiding of each of the high-tension cables, one of which is shown illustrated in Figure 21.8(a). The case of the high-tension transformer is securely earthed (Fig. 21.8(b)) since the electrical safety of the shield is entirely dependent upon the security of this earth point. The braiding of each high-tension cable is connected at one end to the earthed case of the high-tension transformer, and

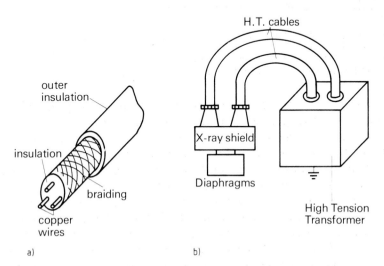

Fig. 21.8 The X-ray shield is made electrically safe by connecting the copper braiding of the high-tension cables to both the shield and the high-tension transformer. The latter is securely earthed.

at the other end to the metal casing of the X-ray shield. The shield is then at earth potential because the braiding is a good conductive link between the two casings.

If a wire within the shield breaks or becomes disconnected, it may be able to touch the shield casing. If the casing is properly earthed, the next exposure will result in a bang and a blowing of fuses, as one end of the secondary of the high-tension transformer will be connected to earth! This is unfortunate, but not so unfortunate as someone touching the casing during an attempted exposure (e.g. screening) if the casing is not earthed!

If one braiding should become disconnected for some reason, then that on the other high-tension cable will ensure that the shield is kept at earth potential. Nevertheless, it is good sense never to touch the casing *during* an exposure as both braidings could have become disconnected! In fact this is good practice, anyway, since the radiation dose to the hands will be minimised, as some X-radiation is always transmitted through the shield (see Ch. 5 on the exponential law). Problems with high-tension cable failures are more likely to be experienced with mobile units than fixed units, in practice, and so special care should be taken with these.

Fuses, switches and circuits breakers

As described above, the earthing of metal parts is necessary in order to prevent the risk of electrical shock. Another essential safety requirement is to be able to isolate the whole of the X-ray unit from the mains supply so that servicing and repair work may be performed without danger. The *mains isolator* or *mains switch* is provided for this purpose, and is enclosed in a strong earthed metal case which is usually fixed to a wall within the same room as the diagnostic unit. However, for specialised installations such as CT scanners and linear accelerators, such an isolator is placed within a separate *plant room* which may also contain high-voltage generators and mains stabilising units. In this case, it is not possible to turn the unit off quickly in an emergency using the mains isolator switch, so *emergency OFF* switches (usually red push-buttons) are positioned within easy reach of the operators at various strategic points. These will break the mains circuit and stop the unit functioning, but some parts of the equipment may still be 'live', however, so that the mains isolator switch must still be used for complete disconnection.

An example of a mains isolator switch is shown in Figure 21.9. The ON/OFF switch operates a sprung 'knife' contact which is able to be in one of two positions only: fully open or fully closed. Also shown in the figure are fuses which 'blow' (i.e. melt and break the circuit) if the electrical current exceeds the rating of the fuses. A fuse is just a length of wire of a given cross-sectional area which is designed to reach its melting point at a particular current. Alloys of lead and tin are frequently used for this purpose. Modern practice is to en-close the fuse wire in a glass or ceramic tube with each end soldered to a metal cap — a *cartridge* fuse. This has the advantage both of easy replacement and of containing the melted fragments within the cartridge, so reducing the fire risk.

3 phases 'in' + earth

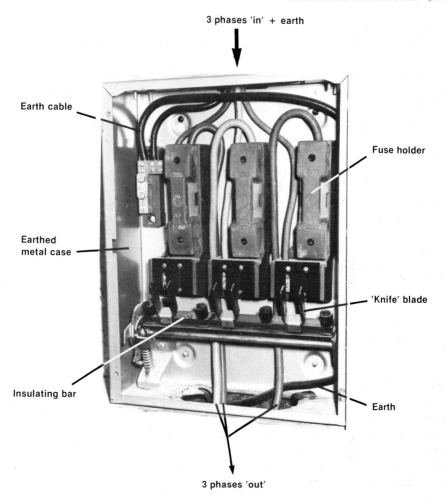

Earth cable

Fuse holder

Earthed
metal case

'Knife' blade

Insulating bar

Earth

3 phases 'out'

Fig. 21.9 A photograph of a 3-phase mains isolator switch. Each U-shaped 'knife' contact connects one of the three phases (from the top of the photograph) through a fuse and then to the X-ray equipment via trunking at the bottom of the earthed metal case.

Fuses of various ratings are used extensively throughout the X-ray circuit in order to protect individual circuits or components. For example, a sudden fault in a power supply unit which results in an excessive voltage being fed to other circuits may result in widespread damage unless each circuit is protected by its own fuse. A fuse within the power supply circuit which 'blows' before these individual fuses would also limit the consequences of such a fault. The use of fuses for circuit protection is inexpensive and efficient, and it is bad practice to replace a blown fuse with one of a higher current rating, and even worse to use a piece of wire or a nail!

Another common method used to protect a circuit against overloading is to use a *circuit-breaker.* This may operate by mechanical means (such as when using a bi-metallic strip) electromagnetically or electronically. The principle of their use is that they may be reset after a momentary surge has caused them to trip so that, unlike a fuse, no replacement is necessary. However, a genuine circuit failure (as opposed to a mains surge) will result in the circuit-breaker tripping again, so that the cause of the trip will need to be established and cured.

It is important to note that neither fuses nor circuit-breakers can prevent possible damage to the X-ray tube resulting from the selection of inappropriate exposure factors, or by allowing insufficient time between exposures. Protection of the tube in these circumstances is performed either by careful use by the radiographer or, in the more sophisticated installations, by additional monitoring and control circuits.

Many mains supplies in hospitals are fairly 'dirty' in that they often have voltage 'spikes' superimposed upon a somewhat ragged sinusoidal waveform (Ch. 15). These effects are caused by other electrical equipment being switched on and off, e.g. lifts, centrifuges, other X-ray units. Such spikes may easily reach several hundred volts over a very short time and may damage sensitive electronic components, such as computer memories and other 'chips'. Other mains problems include *black-outs*, where the supply completely fails, and *brown-outs*, where the mains voltage drops to a lower value for a few seconds. The latter effect can cause computer memories to lose part, or all, of their contents, and a complete black-out can damage a computer disk storage system.

Various levels of protection exist to overcome these problems, from a simple electronic filter circuit on the mains supply to remove the spikes (which are at a higher frequency than the mains, and therefore may be preferentially absorbed), to a constant-voltage transformer (16.5) or other form of automatic mains conditioner, through to an *Uninterruptible Power Supply (UPS)*. A UPS is commonly used to protect sensitive electronic systems, such as computers, since it is important for these systems to have a 'clean' supply. A set of batteries of adequate power is used to generate a clean AC signal via a 'static invertor', which is a circuit to change DC to AC, and the batteries are kept charged by charging them from the rectified 'dirty' mains. In the event of a mains failure, or a 'brown-out', the batteries ensure that the system is kept operating for long enough to either be shut-down in an orderly manner, or until the mains supply is restored, e.g. by a standby generator.

21.3.2 Radiation safety

Radiation safety is important both for the operators of X-ray units as well as patients, and careful attention must be paid to both. The lining of lead foil within the shield (Fig. 21.7) is primarily for the benefit of the operators, although it also increases picture quality by reducing X-ray scatter reaching the film. It should be borne in mind that X-rays are emitted in *all directions* from the focus on the anode, but only those passing through the volume of interest within the patient are actually desired. Hence the reason for the lead lining: it absorbs the great majority of all the X-rays which do not contribute to the radiograph. The anode itself has a high absorption to those X-rays which are emitted into it. However, the absorption of X-rays is exponential in nature

(5.3) and so not all the X-rays are absorbed by the lead lining or anode. It is the usual practice to measure the Exposure rate (Ch. 32) at points 1 metre from the focus when the diaphragms are fully closed and the X-ray unit is operated at its maximum likely combination of kV_p and mA. Such dose rates should not exceed some recommended value.* Obviously, any gap in the lead lining could give rise to an intense, directional beam of radiation which, although incident upon the operator, may not be detected by the operator's film badge or other dosemeter. For this reason it is important that the radiation leakage from X-ray units be checked at periodic intervals by trained personnel (usually physics staff). It is the older units, however, which often prove to be deficient in this respect.

Radiation safety as far as the patient is concerned means receiving only that radiation dose necessary to produce a diagnostically acceptable radiograph. No shield design can correct for inappropriate settings of kV_p or mAs or misaligned beams which require repeat exposures, but it can ensure that a high radiation dose caused by excessive amounts of 'soft' X-rays is eliminated. Such soft X-rays are readily absorbed in the patient but contribute nothing to the radiograph, so producing a quite unnecessary radiation dose to the patient. They are greatly reduced by the use of *filtration*, both 'inherent' and 'additional'. Inherent filtration is the modification of the X-ray spectrum from the anode by its passage through the tungsten deposit on the glass, the glass itself, the oil and the shield aperture (see Fig. 21.7), all of which absorb low-energy X-rays far more than the high-energy X-rays. The additional filtration is provided by a sheet of aluminium placed just outside the shield aperture which absorbs even more of the 'soft' X-rays. The 'total' filtration is just the sum of the inherent filtration and the additional filtration (29.1).

Scattered radiation produced within the patient also contributes to the photographic exposure of the radiograph and to the radiation dose received by the patient. The effect of reducing the X-ray beam field size (i.e. 'coning down') is to reduce the amount of scattered radiation produced within the patient. This has two effects: it reduces the radiation dose received by the patient, and it increases the required exposure factors to some extent. However, the overall effect is one of reduction of radiation dose to the patient, even taking into account the increased exposure factors, so that the selection of the minimum beam size by adjustment of the movable diaphragms shown in Figure 21.7 (or, alternatively, the selection of detachable cones of different sizes) is an important method by which the radiation dose may be reduced to the practical minimum, simply by reducing the field size to cover only the required area. Since this also improves picture quality by reducing the contribution of X-ray scatter to the radiograph, there is an additional advantage in so doing.

---

* 100 mR in 1 hour for older units, and 10 mR in 1 hour for modern units. These figures correspond to $2 \cdot 58 \times 10^{-5}$ C kg^{-1} and $2 \cdot 58 \times 10^{-6}$ C kg^{-1} in 1 hour.

21.4 PRINCIPLES OF OPERATION

It is the author's experience that much confusion exists in the minds of many students concerning the operation of an X-ray tube beyond the simple statement that 'electrons strike the anode and produce X-rays'. Much of the confusion appears to be associated with the difference between the mA and the filament current, and the manner in which the electrons are focused onto the anode. These two topics are discussed under this section, followed by a brief description of the mechanism of X-ray production.

21.4.1 mA and filament current

Figure 21.10 shows a circuit diagram of the X-ray tube and high-tension circuit which has been greatly simplified in order to illustrate the difference between the tube current (mA) and the filament current (I_f). Battery $B1$ is connected across the X-ray tube and battery $B2$ across the filament, and the electron flow is as shown in the figure. At the common part of the two circuits, both electron flows add together to produce (mA + I_f), but the mA is 'lost' to the filament circuit and flows through the X-ray tube, leaving I_f to flow back to $B2$. Thus, a current I_f leaves $B2$ and arrives back at $B2$, so that there is no net gain or loss of electrons in the filament circuit. The same observation applies to the high-tension circuit, since a current mA leaves and arrives at battery $B1$. Thus, the *filament current and mA are not the same*. However, they are related to each other, since a high filament current produces a greater thermionic emission from the filament and hence more electrons which are able to flow through the X-ray tube, i.e. a higher mA. Typical values are: $I_f = 5$ A and tube current = 200 mA, so that the filament current is very much bigger than the mA (25 times in this example). Obviously, the high filament current is required to heat the filament to a sufficient temperature for good thermionic emission to take place (Ch. 18).

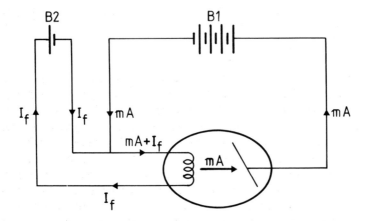

Fig. 21.10 The difference between mA and filament current (I_f) — see text.

Exercise 21.1

Why is it possible to have a filament current without an mA, but not to have an mA without a filament current?

21.4.2 Electron focusing

During conduction, the anode of the X-ray tube is positively charged and the cathode is negatively charged. The electron space charge (18.1.1) emitted by the heated filament is thus repelled from the cathode and attracted towards the anode, since electrons are themselves negatively charged. The situation which would arise if both the anode and cathode were flat plates is shown in Figure 21.11(a). The electric field (9.4) consists of parallel lines starting from the

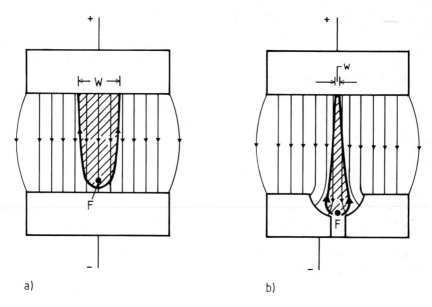

a)   b)

Fig. 21.11 Simplified explanation of the focusing of electrons in an X-ray tube. The concave focusing-cup directs the electrons from thermionic emitter F toward the central axis, so that they strike the anode over a small area.

anode and finishing on the cathode. The 'plume' of electrons from the thermionic emitter F, being charged negatively, travel against the direction of the electric field, striking the anode over a width, W, which is greater than the size of F. This situation therefore produces an unacceptably large focal area on the anode, and recourse is made to a 'focusing-cup' cathode (21.1.2) as shown in Figure 21.11(b). The thermionic electrons from F now experience a force which is always towards the central axis (as well as towards the anode) owing to the shape of the electric lines of force produced by the cup. The 'plume' of electrons is therefore spread over a much smaller width, w, on the anode (smaller than the dimensions of the filament), and the electron beam is said to have been 'focused'. A 'line-focus' is produced (21.1.3).

21.4.3 X-ray production

The production of X-rays is discussed in detail in Chapter 28; it is necessary only to state here that it is the *deceleration* of the electrons in the target which produces the X-rays. This deceleration is caused by the close passage of an energetic electron to a tungsten nucleus, and the whole process of X-ray emission in such circumstances is known as 'Bremsstrahlung' (or 'braking') radiation. Superimposed on the Bremsstrahlung radiation is the 'characteristic' radiation from the tungsten (28.1.1) caused by electron-level changes within the tungsten atoms.

The *intensity, I*, of the Bremsstrahlung, which forms the bulk of the X-radiation, varies with both the energy, E, of the electron beam striking the target, and the atomic number (Z) of the target material, such that

$$I \propto Z . E^2 \qquad \text{Equation 21.1}$$
$$\text{or} \quad I \propto Z . kV^2 \qquad \text{Equation 21.2}$$

since the energy in keV is just the value of the kV at any instant (6.4.3).

The process of X-ray production is very inefficient, however, and about 95–99% of the total energy of all the electrons is converted into heat, which must be rapidly transferred from the focal area in order to avoid damage to the target (8.5.1).

Exercise 21.2

  a.   Draw a stationary anode X-ray tube and explain the function of its parts.

  b.   Repeat the above for a rotating anode X-ray tube.

  c.   List the materials used in the construction of an X-ray tube. Explain why these materials are chosen.

  d.   Write notes on:

  (i) the line-focus principle
  (ii) the heel-effect
  (iii) anode induction motor
  (iv) extra-focal radiation
  (v) electron focusing
  (vi) dual-focus

as applied to an X-ray tube.

  e.   Sketch the X-ray tube with its shield (or housing). What features in your sketch contribute towards

  (i) electrical safety
  (ii) radiation safety?

  f.   What is the purpose of the filament current in an X-ray tube? How is this related to the mA? What is the effect of kV_p on the mA (assuming that the X-ray tube is operating in a perfectly 'saturated region').

g.   Investigate modern developments in X-ray tube design. For example:

(i) electrically gated tubes
(ii) ceramic tubes
(iii) carbon anodes
(iv) high-speed anodes
(v) radial slits in anodes
(vi) field-emission cathodes
(vii) anodes of large surface area
(viii) black anodes
(ix) automatic measurement of anode temperature.

SUMMARY

1.   The X-ray tube (insert) consists of an evacuated glass envelope within which is the anode at one end and the cathode at the other. A positive potential on the anode with respect to the cathode allows electrons to travel from the cathode to the anode at high energy. When they are stopped, X-rays are produced (Bremsstrahlung and characteristic radiation).

2.   The filament is raised to incandescence by a high filament current (3 – 8 A) so as to produce a space charge of electrons around the filament by thermionic emission.

3.   A 'dual-focus' tube has two filaments attached to the cathode: one smaller than the other for 'fine-focus' radiography.

4.   The filament is made of tungsten (or thoriated tungsten) wire because:

a.   it is a good thermionic emitter
b.   it does not vaporise easily
c.   it is rugged.

5.   The 'compound' anode of the stationary anode tube is constructed of copper with a tungsten insert — the 'target'. Tungsten is chosen because:

a.   it has a high atomic number (X-ray intensity $\propto Z$)
b.   high melting point
c.   good electrical conductivity
d.   adequate thermal conductivity
e.   does not vaporise easily
f.   it is fairly easily machined.

6.   The main mechanism of heat loss from a stationary anode tube is *conduction* (see 8.5.1), whilst that from a rotating anode is *radiation* (see 8.5.2).

7.   A 'line-focus' is produced on the anode which is smaller than the size of the filament because of the focusing effect of the 'focusing cup' on the electron beam.

8.   An electrical induction motor is used to rotate the anode by means of a rotating magnetic field which induces currents in the rotor (Lenz's Law). The rotation speed of the anode is just below that of the mains frequency (although

it is also possible to have rotation speeds of two or more times the mains frequency).

9.   Electrical safety is ensured by earthing all metal parts. In particular, the X-ray shield is joined to the earth on the casing of the high-tension transformer via the copper braidings on the high-tension cables.

10.   The use of mains isolating switches enables the X-ray unit to be completely disconnected from the mains supply, so that servicing and repairs may be performed in safety and so that the unit may be switched off in an emergency. Fuses and circuit-breakers protect the X-ray circuits from the consequences of overloading before damage can occur. Systems with sensitive electronic circuits may need further protection from 'dirty' mains by the use of an Uninterruptible Power Supply.

11.   Radiation safety to the operators is ensured by lead lining on the inside of the shield. Radiation dosage to the patient is reduced by the use of the smallest practicable field size and aluminium filters.

12.   mA and filament current are *not* the same.

22. Rating

22.1 DEFINITION OF RATING

The general term 'rating' is used to describe the practical limits inherent in a particular device. For example, if a fuse is 'rated' at a current of 5 A, then any current greater than this will cause it to melt (or to 'blow'). A high-tension transformer is a more complicated device than a simple fuse, of course, and so has a more complicated set of rating conditions (16.6). Similarly, the rating of an X-ray unit (i.e. the tube and associated equipment) depends upon how it is used as well as its construction, and may be defined as follows:

Definition

> The *rating* of an X-ray unit is that combination of exposure settings which the unit can just withstand without incurring unacceptable damage.

Any exposure gives rise to some 'damage' to the X-ray tube, since the anode becomes slightly more pitted and the filament becomes slightly thinner. However, in this context 'unacceptable damage' means that amount of damage which will seriously impair the performance of the unit for further exposures or even to make the unit completely inoperative. For example, single and multiple exposures of short or long duration all have their practical limits above which damage may occur. Thus a short exposure at a very high mA may (unless prevented by interlocks) damage the anode by melting the focal area. Alternatively, a long exposure at a low mA may damage either the anode, the shield or the high-tension transformer (16.6), should any of *their* individual ratings be exceeded. Similarly, multiple exposures, each of which is individually within the rating, may produce sufficient accumulated heat on the anode to cause damage to it. Obviously, the closer the exposures follow each other, the more likelihood there is of anode damage owing to the finite time required by the anode to cool. For this reason single and multiple exposures will be considered separately in this chapter.

22.2 SINGLE EXPOSURES AND RATING CHARTS

22.2.1 Stationary anode tubes

The exposure factors which are under the control of the operator, and those which are not, are shown in Table 22.1.

Table 22.1 Selectable and non-selectable factors for a given X-ray unit.

Selectable factors:	kV_p, mA, exposure time/mAs, focal spot size, single/multiple exposures, radiography/screening
Non-selectable factors:	(a) Stationary anode tube: rectification, thermal capacity of anode/shield, efficiency of heat loss from anode/shield, anode angle, filtration, rating of high-tension cables and transformers (b) Rotating anode tube: — as above, plus: anode diameter, anode rotation speed

For any particular X-ray unit, the second list of quantities in Table 22.1 is unalterable, and a *rating chart* is used which is applicable only to that unit. This chart shows the effect of varying the quantities in the first list, i.e. those which may be altered. A simplified rating chart is shown in Figure 22.1, where a 'rating curve' corresponding to the use of the 'broad focus' (e.g. 2 mm) is shown for 80 kV_p. The curve indicates the upper limit of safety for all combinations of mA and the exposure time for this value of kV_p. Thus, points *below* the line are 'safe', while those above it are 'unsafe' in that they result in unacceptable damage to the X-ray tube. The wide range of possible exposure times shown (0·05 to 20 seconds) makes it convenient to use a logarithmic scale (1.8.1) on the X-axis of the rating curve and enables the effect of shorter exposure times to be shown more clearly.

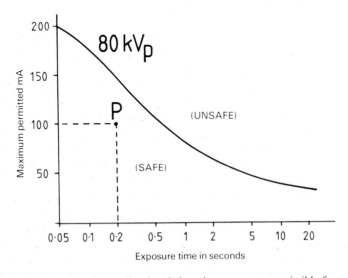

Fig. 22.1 A simplified rating chart. All points below the curve are permissible for radiographic exposures.

The rating curve shows that a higher value of mA may be tolerated for short exposures than for long exposures, and this reflects the fact that the energy of the electron beam may either be delivered to the anode 'all at once' (i.e. at high mA for a short time), or spread over a longer time at low mA. The limiting factor in either case is the anode temperature. In addition, the longer exposures allow more time for the anode to cool (i.e. transfer the heat away from the focal area) during the exposure. The rating curve 'flattens' for these longer exposures because of the significant anode cooling which then occurs.

Example

It is desired to make an exposure at 80 kV_p and 100 mA using the broad focus. Does 20 mAs exceed the rating of the tube?

20 mAs at 100 mA means an exposure time of 0·2s (mAs = mA × t), which corresponds to point P in the figure — well within the tube rating. Note that the maximum exposure time is 0·5 s for this combination.

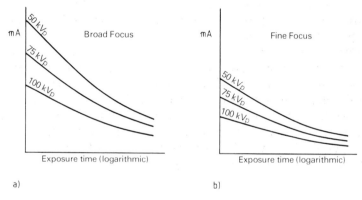

Fig. 22.2 Comparison of rating charts for broad and fine focus selection.

In practice it is much more convenient to include more than one rating curve on each graph, and it is usual to have two rating charts for a dual-focus tube (21.1.2): one for the fine focus and one for the broad focus, as shown in Figure 22.2. Obviously, the rating of the X-ray tube for the fine focus will be lower than that using the broad focus, since the electron beam is focused onto a smaller area, thus causing a higher temperature for the same mA.

Figure 22.2 also shows that larger mA values are permitted as the kV_p is reduced, the difference between the curves being most marked for the shorter exposure times. This is because of the effect of the kV_p on the energy which each electron obtains when accelerating towards the anode. As the kV_p is increased the energy becomes greater, so that the same number of electrons striking the anode per second (the mA) deposits a greater amount of energy. Thus, the maximum permitted value of the mA must be reduced if the kV_p increases in order to avoid depositing so much power on the anode (i.e. energy per second — 6.3.7) that it becomes damaged. The rating charts show this inverse relationship between the mA and kV_p in an easily understandable graphical form.

Insight

For a given exposure time t, the anode may accept a given total energy E from the electron beam without being damaged. The energy of one electron is given by the kV_p value and the total number of electrons is proportional to the mAs,

$$\therefore\quad E \propto kV_p \times mA \times t$$

i.e. $mA \times kV_p = $ constant if t is constant.

Visual inspection of any rating chart will show that, for a given exposure time, halving the kV_p doubles the permissible mA, and so on in agreement with this equation.

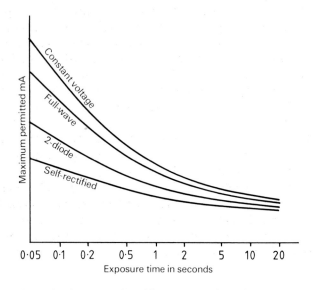

Fig. 22.3 Comparison of rating charts for different types of rectification.

Finally, a rating chart may be used to illustrate the effect of *rectification* on tube rating when using the same X-ray tube. Figure 22.3 summarises the effect of four types of rectification as shown illustrated, where the same focus and kV_p setting is assumed for the four curves. The maximum difference between the curves exists at short exposures, since it is here that the heating effect of individual half-cycles becomes increasingly apparent. As discussed in (20.1.1), the limiting factor with the self-rectified system is that of reverse conduction due to thermionic emission from the target, while that of the other rectification systems is the melting point of the target. The more constant the heat production can be made to occur, the better the target is able to cope — hence the maximum permitted mA for short exposures is always highest for constant voltage rectification. For longer exposures it is the thermal capacity (8.1.2) of the anode which becomes the dominating factor. This is independent of the type of rectification, and so the curves all tend to come together as the exposure times increase. Thus, for short exposures the so-called *critical element* is the surface of the anode, while for long exposures it is the thermal capacity of the anode and the shield and the heat dissipation of the high-tension transformer.

22.2.2 Rotating anode tubes

The rating of stationary anode tubes described in the previous section is significantly less than that of rotating anode tubes. In other words, rotating anode tubes are able to withstand more *power* (either in the form of higher mA of kV_p) without becoming damaged. This, in turn, enables higher intensities of X-rays to be produced, and a greater range of exposure factors to be selected, particularly for short exposures.

The limitations of the stationary anode tube are caused by the relative inefficiency of anode cooling and the melting point of copper (1083°C). These two factors are related because the stationary anode is designed to lose heat primarily by *conduction* (8.5.1) where the good thermal conductivity of copper is an important design feature. However, conduction from the anode is inhibited in the rotating anode tube and the main mechanism of heat loss is *radiation* (8.5.2). The rotating tungsten anode (21.2.1) is often raised to incandescence during an exposure (well above the melting point of copper), radiation heat loss being efficient at these high temperatures (8.2.3).

There are two basic factors which affect the rating of rotating anode tubes (in addition to those described in the previous section): anode diameter and anode rotation speed (Table 22.1). The electron beam lands upon the moving bevelled edge of the anode (the 'track') and therefore deposits heat energy around the *whole* anode, rather than on the same area, as is the case with the stationary anode tube. Thus, the smaller the heat energy deposited upon any particular point of the bevelled edge of the anode, the *greater is the anode*

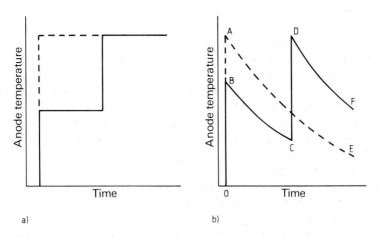

Fig. 22.4 The advantage of a high-speed anode is due to anode cooling. The dotted lines in (a) and (b) represent an anode rotating at one-half the speed of the full line. Without cooling there is no advantage (as shown in (a)), but cooling allows a higher anode 'loading' (OB + CD compared to OA).

rating. There are two ways in which a smaller amount of heat may be deposited (for the same mA and kV_p):

a. using an anode of large diameter for a given rotation speed, or
b. rotating the anode faster.

Both of these changes produce the same effect, in that the anode moves faster, causing fewer electrons to land per unit area of track. For example, a doubling of the rotation speed means that one-half of the heat energy is deposited per unit area for each revolution of the anode, although the same area passes through the electron beam twice as many times for the same exposure time. If there were no cooling between successive heatings of the same point, there would be no advantage in using a faster rotation speed. This point is illustrated in Figure 22.4 where one revolution of the anode is compared to two revolutions in the same time, with and without anode cooling (Fig. 22.4(a) and (b) respectively). In both cases the maximum permitted temperature of the anode surface has been reached during the same time, but the faster anode has enabled this to be reached in two stages with cooling in between. This may be seen by comparing curves OAE and OBCDF in Figure 22.4(b). The cooling effect is shown by curve BC, the increase in rating so produced being (OB + CD) compared to OA.

The effect of doubling the rotation speed is to increase the rating by about 40–50% for short exposure times. The same improvement is obtained by doubling the diameter of the anode. Examples of the rating curves so obtained are shown in Figure 22.5(a) and (b). Note that the maximum permissible mA levels are higher than for the stationary anode tubes (previous section) and that the differences in the rating diminish as the exposure times increase, since it is the overall heat capacity of the anode which is then the dominant factor (or 'critical element').

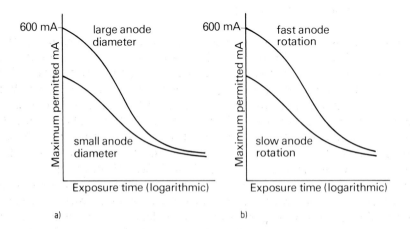

Fig. 22.5 The effect on rating of (a) anode diameter, (b) anode speed.

22.3 MULTIPLE EXPOSURES

22.3.1 Anode cooling curve

If exposures occur sufficiently close together so that the anode has not had time to cool almost completely, then the rating charts discussed in the previous section must be used with great caution, since subsequent exposures may well take the temperature of the tungsten target above its permitted level. However, the rating charts may be used with the *anode cooling curve* to predict the safety of any combination of exposures. An example of a cooling curve is shown in Figure 22.6 where Heat Units (6.4.4) are plotted against time. The anode of a particular X-ray tube has a given mass and heat capacity (the heat energy required to raise it by one degree — 8.1.2) — there is thus a quantity of heat

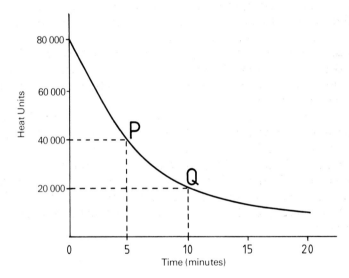

Fig. 22.6 An example of an anode cooling curve.

which would take the whole anode to its maximum desirable operating temperature. This quantity is referred to as the *heat storage capacity* of the anode and is expressed in Heat Units. The cooling curve in the figure is the number of Heat Units left after a given time, assuming that the anode has received its maximum permitted number of Heat Units at $t = 0$. Suppose, for example, that an exposure of 80 kV$_p$, 250 mA and 2 s has just been made. This corresponds to $80 \times 250 \times 2 = 40\,000$ Heat Units, which is point P in the figure. The anode then loses heat as given by the curve below P, such that 5 minutes later it has managed to cool to 20 000 Heat Units (point Q).

The use of the cooling curve in any proposed combinations of exposures is straightforward, if somewhat tedious, for short exposures times, i.e. when the anode cooling *during* an exposure may be neglected. If this is not the case, anode *heating* curves are used as described below. Examples of calculations used in practice are given at the end of the next section.

22.3.2 Anode heating curves

For a long exposure, as in fluoroscopy, the cooling which occurs during the exposure itself becomes important. The anode initially heats up quite quickly, but tends towards *thermal equilibrium* (8.2), which occurs when the rate of heat generated on the anode by the electron beam is exactly balanced by the rate of the heat loss from the anode. Examples of anode heating curves are shown in Figure 22.7, where the number of Heat Units stored by the anode at any moment is plotted against time. The maximum heat storage capacity of the anode is assumed to be 100 000 Heat Units and three different exposures are shown i.e. one at 1 000 Heat Units per second which exceeds the heat capacity of the anode quite quickly, one at 500 Heat Units per second which levels off at the maximum permitted value, and one at 100 Heat Units per second, which produces thermal equilibrium with the anode at a much lower temperature. Obviously, both the heating curves and cooling curve may be shown on the same graph for convenience.

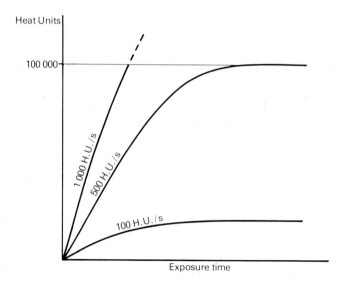

Fig. 22.7 An example of a series of anode heating curves. The maximum thermal capacity of the anode is 100 000 Heat Units and this may be exceeded if the rate of heat production is sufficiently high.

22.3.3 'Angiographic' rating charts

The calculations shown in the next section are examples of the use of the simple rating charts and cooling curves explained above. In the case of rapid sequential imaging, as in angiography, the obvious and usual practice is to keep to one of a series of set procedures which is known not to exceed the rating of the X-ray unit. Any proposed deviation from these known procedures may need some preliminary calculations in order to determine whether it is within the rating. However, it is more convenient to use a special angiographic rating chart which, in its simplest form, relates the number of exposures per second and the total number of exposures to the maximum permitted number of Heat units per exposure. Such rating charts are calculated and verified by the manufacturers of the equipment and go some way in avoiding the possibility of arithmetical slips which are almost inevitable when the calculation is performed under pressure of time, for example.

The physical principles behind such angiographic rating charts are no different from those discussed above. Thus, they are not discussed further in this book, but the reader is recommended to study and compare all types of rating charts in use in his or her place of work.

22.3.4 Worked examples

a.   short exposure times

This class of calculation assumes that the cooling that takes place during an exposure is negligible, so that the heating curves described in the last section are not used. Examples are further sub-divided into rapid sequential exposures (e.g. angiography) and sequential exposures with an appreciate time-lag between them.

If an angiographic rating chart is not available, and the combination of exposure factors is not part of a routine procedure then the procedure for rapid serial exposures is as follows:

(i)   the rating chart is first consulted to verify that an *individual* exposure is permitted

(ii)   the total number of Heat Units is calculated for the complete investigation and compared to the rating chart for the *same overall time*

(iii)   if (ii) is within the rating, the investigation may proceed.

If, to take a specific example, it is desired to make a series of 10 exposures at 80 kV_p, 100 mA and exposure times of 0·2 s at 0·5 s intervals, then; (i) the appropriate rating chart (e.g. Fig. 22.1) indicates that an individual exposure is permissible, (ii) the total number of Heat units is $10 \times 8 \times 100 \times 0·2$ = 16 000. The rating chart shows that the total number of Heat Units permitted over a total time of 5 s is $45 \times 80 \times 5 = 18\,000$, which is greater than 16 000, so the exposures are permitted. This method of calculation errs on the side of safety, as no account is made of anode cooling between exposures.

Other types of multiple exposures make use of the anode cooling curve, as in the following numerical example:

Is it permissible to give six exposures of 80 kV_p, 300 mA, 1·0 s at 30 s intervals (using the cooling curve shown in Fig. 22.6)?

Each exposure generates $80 \times 300 \times 1 = 24\,000$ Heat Units, and we may construct Table 22.2 to show the effect of each exposure. Note that the numbers in the last column are the residual amounts of heat immediately prior to the next exposure, and are obtained from the cooling curve of Figure 22.6. These numbers are added to the Heat Units from each individual exposure to give the total figure after each exposure in the sequence, as shown in the second column of Table 22.2. As in the case of the previous example, the calculation does not take any account of the cooling during an exposure, and so is a conservative estimate of the capabilities of the tube. However, such a 'safety factor' is obviously desirable, in the interests of tube longevity!

Table 22.2 Example of use of anode cooling curve

Exposure no.	HUs after exposure	HUs after further 30 s
1	24 000	22 000
2	22 000 + 24 000 = 46 000	43 000
3	43 000 + 24 000 = 67 000	62 000
4	62 000 + 24 000 = 86 000! (i.e. rating exceeded)	

Note: All values are taken from Figure 22.6 and are approximately only.

b. long exposure times

The practical situation where multiple long exposures are undertaken is in 'screening', where the rating of the tube is rarely even approached (particularly with image intensification), and the anode is usually used stationary in order to prolong the life of the anode bearings. Thus, this section is of theoretical interest only and the type of calculations involved are only briefly outlined. The method is simple, and requires the alternate use of the appropriate heating curve (as typified by Fig. 22.7) and the cooling curve for the particular X-ray tube. In the case of Figure 22.7 the anode can never exceed its rating if the exposure delivers heat at a rate less than 500 Heat Units per second, since thermal equilibrium below the maximum permitted value of anode temperature always occurs. However, this is not to say that the ratings of either the shield or the high-tension transformer will not be exceeded. In particular, inadequate ventilation of the shield reduces its heat loss to the surrounding air, and consequently reduces the heat loss from the anode to the oil in the shield for a stationary anode tube. The microswitch in the bellows (21.3) will operate before damage to the shield or anode can occur, however, for these long exposures.

Exercise 22.1

a. What is meant by the *rating* of an X-ray tube? Illustrate your answer with a sketch of a rating chart, explaining the important features of such a chart.

b. How does the rating of an X-ray tube depend upon

(i) the focal spot size
(ii) the kV_p
(iii) the exposure time
(iv) the rectification.

c. What is meant by the term *critical element* when applied to the rating of an X-ray tube. Make a list of the critical elements appropriate for exposures of different lengths. Explain your choices.

d. Why are the curves of a typical rating chart further apart at short exposure times, and closer together at long exposure times?

e. Write briefly on:

(i) Heat Units
(ii) Anode cooling curve
(iii) Anode heating curve.

f. Under what circumstances can a single exposure which is itself within the rating of an X-ray tube nevertheless do damage to the tube?

g. Describe the use of an angiographic rating chart used in your department.

SUMMARY

1. All exposures produce tube damage, but the *rating* of an X-ray tube corresponds to the combinations of exposure settings which the tube is just able to withstand. Higher exposures result in unacceptable (or even total) damage.
2. A rating chart describes the relationships between the exposure settings (kV_p, mA, time, focal spot size) which result in the rating being reached. See Figure 22.2.
3. The factors beyond the control of the radiographer which affect the rating include the rectification, efficiency of heat loss from the anode, heat capacity of anode, diameter of and speed of rotating anode.
4. The differences in the rating from the sources in 2 and 3 above are most significant at very short exposure times, where the variation of deposited electron energy over each half-cycle of the electrical supply becomes important.
5. All the rating curves for a particular tube tend together at the longer exposures (5 s and above), since the heat capacity of the anode then becomes paramount and the other factors relatively unimportant.
6. The rotating anode tube has a significantly higher rating than a stationary anode tube (approx. 3–5 times greater) because of its more efficient heat loss (radiation rather than conduction) and the use of a moving 'track' so that the energy is deposited over a larger area on the anode. The moving track appears stationary to the radiograph, of course.
7. The rating of the oil and shield, and that of the high-tension transformer, are also important in practice, particularly for the longer exposures where there may be difficulties of adequate heat loss, i.e. they may overheat.
8. A single exposure may not exceed the rating of an X-ray tube, but the same exposure repeated several times may do so, owing to the incomplete anode cooling between the exposures. Thus the rating charts should be used in

conjunction with the anode cooling curve to establish whether a particular combination of exposures is within the rating of the tube. Examples of this, and the use of the anode heating curves, are given in the text.

9. The particular part of the X-ray unit which is close to its maximum rating is called the 'critical element'. For short exposures, the critical element is the surface of the anode. As the exposure times increase, the critical element becomes in turn the anode thermal capacity, the anode bearings, the shield heat loss and thermal capacity, and the temperature of the HT transformer.

Part D
ATOMIC PHYSICS

23. Laws of physics (modern)

23.1 CLASSICAL VERSUS MODERN

The classical laws of physics discussed in Chapter 7 have been sufficient for all the previous chapters. However, in the following chapters on atomic and radiation physics, some important aspects of modern physics must be introduced in order to explain many of the phenomena discussed. The purpose of this chapter is to describe those principles (or laws) of modern physics which are relevant to our needs.

'Modern' physics started at the turn of the twentieth century with the 'quantum hypothesis' of Planck in 1900, in which it was conjectured that radiation energy could only be absorbed or emitted by a body at discrete values of energy, i.e. that the energy of the process had to take on certain values and was therefore not continuous. Other dates of interest to us include the mass–energy relationship of Einstein in 1905, the atomic model by Bohr in 1913 and the 'de Broglie wavelength' of particles in 1924. There have been enormous technical and theoretical strides since these discoveries, but they form part of the firm experimental foundation upon which modern physics is built.

The essential differences between classical and modern physics concern the way in which matter and energy are regarded. In classical physics, matter and energy are completely separate entities, so that a Conservation Law is used for each (7.1 and 7.2). Similarly, matter is supposed always to behave like matter and waves always to behave like waves, and the one cannot behave like the other (e.g. a particle of matter cannot possess a wavelength). However, there are no such rigid boundary lines in modern physics. In particular, the work of Einstein showed that matter may be thought of as being 'stored' or 'locked-up' energy which may be transformed back into energy under the right conditions. This principle is known as 'mass–energy equivalence', and is discussed below (23.2.1). In addition, it was found that particles of matter *do* sometimes behave like waves and *vice versa*, and this principle is called the 'wave-particle duality' (23.4).

With these concepts in mind, the laws of modern physics may be considered in more detail in the remainder of this chapter.

23.2 CONSERVATION OF ENERGY

Statement
    The total energy in a system is constant.

This formula may be written more descriptively as:

Sum of all (rest energies + kinetic energies + potential energies) = constant for a given system.

A 'system' may be two particles, the whole Earth or even the Universe. It is a region outside which the influence of other particles or bodies is negligibly small. However, the use of the word 'energy' in the above law embraces the contribution of matter to the total energy present in the particular system under consideration. This concept of 'mass–energy' is described below.

23.2.1 Mass–energy equivalence

Einstein showed that the mass, m, of a body and its total energy, E (but not including potential energy), are related by the simple formula:

$$E = mc^2 \qquad\qquad \text{Equation 23.1}$$

where c is the velocity of light. The units of this equation are E in joule, m in kg and c in m s^{-1}. Thus, the energy of a body is proportional to its mass, since c is a constant. If the mass of a stationary body (i.e. the 'rest mass') is m_0, the energy within the body is just $E_0 = m_0 c^2$. Similarly, the energy E_v when the body moves at a velocity v is $E_v = m_v c^2$ where m_v is the mass of the body when moving at this velocity. Since the body has a greater energy when moving than when stationary, m_v must be greater than m_0, i.e. a *body increases in mass as it travels faster*. This is, like other of Einstein's findings, not a matter of common experience since it is only measurable for bodies travelling at a signifcant fraction of the velocity of light. The mass which they then possess is termed the 'relativistic mass'. Classical physics is of course violated by Equation 23.1, which however has a wealth of confirmatory experimental evidence.

The law of conservation of energy stated above is sometimes referred to as the law of conservation of *mass–energy*, because of this concept of equivalence between mass and energy. It is not infrequent that the mass of an atomic particle is expressed in MeV (a unit of energy), for example, as this can have practical advantages. An example of this is the mass of an electron which may either be expressed as $9 \cdot 1 \times 10^{-31}$ kg or $0 \cdot 511$ MeV.

Exercise 23.1
Given that $c = 3 \times 10^8$ m s^{-1} and 1 J $= 6 \cdot 24 \times 10^{18}$ eV, substitute the mass of the electron in kg in Equation 23.1 and verify that $E = 0 \cdot 511$ MeV.

Insight
If a body of rest mass m_0 moves at velocity v, then Einstein's Relativity Theory predicts that the mass at velocity v, m_v, is given by

$$m_v = \frac{m_0}{\sqrt{1 - \dfrac{v^2}{c^2}}} = m_0\left(1 - \frac{v^2}{c^2}\right)^{-1/2}$$

i.e. $m_v = m_0 \left(1 + \dfrac{v^2}{2c^2} \right)$ approximately (i.e. for small v)

Now, as shown above, 'resting' energy $= m_0 c^2$ and 'moving' energy $= $ '$m_v c^2$' so that (by substitution)

$$\text{moving energy} = m_0 c^2 \left(1 + \dfrac{v^2}{2c^2} \right)$$

Thus, the net energy due to movement (i.e. the kinetic energy) is just the difference between the 'rest' energy and the 'moving' energy,

i.e. $m_v c^2 - m_0 c^2$

i.e. $m_0 c^2 \left(1 + \dfrac{v^2}{2c^2} \right) - m_0 c^2$

i.e. $\frac{1}{2} m v^2$

so verifying Newton's expression for the kinetic energy of a moving body (Equation 7.4), but only for velocities which are small compared to the velocity of light.

In conclusion, therefore, energy and mass are to be considered as two manifestations of the same thing, and may be changed from one to the other in the appropriate circumstances, as the following two examples show:

a.   The forces that hold an atomic nucleus together are obtained by some of the matter being converted to energy (25.2.1). Thus, a nucleus weighs less than the sum of the individual weights of the particles which make up the nucleus!

b.   A gamma ray whose energy is in excess of 1·02 MeV may, in the proximity of a nucleus. spontaneously 'disappear' and create two particles of matter: a negative electron and a positive electron ('positron'). This process is known as 'pair production' (30.6). The positron so created will eventually meet an electron and both will disappear, producing two gamma rays of 0·51 MeV. This example therefore shows first the creation of matter from electromagnetic energy, then the creation of energy from matter.

23.3 CONSERVATION OF MOMENTUM

The law of conservation of momentum is sometimes referred to as the 'most general law in physics', being even more fundamental than the law of conservation of energy, and may be simply stated as:

STATEMENT
   The total linear momentum in a system is constant.

The word 'system' is used in the same manner as in the previous section.
   An alternative manner of expressing this law is:

Sum of (mass × velocity) = constant

Here, it is the *relativistic* mass (23.2.1) which is implied, i.e. the mass of any body moving at velocity v. For example, momentum is conserved in the Compton scattering process (where an electron removes some of the momentum of an incoming photon) and in photoelectric absorption (where some momentum is imparted to the whole atom). These are explained in Chapter 30.

23.4 WAVE–PARTICLE DUALITY

In addition to the 'mass–energy equivalence' principle outlined in section 23.2.1, modern physics also blurs the rigid distinction which existed in classical physics between a particle and a wave. We shall take these in turn.

23.4.1 Waves as particles

Classical physics was very successful at explaining many phenomena associated with electromagnetic radiation (e.g. diffraction and interference) by assuming such radiation to be made up of periodic waves travelling at the speed of light, c, such that $c = v\lambda$, where v is the frequency of vibration of the radiation and λ is its periodic wavelength (24.1.1). However, the Compton and photoelectric effects as mentioned above (23.3) were not easy to explain on this wave principle. It was only when it was considered that sometimes electromagnetic radiation behaved as 'packets' of energy with an associated momentum that such effects could be explained. Such a wave packet is called a *photon* or a *quantum*, and Quantum Theory predicts that:

    a.   the quantum will have an energy, E, given by:

$$E = \boldsymbol{h}v \qquad\qquad\qquad \text{Equation 23.2}$$

where $\boldsymbol{h}$ is a constant, known as 'Planck's constant', and v is the frequency of vibration of the associated wave. We shall have occasion to use this formula often in this section on atomic physics.

    b.   the quantum will have a momentum, p, given by:

$$p = \frac{\boldsymbol{h}v}{c} \qquad\qquad\qquad \text{Equation 23.3}$$

(This equation may be derived from Equation 23.2 and $E = mc^2$, for $mc = E/c = \boldsymbol{h}v/c$ and mc is just the momentum, p, of a body moving at the velocity of light, i.e. an electromagnetic quantum.)

    Thus, the electromagnetic wave may also behave like a particle, possessing energy and momentum.

23.4.2 Particles as waves

Moving particles of matter, large or small, have both kinetic energy and momentum. Do they ever behave as though they are waves, though? Perhaps the most dramatic example of particles behaving like waves is in the operation of an electron microscope, where high-energy electrons are passed through, or scattered from, a sample. A very highly magnified imaged of the sample is obtained, it now being possible to distinguish between individual gold atoms! The reason for such incredible performance lies in the very small wavelength associated with the individual electrons. The smaller the wavelength of radiation used (24.1.1), the finer the detail it is possible to see, whether it be 'optical' or 'electron' microscopy.

Another example of particles having wave-like properties is the well-known neutron diffraction experiments used to establish the structural details of various crystals. Here, the neutrons are scattered at preferred angles from the crystal, rather like light from a diffraction grating.

De Broglie proposed the following relationship to exist between the momentum, p, of the particles and its associated wavelength, λ:

$$p = \frac{h}{\lambda}$$

Equation 23.4

λ is called the 'de Broglie' wavelength, the existence of which has been abundantly verified by experiment.

Note the *inverse* relationship between the momentum of the particle and its associated wavelength. Thus. the wavelength decreases as the momentum increases, and *vice versa*. For example, the de Broglie wavelength associated with an electron moving at one-half of the velocity of light is about 4×10^{-12} m, which is less than the diameter of a hydrogen atom (100×10^{-12} m): When the velocity of an electron is one-hundredth of that of light, the de Broglie wavelengths is at the larger value of 240×10^{-12} m, which is in the X-ray range of wavelengths (24.2) and may be used to investigate the structure of crystals as in the case of neutrons mentioned above.

The aspects of the principles of 'wave–particle duality' outlined in the above two sections which concern the following chapters are mainly those of waves behaving as quanta rather than particles behaving as waves. This is particularly the case when considering the effects of changes in the electron orbits of atoms (25.5) and X-ray interaction with matter (Ch. 30).

23.5 HEISENBERG'S UNCERTAINTY PRINCIPLE

Heisenberg's Uncertainty Principle is not of such importance to an understanding of radiology as either of the principles of Mass–Energy Equivalence or Wave–Particle Duality described above. In fact, this section may be omitted by the reader if so desired, as it is somewhat more advanced, and is only referred to in the section on alpha decay (26.5). Its inclusion, however, does show another fundamental difference between classical and modern physics, an understanding of which may be conceptually helpful to the reader.

In classical physics, it is possible in *principle* to measure exactly a number of quantities concerning the state of a body, for example its energy, position and momentum. Furthermore, if it were possible for measuring apparatus to be built which produced no errors of measurement (i.e. with infinite precision), it would be likewise possible to measure exactly several of these quantities *simultaneously*.

According to modern physics, however, we have seen that it is not possible to treat quantities like mass and energy, or matter and waves, as being totally independent of each other. The Uncertainty Principle is an extension of the principle of wave–particle duality, and concerns the maximum possible precision which may be obtained in ideal circumstances when measuring two quantities simultaneously. The central point is that measuring one quantity (e.g. momentum of a particle) affects another quantity (position of the particle), so that it is never possible to measure both simultaneously with complete accuracy. This is different in principle from the case of classical physics, where perfect instruments are assumed to produce perfect results. Effects due to the Uncertainty Principle are too small to be observed in everyday life, of course, and concern mainly atomic and nuclear systems.

Exercise 23.2
a.   Why is there no law of conservation of matter in modern physics? Hence explain what is meant by 'mass–energy equivalence'.
b.   Describe the following terms:

(i) rest mass
(ii) relativistic mass
(iii) quantum (or photon)
(iv) de Broglie wavelength.

c.   Give an example of matter being transformed into energy and *vice versa*.
d.   Using Einstein's relationship: $E = mc^2$, calculate the mass–energy of a proton if the proton mass $= 1\cdot67 \times 10^{-27}$ kg and $c = 3 \times 10^8$ m s^{-1}.
e.   What is meant by 'wave–particle duality'? Give an example of a wave behaving as a particle and a particle behaving as a wave. What is the energy in joule of an X-ray of frequency 3×10^{18} Hz (cycles s^{-1}) (use $E = hv$, where $h = 6\cdot63 \times 10^{-34}$ J s).

SUMMARY

1.   Classical physics propounds three conservation laws: of mass, energy and momentum.
2.   Modern physics has two corresponding conservation laws: of energy and momentum.
3.   'Mass–energy equivalence' relates energy (E) and mass (m) by $E = mc^2$. Mass may be 'converted' to energy and *vice versa* (examples in text).
4.   'Wave–particle duality' refers to the fact that electromagnetic waves may

sometimes behave as if they were packets of energy and momentum called *photons* or *quanta*. Similarly, particles may sometimes behave like waves of a definite wavelength. The relationships are $E = \boldsymbol{h}v$ and $\lambda = \boldsymbol{h}/p$ respectively, where $\boldsymbol{h}$ is 'Planck's constant' and λ is the 'de Broglie wavelength'. (Examples in text.)

24. Electromagnetic radiation

24.1 PROPERTIES OF ELECTROMAGNETIC RADIATION

There are three types of radiation to which we are subject in our everyday lives: sound, radiation due to particles (e.g. cosmic rays) and electromagnetic radiation. Concerning sound radiation, it is a matter of common experience that the ear is not equally sensitive to the whole range of frequencies (or pitch) of sound waves, since bats (for example) are able to hear much higher pitches than us. In a similar manner, we are not equally sensitive to the whole of the range of electromagnetic radiation. We see the world around us by means of a very narrow range of the electromagnetic spectrum ('light'), feel heat from the sun from another part ('infra-red') and become sun-tanned by yet another part ('ultra-violet)'). In addition, 'microwave' ovens may cook our food, radio waves carry radio and television programmes and X-rays be used to produce

Table 24.1 Properties of electromagnetic radiation

General properties

Waves composed of transverse vibrations of electric and magnetic fields
Vibrations have a wide range of frequencies and wavelengths, but always travel in vacuum at the speed of light (3×10^8 m s^{-1})
Unaffected by electric or magnetic fields
May be polarised, i.e. to vibrate in one plane only
Able to produce constructive or destructive interference
Carries energy and momentum

Interaction with matter

Type	Comment
Emission	Most efficient from 'black body' (8.2.4)
Reflection	Not for high energies (X- and γ-radiation)
Refraction	Not for high energies (X- and γ-radiation)
Transmission	Different materials are transparent to different wavelengths
Absorption	Always exponential (5.3)
	Photoelectric from u.v. to γ-radiation
	Compton scatter by X- and γ-radiation
	Pair production for energies greater than 1·02 MeV
Fluorescence	Electron vacancies caused by photon produce fluorescent radiation — wavelength is always greater than incident wavelength
	Many fluorescent photons may be produced from one incident photon

radiographs. The general properties of all these electromagnetic radiations are identical, however, and it is only the differences they exhibit in their interaction with matter which enables them to be used for such widely different purposes. Table 24.1 summarises the general properties of all electromagnetic radiations and also outlines some of the ways (relevant to our purposes) in which they interact with matter. For example, all electromagnetic radiation is propagated in straight lines, which has important consequences, such as the Inverse Square Law (Ch. 4). Further, such radiation is able to travel through a vacuum, so enabling heat and light to reach us from the sun, and the X-radiation from the anodes of X-ray tubes to pass through the vacuum inside the tubes. As discussed in the previous chapter, there is a wave-particle duality (23.4) which exists between electromagnetic radiation and matter. This is expanded further in the following sections.

24.1.1 Wave-like properties

As the term 'electromagnetic' suggests, electromagnetic radiation consists of both electric and magnetic fields. These fields are at right-angles both to each other and to the direction of travel, as shown in Figure 24.1. Thus both the electric and magnetic *vectors* (6.3.1), as shown in E and B in the figure, vibrate *transversely* to the direction of propagation of the wave. (This is in contrast to sound radiation, in which pressure waves move in the same direction as that of the propagation — i.e. *longitudinal* waves.) In addition, the vectors vary in strength in a sinusoidal manner (15.2), as illustrated in the figure. Thus, if we draw the variation of the electric vector (for example), a sinewave results, as

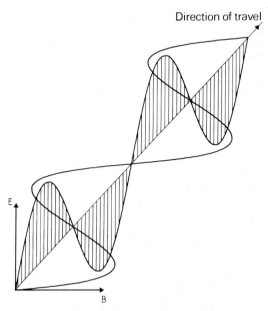

Fig. 24.1 Electromagnetic radiation depicted as a wave consisting of alternating electric and magnetic vectors vibrating at right-angles to each other and to the direction of motion of the wave.

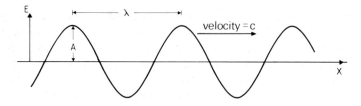

Fig. 24.2 An electromagnetic 'sine-wave' of amplitude A and wavelength λ travelling at the velocity of light, c (3×10^8 m s^{-1}).

shown in Figure 24.2. The periodic variation of the vectors, as shown in the figure, is the reason why electromagnetic radiations are often referred to as electromagnetic 'waves', and such was thought to be the whole explanation of their behaviour by classical physics (23.4). The parameters which are of importance in describing a particular wave are:

a. the *cycle* — one complete waveform
b. the *wavelength* — the distance travelled in completing one cycle
c. the *frequency* — the number of cycles per second, or Hz
d. the *velocity* — the speed of light, c, in a vacuum
e. the *amplitude*, A — the magnitude of the peak of the waveform.

There is a simple relationship which exists between the velocity, wavelength and frequency, for if there are v cycles per second, and each cycle is of length λ, then in one second the wave must travel a distance $v \times \lambda$. However, the 'distance travelled per second' is just the velocity, c, so that we have:

$c = v\lambda$ Equation 24.1

   in a vacuum

As Table 24.1 shows, all electromagnetic radiation travels at the velocity of light in a vacuum, so that what distinguishes one 'ray' from another is the individual values of frequency and wavelength. For example, 'blue' light has a wavelength of approximately 400 nm (n = 'nano' — see 1.6) and a frequency of 7.5×10^{14} Hz, while 'red' light has a wavelength of about 800 nm and a frequency of 3.75×10^{14} Hz. Hence the greater the frequency, the smaller the wavelength and *vice versa*.

Insight

    Chapters 12 and 14 have shown that is possible to produce both a magnetic field from moving electric charges (electromagnetism) and an electric field from a changing magnetic flux (electromagnetic induction). It may be shown mathematically that a changing electric field can sustain a changing magnetic field, and *vice versa*, *if* they both travel at the velocity of light. This is the basis both for the linear propagation of such electromagnetic waves and for the fact that the wave does not gradually diminish in amplitude with time.

    Electromagnetic radiation is therefore a self-sustaining interaction of electric and magnetic fields travelling at the speed of light.

In a transparent medium the waves travel at a velocity **v**, given by $c = n v$, where n is a constant for a given incident wavelength and is known as the 'refractive index'. The frequency of vibration is unaltered in the medium, but the wavelength is reduced owing to the reduction of the velocity of the wave, i.e. the wave will have travelled a shorter distance to complete a cycle. If the wavelength in the medium is λ', then equation 24.1 becomes:

$$\mathbf{v} = v\lambda'$$

Substituting the value of v from $c = n\mathbf{v}$, we obtain:

$c = n v \lambda'$
　　　in a medium of refractive index n

Equation 24.2

Two further important properties of electromagnetic radiation which are a consequence of its wave-like nature are *polarisation* and *interference*. A beam of light from a bulb, for example, consists of many millions of waves whose electric vectors are pointing in random directions with respect to each other. If the beam is passed through a 'polarising' substance (e.g. a tourmaline crystal), then it is found that it transmits best those waves whose electric vectors are pointing in one direction, and completely absorbs those at right-angles to this direction. The emergent light is said to have been *plane polarised*, i.e. its vibrations are all in one plane. It was evidence such as this which showed that electromagnetic radiation consisted of *transverse* rather than *longitudinal* vibrations.

Further evidence of the wave-like properties of electromagnetic radiation comes from the phenomenon of interference, where the amplitudes of two 'coherent' beams (i.e. two beams which are 'in phase' with each other — see 15.4.1) are added together to form the resultant amplitude at any point, in the same way that ripples in a pool of water may superimpose on each other to become bigger or smaller. Such interference effects are relevant to radiography in applications such as holographic imaging by X-rays — well outside the scope of this book and so not pursued further!

24.1.2 Particle-like properties

The advent of modern 'quantum physics' (23.4.1) has enabled many previously unexplained phenomena associated with electromagnetic radiation to be understood in terms of 'quanta' or 'photons' of radiation which possess discrete levels of energy and momentum. Electromagnetic radiation may therefore behave in two different ways: like a pure wave, as in interference etc., and as a *particle* having momentum and energy. This 'wave-particle duality' is discussed in more detail in Chapter 23, the results of which may be summarised here. The energy, E, of a quantum is proportional to the frequency of the associated wave, such that

---

$E = \mathbf{h} v$

Equation 24.3

---

where h is a constant, known as 'Planck's constant'. The momentum, p, of the quantum is also proportional to the frequency, and is given by:

$$p = \frac{h\nu}{c}$$ Equation 24.4

where c is the velocity of light in vacuum.

These concepts are essential to an understanding of both the photoelectric and Compton effects (Ch. 30).

A useful formula relating energy and wavelength is obtained simply by using Equation 24.3 and substituting $\nu = c/\lambda$ from Equation 24.1,

i.e. $E = \frac{hc}{\lambda}$

where $h = 6\cdot62 \times 10^{-34}$ J s, $c = 3\cdot0 \times 10^8$ m s^{-1} and E is expressed in joule. It is more convenient to our purpose to express E in keV, however, and the conversion factor is 1 keV $= 1\cdot6 \times 10^{-16}$ J, and substitution of all these values in the above equation results in the expression

$$E = \frac{1\cdot24}{\lambda}$$ Equation 24.5

where E is in keV and λ is in nanometers. For example, an X-ray of energy 100 keV has a wavelength of $1\cdot24/100$ nm, i.e. $0\cdot0124$ nm (or $1\cdot24 \times 10^{-11}$ m). Lengths as small as this are difficult to imagine, being about one-hundred-millionth of a millimetre! This is less than the diameter of an atom (about 10^{-10} m) but greater than the diameter of an atomic nucleus (about 10^{-14} m).

24.2 THE ELECTROMAGNETIC SPECTRUM

The previous section has shown that electromagnetic radiation may have a very large range of wavelengths, i.e. a *spectrum* of wavelengths (and frequencies). It is convenient to split up such an electromagnetic spectrum into bands which are broadly categorised by their interaction with matter and hence the uses to which such bands may be put. This is illustrated (in simplified form) in Figure 24.3, which also shows the wavelengths, frequencies and energies corresponding to the approximate boundaries between the various bands. The small wavelengths occur at high frequencies and energies, as previously discussed.

The common factor which links the types of interaction between electromagnetic radiation and matter is that the *value of wavelength determines the size of the objects* with which it will directly interact. Thus, radio waves (long wavelengths) are both transmitted and received by relatively large conductors; infra-red radiation interacts with whole atoms and molecules (giving them kinetic energy, or heat); visible and ultra-violet light interact with the outer

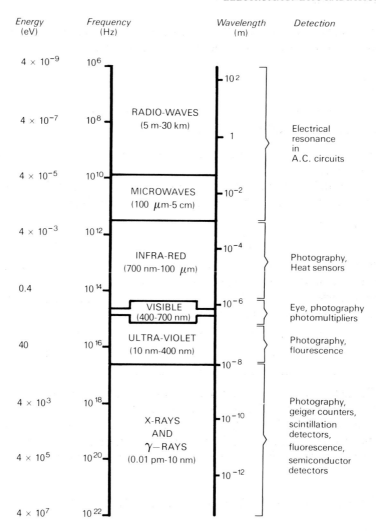

Fig. 24.3 The electromagnetic spectrum (not drawn to scale). Typical values of wavelengths, frequencies and photon energies for different bands of the spectrum are shown, together with some methods used in their detection. (*Note:* 1 Hz = 1 cycle per second; 1 pm = 10^{-12} m etc.)

electron orbits of an atom; X-rays and γ-rays interact with the inner electron orbits of an atom; and very high energy gamma rays (having very short wavelengths) interact with the tiny nuclei of atoms.

Table 24.1 gives some examples of the types of interaction which occur together with brief comments. For example, refraction is a phenomenon associated with the outer electron orbits of atoms. It is therefore most efficient for those wavelengths which are able to interact with such electrons, i.e. those of ultra-violet and above. Smaller wavelengths (higher energies) become progressively less affected by the outer atomic orbits, although it is just possible to show refraction effects for low-energy X-rays. The other comments in the table also show the dependence of each effect on the energy of the incident radiation, due to the principle outlined above. Those interactions due to X-rays (which are, of course, most relevant to this book) are discussed in Chapter 30.

24.3 ELECTROMAGNETIC RADIATION AND RADIOGRAPHY

The process of taking a radiograph results in the emission of radiation whose wavelengths and energies are from three different parts of the electromagnetic spectrum described in the previous section. These are summarised in Figure 24.4.

The anode emits both heat and light in addition to X-rays. The latter is composed of the Bremsstrahlung continuous spectrum upon which is super-

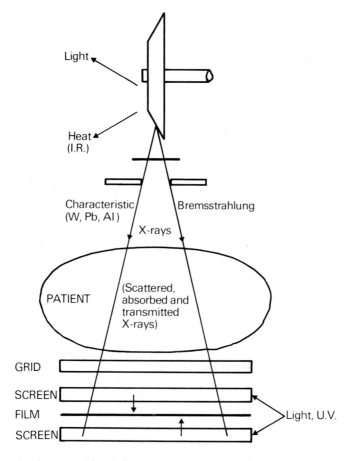

Fig. 24.4 The production of radiation from different parts of the electromagnetic spectrum as a result of a radiograph being taken.

imposed the characteristic radiation due to the tungsten target. The absorption processes within the aluminium filter and lead collimators produces additional characteristic radiation due to these elements (although of low intensity). The passage of the X-rays through the patient produces a minute amount of heat radiation (32.2.1) and characteristic radiation of calcium (for example), although the latter is of too low an energy to contribute to the production of the radiographic image. In addition, the scattering of the incident radiation by the patient's tissue results in the production of radiation of lower energy (longer wavelength). The grid also contributes to scatter and characteristic radiation, and the screens produce fluorescent radiation within the u.v. and visible range of wavelengths, together with a very small quantity of heat.

Further examples of the occurrence and use of electromagnetic radiation in diagnostic radiology include the light emitted by the fluorescent of cathode ray tubes, image intensifiers or 'viewers', and also radioactive decay where both quanta of X and/or gamma rays may be emitted from the radioactive substance.

Exercise 24.1

a.   Explain the following terms in relation to electromagnetic radiation:

(i) electric vector
(ii) magnetic vector
(iii) sinusoidal variation
(iv) wavelength
(v) frequency
(vi) transverse propagation.

b.   Discuss briefly the phenomena of *polarisation* and *interference* of electromagnetic radiation. How would you demonstrate both by simple experiments?

c.   Why do high-energy X-rays have small wavelengths and low-energy X-rays have longer wavelengths? How is the energy of a quantum related to its frequency?

d.   What is the wavelength of an X-ray of energy

(i) 10 keV
(ii) 50 keV
(iii) 20 MeV?

e.   What is the minimum wavelength of a quantum in an X-ray beam which has been produced with $100 \, kV_p$ across the X-ray tube?

SUMMARY

1.   Electromagnetic radiation consists of vibrating electric and magnetic fields which are able to pass through a vacuum at the speed of light.

2.   The general properties of electromagnetic radiation and its interactions with matter are summarised in Table 24.1.

3.   The periodic variation of the wave-like nature of electromagnetic radiation leads to the concepts of wavelength λ and frequency v, which are related to velocity by $c = v\lambda$ in a vacuum.

4.   Electromagnetic radiation also exhibits particle-like behaviour as explained by quantum physics. In particular, each 'quantum' has an energy $E = hv$ and a momentum $p = hv/c$, where h is 'Planck's constant'.

5.   The relationship between the energy of a quantum and its wavelength is given by

$$E(\text{keV}) = \frac{1 \cdot 24}{\lambda \, (\text{nm})}$$

25. Elementary structure of the atom

25.1 INTRODUCTION

The reader is advised to study the previous two chapters on modern physics and electromagnetic radiation before embarking upon this chapter.

Any attempt by Man to understand his surroundings must include the study of what matter is actually 'made of'. The atom, as the fundamental 'building block' of matter in the world around us, has therefore been the subject of a great deal of study (both experimentally and theoretically) by physicists, and a picture of increasing complexity has emerged. However, the relatively simple 'planetary model' of the atom consisting of solid electrons orbiting a central nucleus can be used to explain many atomic phenomena satisfactorily. In addition, it has the advantage of being easy to imagine, and is therefore the atomic model used in this chapter. Modern quantum physics (Ch. 23) has been 'grafted' onto the planetary model where appropriate in some of the sections and Insights in the chapter (e.g. electron orbit changes — 25·5).

The planetary model of the atom is due to Rutherford (in 1911), and it describes the atom as consisting of a central, small positively charged body (the 'nucleus') around which the negatively charged electrons move in defined orbits. This is pictured in Figure 25.1, where an atom of carbon is illustrated.

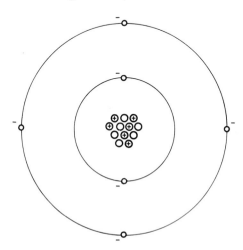

Fig. 25.1 The basic structure of a carbon atom. A central nucleus contains 6 protons (positively charged) and 6 neutrons — i.e. 12 nucleons altogether. Six electrons orbit the nucleus in defined orbits. The atom is neutrally charged owing to equal numbers of protons and electrons.

The nucleus of carbon consists of 12 'elementary particles': 6 protons and 6 neutrons. These are bound together in an incredibly tiny volume of very large density (about three thousand million million times greater than water). The electrically neutral carbon atom has 6 orbiting electrons to match the 6 protons in the nucleus. These electrons are arranged in 'shells', called '$K, L, M, \ldots$' starting from the inner shell. The K shell can only contain 2 electrons, and the L shell of the carbon atom contains the remaining four. Different types of atom contain differing numbers of protons and neutrons in the nucleus and a differing electron configuration, as explained in sections 25.3 and 25.4. The atom consists largely of space since the particles themselves are so tiny. For example, if the atom is pictured as being as big as a house, the size of the nucleus is about that of a pin-head, although it contains about 99·95% of the total mass of the atom! The masses and charges of the particles considered in this and other chapters are summarised in Table 25.1.

Table 25.1 Masses and charges of some atomic particles

Particle	Symbol	Rest mass (kg)	Rest mass (amu)*	Rest energy (MeV)	Charge†	Comments
Proton	p	$1\cdot672 \times 10^{-27}$	$1\cdot007$	938	+1	'Nucleons', i.e. present in atomic nuclei
Neutron	n	$1\cdot675 \times 10^{-27}$	$1\cdot009$	939	0	
Alpha particle	α	$6\cdot645 \times 10^{-27}$	$4\cdot003$	3725	+2	2 protons and 2 neutrons — a helium nucleus. Ejected in α decay
Electron	e^- or β^-	$9\cdot109 \times 10^{-31}$	$0\cdot00055$ (or 1/1820)	$0\cdot511$	−1	Form stable 'discrete' orbits around nuclei
Positron	e^+ or β^+	$9\cdot109 \times 10^{-31}$	$0\cdot00055$ (or 1/1820)	$0\cdot511$	+1	'Anti-particle' of electron — produces annihilation radiation when meet
Pi meson	π^+	$2\cdot480 \times 10^{-28}$	$0\cdot150$	139	+1	Keep nucleus together (π^0 and π^- also exist)
Neutrino	ν	0	0	0	0	Emitted during β-decay and 'electron-capture' Very weakly absorbed by matter
Photon or $h\nu$ quantum	—	—	—	—	0	Travels at the velocity of light, with energy $= h\nu$ and momentum $= h\nu/c$ Forms the electromagnetic spectrum

* 1 amu is 1 'atomic mass unit', which is 1/12 of mass of neutral $^{12}_{6}C$ atom
† A charge of +1 is $+1\cdot602 \times 10^{-19}$ coulomb

Insight

Rutherford carried out some elegant experimental work connected with the scattering of α-particles by atoms, and concluded that the only explanation whereby α-particles could be scattered over such wide angles as he found experimentally was given by assuming the atom to consist of a small heavy positively charged nucleus with orbiting electrons. The alternative model whereby all the atomic particles were contained in the same small volume was unacceptable because of the small scattering that would have been produced on the α-particles.

25.2 THE ATOMIC NUCLEUS

The number of protons and neutrons contained in an atomic nucleus determines both the mass and the charge of the nucleus and the particular configuration of electron orbits around it. There are several important terms which recur in this and ensuing chapters which require definition at this stage. These terms are helpful to the understanding of atomic structure and are defined in Table 25.2. To take an example, the most abundant naturally occurring stable *isotope* of carbon has 6 protons and neutrons in the nucleus, as shown previously in Figure 25.1. The *atomic number* (Z) is therefore 6, the atomic *mass number* (A) is 12 and the whole atom may be written as $^{12}_{6}C$. Thus $^{12}_{6}C$ is an example of a *nuclide*: one which contains 6 protons and 6 neutrons. In

Table 25.2 Terms used to describe a nucleus

Term	Symbol	Definition
Nucleon	—	A proton or neutron within the nucleus
Atomic number	Z	The number of protons in the nucleus
Atomic mass number	A	The total number of nucleons within the nucleus
Neutron number	N	The number of neutrons within the nucleus
Nuclide	—	A nucleus with particular values of Z and A
Element	E	A nucleus with a given value of Z
Isotope (of an element)	—	Any nucleus which contains the same number of protons as a given nucleus (i.e. same Z)
Isobar	—	Any nucleus which has the same atomic mass number as another nucleus (i.e. same value of A)
Radionuclide or 'radioisotope'	—	Any nuclide which is radioactive

general, an element E is written as $^{A}_{Z}E$. An *isotope* of $^{12}_{6}C$, which is also naturally occurring but less abundant, has 7 neutrons in the nucleus (i.e. 1 more than before) and may be written as $^{13}_{6}C$. Note that it is not necessarily the case that 'isotopes are radioactive', as this example shows, since $^{12}_{6}C$ and $^{13}_{6}C$ are both isotopes of carbon, neither of which is radioactive. The definition of an isotope in Table 25.2 does not imply any associated radioactivity. An isotope of carbon which *is* radioactive is the well-known 'carbon-14', or $^{14}_{6}C$. Being carbon, the nucleus still contains 6 protons, but there are now 8 neutrons rather than 6. As a radioactive nuclide, $^{14}_{6}C$ is an example of a *radionuclide*, or (less satisfactorily) a 'radioisotope'. It decays by the emission of electrons from the nuclei (beta decay — 26.3).

Exercise 25.1

a. What elements do the following symbols represent, and how many protons and neutrons are contained in each nucleus?

$${}_{1}^{1}H, \ {}_{1}^{2}H, \ {}_{2}^{4}He, \ {}_{29}^{63}Cu, \ {}_{53}^{131}I, \ {}_{74}^{184}W, \ {}_{88}^{226}Ra, \ {}_{92}^{235}U, \ {}_{92}^{238}U$$

b. Write the appropriate symbols for an element containing:

(i) 1 proton and 2 neutrons

(ii) 2 protons and 2 neutrons.

25.2.1 The stability of the nucleus

What is it that prevents the nucleus from flying apart? After all, the nucleus should be quite unable to 'stick together' because of the mutual repulsion of like positive charges (9.1), since the protons are the only charged particles within the nucleus. The neutrons, being electrically neutral, have no electrostatic effect.

In practice, some nuclei are so stable as to possess no measureable radioactivity whatever (e.g. ${}_{6}^{12}C$) while others decay with a half-life (5.2.2) of less than a millionth of a second. The nucleus may therefore be visualised as a *dynamic*, rather than a *static*, entity where opposing forces are acting: a force which tends to keep the nucleus intact and a force tending to disrupt it. Thus, a stable nucleus is one in which the disruptive forces never succeed, and an unstable nucleus is one in which they do succeed. The nucleus is then said to 'decay'. It is not possible to predict the exact moment when any particular nucleus will decay, as it is a matter of probability rather than certainty. However, the 'law of radioactive decay' (5.2) is obeyed when there is a large number of such unstable nuclei.

The forces which hold a nucleus together are quite unlike the forces of gravity, magnetism and electrostatics with which we are familiar. They are known as 'short-range forces' and act over distances of about 10^{-15} meter, over which range they are much more powerful than the forces of electrostatic repulsion. The energy expended in keeping the nucleus together is known as the *Binding Energy* (BE). If the BE is divided by the number of nucleons within the nucleus, then a figure of about 8·4 MeV is obtained for most nuclei — this is known as the 'binding energy per nucleon'.

Nuclei containing even numbers of protons and neutrons exhibit the greatest stability, leading to the concept that nuclear 'shells' exist in somewhat the same manner as electron shells around the nucleus — a completed shell being particularly stable. However, further treatment of nuclear shells is beyond the scope of this book.

Insight

The π-meson is a particle with a mass between that of an electron and a nucleon (i.e. proton or neutron) and is thought to be responsible for the forces holding the nucleons together. These 'short-range' forces are

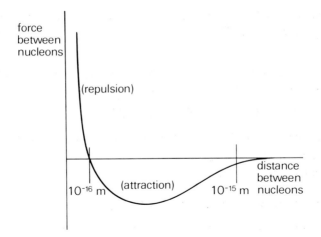

Fig. 25.2 'Short-range' forces between nucleons. A strong attraction between 10^{-15} and 10^{-16} m holds the nucleus together.

known as *exchange forces* and result in an adjacent proton and neutron (for example) changing continually into a neutron and proton and back again! This may be written as:

$$p_1 + n_1 \rightarrow n_2 + \pi^+ + n_1 \rightarrow n_2 + p_2$$

The π^+-meson has left the original proton p_1, leaving it as a neutron, and has formed a proton p_2 from the original neutron n_1. The proton and neutron are therefore continually changing their position. Negative and neutral π-mesons exist and are also exchanged between the nucleons.

A graph of the short-range forces between nucleons is as shown. A strong force of attraction is evident below about 10^{-15}m which changes to a force of repulsion at about 10^{-16}m. The nucleons are thus kept apart by about 5×10^{-16}m. The Binding Energy between the nucleons is obtained by the transformation of matter into energy as given by Einstein's equation: $E = mc^2$. Each nucleon 'weighs' about 931 MeV, and about 8·4 MeV of this is used for its Binding Energy to nearby nucleons. Thus, each nucleus weighs less than the sum of the individual weights of its nucleons, a finding which is verified by experiment.

25.3 ELECTRON ORBITS

Consider an atom of hydrogen as depicted in Figure 25.3. It is assumed that the solitary electron is on a circular path around the nucleus. It may be shown that a body moving in a circle of radius r at a velocity v has an acceleration of v^2/r towards the centre of the circle. Such an acceleration should, according to classical physics, result in the emission of electromagnetic radiation (see Insight in 8.2.4) from the charged electron, so that the electron would lose energy, fall toward and eventually collide with the nucleus (path 2 in Fig. 25.3). In practice, of course, electron orbits do not behave in this manner, or atoms as

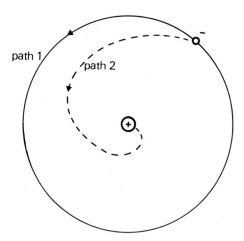

Fig. 25.3 A stable, discrete electron orbit (path 1) compared to a 'decaying' electron (path 2) as predicted by classical physics.

we know them would not exist! The electrons orbit the nucleus only in stable paths (e.g. path 1) — the so-called 'discrete' orbits. Further, these orbits are grouped in 'shells', where there is a particular maximum number of electrons in each shell and the energy of the electrons in each shell is approximately the same. The electrons 'fill-up' the inner shells first, since the energies of the inner shells are less than the outer shells.

Table 25.3 shows the maximum permitted number of electrons in each shell, from the inner K shell to shell N. The shell number, n, starts from $n = 1$ for the K shell, and is known as the 'principal quantum number'. Atoms with completed electron shells are chemically very stable (i.e. non-reactive). For example, the inert gas neon ($^{20}_{10}Ne$) has full K and L shells as illustrated in Figure 25.4. The fact that the L shell is full makes neon chemically non-reactive, in contrast to the next element sodium which has one electron in the M shell. This solitary electron makes sodium very chemically reactive in that it readily 'gives' the electron to other atoms and becomes a positive 'ion' with the appearance of an outer closed shell.

Table 25.3 Numbers of electrons in atomic shells

Principal quantum no. or Shell no. (n)	Shell letter	Maximum no of electrons	$2n^2$
1	K	2	2
2	L	8	8
3	M	18	18
4	N	32	32

Note that the maximum number of permitted electrons in each shell is given by $2n^2$

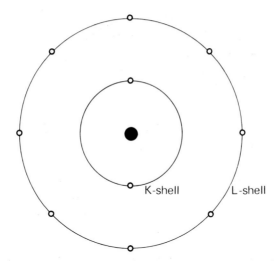

Fig. 25.4 An atom of neon, showing both K and L shells containing their maximum number of premitted electrons. This makes neon particularly chemically stable.

Thus it is the nucleus which determines the mass of an element, but it is the orbiting electrons which determine its chemical reactivity, as described further in the next section.

The outer shells also contain stable sub-shells within them. Argon has an atomic number of 18, and has an electron configuration of 2, 8, 8 in the K, L and M shells. The K and L shells are therefore full (see Table 25.3) but the M shell only contains 8 of a possible maximum of 18 electrons, and yet argon is chemically inert. An outer sub-shell of 8 electrons is particularly chemically stable, a fact which is confirmed by the next inert gas krypton which has an electronic configuration of 2, 8, 18, 8.

Insight

The wave-particle duality of matter (23.4) may be used to explain the existence of discrete electron orbits if it is assumed that an orbiting electron had a 'de Broglie' wavelength which is able to fit around the circumference of the orbit an exact number of times. This fixes the size of each orbit. The necessary condition for this to occur is $n\lambda = 2\pi r$ where n is a whole number. Now λ is the 'de Broglie' wavelength (23.4.2) of the electron of momentum p, and is given by $\lambda = h/p$.

Thus we have $\dfrac{nh}{p} = 2\pi r$ or $pr = \dfrac{nh}{2\pi}$

or, the angular momentum (momentum × radius) must be multiple of $h/2\pi$, as first originally postulated by Bhor (1913) on an empirical basis. There is now no question of any electromagnetic radiation occurring from an electron orbit, and this example serves to show that the concepts of quantum physics may be used to described atomic phenomena which are not explicable by classical physics.

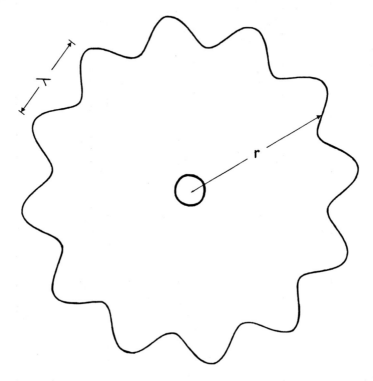

Fig. 25.5 The use of a de Broglie wave to explain the existence of discrete orbits (see Insight).

25.4 PERIODIC TABLE OF THE ELEMENTS

If the elements are arranged in order of increasing atomic number, it may be shown that their chemical properties (such as valency) and physical properties (such as specific heat capacity) tend to recur in a periodic manner. Arranging the elements in these similar groups produces a Periodic Table, as shown in Table 25.4. The chemical similarity of elements in each group may be explained by reference to their electronic structure, as shown in Table 25.5. It has already been noted that as the number of electrons increases with the value of atomic number, each electron takes an orbit of the lowest possible energy. If this was not so it would be able to perform a quantum jump 'downwards' (25.5) to a lower energy level.

There are two rules which determine the way in which the electron shells are gradually built up as the atomic number increases:

    a.   shell number n cannot contain more than $2n^2$ electrons
    b.   the outer shell cannot contain more than 8 electrons.

These are known as the 'Bury-Bohr' rules after their co-discoverers, and ensure that the orbit of minimum energy is filled first.

One additional constraint is required in order that the electrons fill the orbits in the correct manner, and that is that *no two electrons may have*

Table 25.4 — The Periodic Table

Group / Period	0	I	II	III	IV	V	VI	VII	VIII
1	He 4·003 — 2	H 1·008 — 1							
2	Ne 19·992 — 10	Li 7·016 — 3	Be 9·012 — 4	B 10·013 (19·6%), 11·009 (80·4%) — 5	C 12·000 — 6	N 14·003 — 7	O 15·995 — 8	F 18·998 — 9	
3	A 39·962 — 18	Na 22·989 — 11	Mg 23·985 (78·7%), 25·983 (11·2%) — 12	Al 26·982 — 13	Si 27·977 — 14	P 30·974 — 15	S 31·972 — 16	Cl 34·969 (75·5%), 36·966 (24·5%) — 17	
4	Kr 83·912 (57%), 85·911 (17·4%) — 36	K 38·964 — 19	Ca 39·963 — 20	Sc 44·956 — 21	Ti 47·948 — 22	V 50·944 — 23	Cr 51·944 — 24	Mn 54·938 — 25	Fe 55·935 — 26 Co 58·933 — 27 Ni 57·935 (67·9%), 59·931 (26·2%) — 28
4 (b)		Cu 62·929 (69%), 64·928 (31%) — 29	Zn 63·929 (49%), 65·926 (28%) — 30	Ga 68·926 (60%), 70·925 (40%) — 31	Ge 71·922 (27·5%), 73·921 (36·5%) — 32	As 74·922 — 33	Se 77·917 (23·5%), 79·917 (49·5%) — 34	Br 78·918 (50·5%), 80·916 (49·5%) — 35	
5	Xe 128·9 (26%), 131·9 (27%) — 54	Rb 84·912 (72%), 86·909 (28%) — 37	Sr 87·906 — 38	Y 88·905 — 39	Zr 89·904 (51%), 93·906 (17%) — 40	Nb 92·906 — 41	Mo 95·905 (16%), 97·906 (24%) — 42	Tc — — 43	Ru 101·90 (31%), 103·91 (19%) — 44 Rh 102·9 — 45 Pd 105·9 (27%), 107·9 (27%) — 46
5 (b)		Ag 106·9 (52%), 108·9 (48%) — 47	Cd 111·9 (24%), 113·9 (29%) — 48	In 114·9 — 49	Sn 117·9 (24%), 119·9 (33%) — 50	Sb 120·9 (57%), 122·9 (43%) — 51	Te 127·9 (32%), 129·9 (35%) — 52	I 126·9 — 53	
6	Rn — — 86	Cs 132·9 — 55	Ba 136·9 (11%), 137·9 (72%) — 56	'Rare Earths' (57–71)	Hf 177·9 (27%), 179·9 (35%) — 72	Ta 180·9 — 73	W 183·9 (30%), 185·9 (28%) — 74	Re 184·9 (37%), 186·9 (63%) — 75	Os 189·96 (26%), 191·96 (41%) — 76 Ir 190·96 (37%), 192·96 (63%) — 77 Pt 193·96 (33%), 194·96 (34%) — 78
6 (b)		Au 196·97 — 79	Hg 198·9 (17%), 201·97 (30%) — 80	Tl 202·97 (30%), 204·97 (70%) — 81	Pb 205·97 (24%), 207·97 (52%) — 82	Bi 208·98 — 83	Po — — 84	At — — 85	
7		Fr — — 87	Ra — — 88						

Note: The atomic masses are based upon the 1 amu, which is $\frac{1}{12}$ of the mass of a neutral $^{12}_{6}\text{C}$ atom. Only the two most abundant isotopes are shown for each element if the abundancies exceed 10%.

Table 25.5 Electron configuration of the elements

Element	Symbol	Atomic no.	K	L	M	N	O	P	Q
Hydrogen	H	1	1						
Helium	He	2	2						
Lithium	Li	3	2	1					
Beryllium	Be	4	2	2					
Boron	B	5	2	3					
Carbon	C	6	2	4					
Nitrogen	N	7	2	5					
Oxygen	O	8	2	6					
Fluorine	F	9	2	7					
Neon	Ne	10	2	8					
Sodium	Na	11	2	8	1				
Magnesium	Mg	12	2	8	2				
Aluminium	Al	13	2	8	3				
Silicon	Si	14	2	8	4				
Phosphorus	P	15	2	8	5				
Sulphur	S	16	2	8	6				
Chlorine	Cl	17	2	8	7				
Argon	A	18	2	8	8				
Potassium	K	19	2	8	8	1			
Calcium	Ca	20	2	8	8	2			
Scandium	Sc	21	2	8	9	2			
Titanium	Ti	22	2	8	10	2			
Vanadium	V	23	2	8	11	2			
Chromium	Cr	24	2	8	12	2			
Manganese	Mn	25	2	8	13	2			
Iron	Fe	26	2	8	14	2			
Cobalt	Co	27	2	8	15	2			
Nickel	Ni	28	2	8	16	2			
Copper	Cu	29	2	8	18	1			
Zinc	Zn	30	2	8	18	2			
Gallium	Ga	31	2	8	18	3			
Germanium	Ge	32	2	8	18	4			
Arsenic	As	33	2	8	18	5			
Selenium	Se	34	2	8	18	6			
Bromine	Br	35	2	8	18	7			
Krypton	Kr	36	2	8	18	8			
Rubidium	Rb	37	2	8	18	8	1		
Strontium	Sr	38	2	8	18	8	2		
Yttrium	Y	39	2	8	18	9	2		
Zirconium	Zr	40	2	8	18	10	2		
Niobium	Nb	41	2	8	18	12	1		
Molybdenum	Mo	42	2	8	18	13	1		
Technetium	Tc	43	2	8	18	14	1		
Ruthenium	Ru	44	2	8	18	15	1		
Rhodium	Rh	45	2	8	18	16	1		
Palladium	Pd	46	2	8	18	18			

Table 25.5 *(continued)*

Element	Symbol	Atomic no.	K	L	M	N	O	P	Q
Silver	Ag	47	2	8	18	18	1		
Cadmium	Cd	48	2	8	18	18	2		
Indium	In	49	2	8	18	18	3		
Tin	Sn	50	2	8	18	18	4		
Antimony	Sb	51	2	8	18	18	5		
Tellurium	Te	52	2	8	18	18	6		
Iodine	I	53	2	8	18	18	7		
Xenon	Xe	54	2	8	18	18	8		
Caesium	Cs	55	2	8	18	18	8	1	
Barium	Ba	56	2	8	18	18	8	2	
Lanthanum	La	57	2	8	18	18	9	2	
Cerium	Ce	58	2	8	18	20	8	2	
Praseo- dymium	Pr	59	2	8	18	21	8	2	
Neodymium	Nd	60	2	8	18	22	8	2	
Prometheum	Pm	61	2	8	18	23	8	2	
Samarium	Sm	62	2	8	18	24	8	2	
Europium	Eu	63	2	8	18	25	8	2	
Gadolinium	Gd	64	2	8	18	25	9	2	
Terbium	Tb	65	2	8	18	26	9	2	
Dysprosium	Dy	66	2	8	18	27	9	2	
Holmium	Ho	67	2	8	18	28	9	2	
Erbium	Er	68	2	8	18	29	9	2	
Thulium	Tm	69	2	8	18	30	9	2	
Ytterbium	Yb	70	2	8	18	31	9	2	
Lutecium	Lu	71	2	8	18	32	9	2	
Hafnium	Hf	72	2	8	18	32	10	2	
Tantalum	Ta	73	2	8	18	32	11	2	
Tungsten	W	74	2	8	18	32	12	2	
Rhenium	Re	75	2	8	18	32	13	2	
Osmium	Os	76	2	8	18	32	14	2	
Iridium	Ir	77	2	8	18	32	15	2	
Platinum	Pt	78	2	8	18	32	17	1	
Gold	Au	79	2	8	18	32	18	1	
Mercury	Hg	80	2	8	18	32	18	2	
Thallium	Tl	81	2	8	18	32	18	3	
Lead	Pb	82	2	8	18	32	18	4	
Bismuth	Bi	83	2	8	18	32	18	5	
Polonium	Po	84	2	8	18	32	18	6	
Astatine	As	85	2	8	18	32	18	7	
Radon	Rn	86	2	8	18	32	18	8	
Francium	Fr	87	2	8	18	32	18	8	1
Radium	Ra	88	2	8	18	32	18	8	2
Actinium	Ac	89	2	8	18	32	18	9	2
Thorium	Th	90	2	8	18	32	18	10	2
Protactinium	Pa	91	2	8	18	32	18	11	2
Uranium	U	92	2	8	18	32	18	12	2

precisely the same orbit. This is known as the Pauli Exclusion Principle, and ensures that all atomic electrons have different energies, even those of the same shell. If it were possible for the electrons to take exactly the same orbits, then no shells would need to exist and the chemical properties of the elements would therefore be quite different.

For example, the two electrons forming the K-shell of an atom are not at precisely the same energy, for they spin in opposite directions as they orbit the nucleus, and hence inhabit slightly different orbits. These two electrons complete the K-shell (Bury-Bohr rule *a* above), so that further electrons must start to fill up the L-shell at a greater distance from the nucleus and at a higher energy. These L-shell electrons have slightly different energies from each other, and eight of them complete the shell (i.e. $2n^2 = 8$ when $n = 2$).

The K and L shells are thus completed in sequence, but the M shell (which can contain $2n^2 = 18$ electrons) reaches 8 electrons and then puts the 9th and 10th electrons in the N shell before continuing to add to its own shell. This corresponds to elements argon, potassium, calcium and scandium in Table 25.5. This procedure is repeated whenever there are 8 electrons in the outer orbit, and may result in the inner shells being completed first (e.g. elements 57–70). Elements corresponding to the filling of inner orbits are known as 'transition' elements and form sub-groups within their columns in Table 25.4 (not shown, for clarity). The manner in which quantum mechanics is able to explain the electronic configuration of the elements is described in Appendix VIII.

As mentioned above, the number of electrons in the outer orbit determines the chemical reactivity of an element. The ability of one atom to join to another is called *valency* and the electron linkage between them is a *valency bond*. There are two basic types of such bonds: 'ionic' and 'covalent' bonds. Both types of bond produce an effectively closed shell in each atom, which configuration is chemically more stable. An example of an ionic bond and a covalent bond is shown in Figure 25.6. An ionic bond is caused by an electron being totally transferred from one atom to another and forming charged atoms (ions) in consequence. These are then attracted to each other electrostatically, thus forming the bond. A covalent bond is formed by the sharing of electrons so that each atom appears to increase its number of electrons, forming an apparent closed shell.

25.5 ELECTRON ORBIT CHANGES

The previous two sections have shown that electrons may take up only fixed, or 'discrete', orbits around the atomic nucleus. Further, that the inner orbits are filled before the outer orbits, since this constitutes the lowest energy state of the atom as a whole. An atom in this condition is said to be in its *ground state*, since it cannot have an electron configuration of lower energy than this. However, this is not to say that any particular atom at a given moment of time will be in its ground state, since atomic collisions or interactions with electromagnetic radiation may have raised the energy of one of its

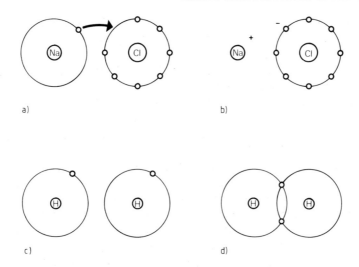

Fig. 25.6 Ionic valency bond (or 'electrovalency') caused by the transfer of an electron from one atom to another — NaCl in (a) and (b). A covalent bond ('covalency') between two hydrogen atoms is shown in (c) and (d).

electrons so that it is able to take up an orbit of higher energy further from the nucleus. Alternatively, an orbiting electron may receive sufficient energy to be able to completely escape from the atom. These two processes are called *excitation* and *ionisation* respectively, and are considered in the next section.

25.5.1 Photoelectric absorption and excitation

Consider an atom as shown in Figure 25.7(a) where the innermost electron has received sufficient energy to be able to perform a 'quantum jump' to a higher orbit. The figure shows a quantum of electromagnetic radiation as the cause of this jump, but it could equally well have been caused by the close passage of a charged particle (e.g. electrons striking the tungsten target of an X-ray tube) or interatomic collisions due to heat. If we denote E_1 as the original energy of the orbiting electron and E_2 as its final energy, then the energy of the quantum ($h\nu$) is given by

---

$$h\nu = E_2 - E_1$$ Equation 25.1

A quantum with less energy than this value will not be able to cause the quantum jump of the electron at all, and a quantum with more energy may be able to raise the electron to an even higher orbit if its energy is just right. This effect is known as *excitation*. This 'excited' electron is then able to return to its original orbit, releasing a quantum of electromagnetic radiation (25.5.3).

If a quantum has sufficient energy it is able to ionise the atom by completely

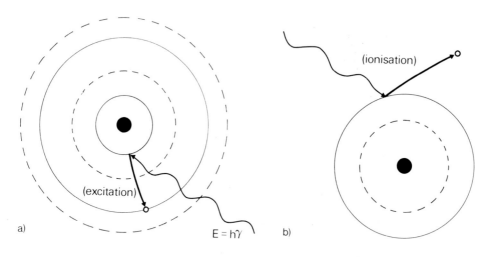

Fig. 25.7 (a) Excitation, and (b) ionisation caused by an incoming photon.

removing the electron from it. In this case, the electron is then 'free' and has a kinetic energy given by:

$$KE = \boldsymbol{h}v - B \qquad \text{Equation 25.2}$$

where $\boldsymbol{h}v$ is the energy of the quantum and B is the *binding energy* of the electron, which is defined as the work done in removing the electron from the atom. The amount of energy left after performing this work is that carried by the electron as kinetic energy. Figure 25.7(b) illustrates the process of ionisation.

The ionisation caused by the absorption of electromagnetic radiation is called *photoelectric absorption*, where the incoming photon completely disappears in ejecting an electron from the atom. The practical effect of photoelectric absorption on an X-ray beam is discussed in more detail in section 30.7.

In a crystalline solid, photoelectric absorpton may result in an electron being able to jump from the valence band up to the conduction band (10.1). If this occurs at the surface of the substance, the kinetic energy given to the electron may be sufficient for it to overcome the surface 'work function' (18.1) and escape from the body. This is very similar to the case of the thermionic emission of electrons (Ch. 18). The emission of electrons from the surface of a substance as a result of irradiation by electromagnetic waves is known as *photoelectric emission* or the photoelectric *effect*. It is caused by photoelectric *absorption*, and the term 'photoelectric effect' is often used to refer to both processes. However, there is a difference between the photoelectric emission of an electron from an *atom* and from a *solid body*, as the atom in question could be well away from the surface of the body so that the electron could not possibly escape from the body as a whole.

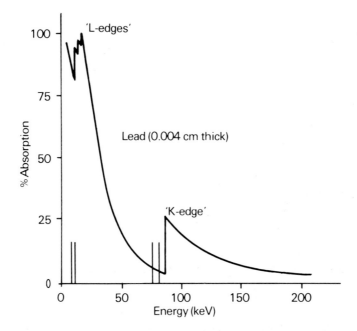

Fig. 25.8 The absorption of electromagnetic radiation by 0·004 cm of lead, the thickness being arbitrary and chosen only so as to produce a satisfactory appearance on the graph. 'Percentage absorption' on the Y axis means the percentage of incident photons absorbed in the lead. The position of each absorption 'edge' corresponds to the energy of photoelectric absorption for the electron shell in question. Also shown are the K and L lines of characteristic radiation — note that these are slightly less energetic than the corresponding edge.

25.5.2 Absorption spectra

If a thin monoenergetic* beam of X-rays is incident upon a slab of lead (say) and the energy of the beam is varied, then the amount which is absorbed in the lead varies in quite a dramatic manner, as shown in Figure 25.8. This type of graph is known as an *absorption spectrum* and may be plotted against wavelength or energy. Also, other parts of the electromagnetic spectrum (24.2) may be used (e.g. light through transparent materials), but the example of Figure 25.8 is chosen as being particularly relevant to this book. Low-energy X-rays are absorbed readily in lead by photoelectric absorption by the outer electron orbits. As the energy increases, the orbits which are able to participate in photoelectric absorption increases one at a time towards the inner K shell. Thus, although the increasing energetic X-ray beam becomes more penetrating (i.e. less is absorbed) for a particular electron shell, an increasing number of inner shells are 'activated' suddenly in turn. Thus, the general appearance of Figure 25.8 is one of a smoothly decreasing absorption distorted by sudden increases of absorption when photoelectric absorption is able to occur at the

* 'Monoenergetic' — all the X-ray photons have the same energy.

next inner shell. The energies where this occurs are known as *edges*; in particular the K edge of lead is at 88 keV and corresponds to the energy required to remove an electron from the K shell and ionise the lead atom. The L edge is composed of 3 separate edges, as shown in the figure, and correspond to 3 subshells within the L shell, each of which is at a slightly different energy.

A better way of presenting the absorption of an element to electromagnetic radiation is to draw a graph of the 'mass absorption coefficient' against energy (30.1). This is superior to Figure 25.8, where a particular thickness of lead is assumed.

25.5.3 Emission spectra (characteristic radiation)

The processes of excitation and ionisation described in the above two sections result in a vacancy in one of the lower electron shells, i.e. the shell from which the electrons was removed. This is very quickly filled by one of the outer electrons undergoing a 'quantum jump' downwards and emitting a quantum of electromagnetic radiation in the process. The energy of the quantum emitted is given by:

$$hv = E_1 - E_2 \hspace{4cm} \text{Equation 25.3}$$

where E_1, E_2 are the initial and final energies of the orbiting electron. (This equation is just the reverse of Equation 25.1, owing to the emission, rather than the absorption, of a quantum.) However, in making this quantum jump, the electron leaves its own vacancy which may be filled by jumps from electron orbits even further out. In this way, a *cascade* of 'dropping' electrons may be produced, with each one emitting a photon of energy as given by Equation 25.3. This process produces what is known as the 'emission spectrum' of the substance. It is also called the 'characteristic radiation' and 'fluorescent radiation'. The term 'characteristic' is used since the energies of the emitted radiation are characteristic of (i.e. unique to) a particular element or substance.

If it is assumed that an electron from the K shell of a lead atom has been removed, then the situation is as shown in Figure 25.9. The most probable quantum jump is from either of the L, M, N shells to the K shell as shown by the arrows in the figure. These jumps are referred to as K_α, K_β, K_γ,... *transitions*. Assuming a K_α transition has taken place (emitting the appropriate 'K_α-line' photon), then a vacancy exists in the L shell which may be filled by one of the L_α, L_β, etc. transitions, as shown by the dotted lines in Figure 25.9. The 'line spectra' of such K and L emission is shown in Figure 25.8 by the lines just below the K and L edges respectively. This is because the energy difference between the K and L shells (which is the energy of the emitted characteristic photon) is less than the energy difference between the K shell and ionisation (i.e. the energy of the 'edges'). Thus an element is 'relatively transparent' to its own characteristic radiation. This fact may be used to advantage, for example, in mammography where X-rays from a molybdenum target are passed through a molybdenum filter, so filtering out almost all X-ray energies apart from the

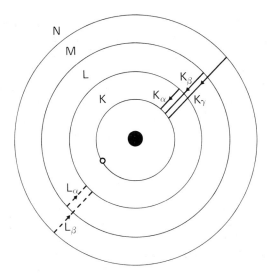

Fig. 25.9 The production of characteristic radiation. The K lines are formed by quantum jumps down to the K shell etc. Note that (for example) the energy of the K_a line must be less than the binding energy of the K shell, so that the K lines are always less energetic than the K edge (see previous figure).

K lines. The almost monoenergetic beam produced with this arrangement gives a low radiation absorbed dose (32.1) in the breast because of the absence of low-energy X-rays.

Exercise 25.2.

a. Describe the elementary structure of the atom. What distinguishes one element from another?

b. Explain what is meant by:

   (i)   a nuclide
  (ii)   a radionuclide
 (iii)   an isotope
 (iv)   an isobar
  (v)   atomic number
 (vi)   atomic mass number
(vii)   discrete electron orbit
(viii)   electron shells
 (ix)   electron binding energy.

c. Explain the term 'characteristic radiation', with reference to the 'K lines' and 'L lines' seen on an X-ray spectrum.

d. Describe the process of photoelectric absorption. How is this related to photoelectric emission?

e. Sketch a graph of the 'absorption spectrum' of lead and explain its shape.

f.   Why is an element 'relatively transparent' to its own characteristic radiation? (*Hint:* Sketch an X-ray spectrum from a molybdenum target and superimpose the absorption spectrum of molybdenum on the same graph. Hence show how the *K* lines are transmitted through a molybdenum filter and the other energies are strongly absorbed.)

SUMMARY

1.   The atom consists of a central positively charged nucleus around which negatively charged electrons orbit.

2.   The nucleus contains protons and neutrons (the 'nucleons') held together by 'short-range' forces. The energy required to hold the nucleus together (about 8.4 MeV per nucleon) is achieved by a loss of mass of the nucleons as determined by Einstein's formula $E = mc^2$. The nucleus thus weighs less than the sum of the individual weights of the protons and neutrons.

3.   Electrons can only take up clearly defined orbits around the nucleus, known as 'discrete' orbits. No electromagnetic radiation is emitted from these orbits, in contradiction to classical physics.

4.   Electrons arrange themselves in groups, or 'shells', around the nucleus, where members of the same shell carry approximately the same energy. The shells are numbered as $n = 1, 2, 3, \ldots$ from the inner orbits outwards and/or called the *K*, *L*, *M*, ... shells.

5.   There is a maximum number of permitted electrons in each shell as given by $2n^2$, so that the completed *K*, *L*, *M*, ... shells have 2, 8, 18, ... electrons. The shells fill up from the inner orbits outwards, as this corresponds to the lowest energy state for the atom.

6.   The nucleus of an atom determines its atomic weight while the configuration of its electron orbits determines its chemical properties. A completed shell or subshell is chemically non-reactive while an incomplete shell enables 'bonds' to form between atoms. Such 'valency' is determined by the number of electrons in the outer orbit of the atom.

7.   The elements may be grouped in a Periodic Table where the elements in the same group have similar chemical and physical properties. This is a consequence of the similar configuration of the electron shells in each group.

8.   An electron may perform a 'quantum jump' either into a higher or a lower orbit. In each case the energy difference between the two orbits is equal to **h**v, the energy of the photon absorbed or emitted.

9.   Photoelectric absorption occurs when a photon gives up all its energy to an orbiting electron, thus raising it to a higher orbit (excitation) or removing it from the atom completely (ionisation). Photons of low energy affect the outer orbits, while increasing photon energy affects the inner orbits in turn until the innermost *K* shell is reached. This may be plotted as an absorption spectrum (see Fig. 25.8).

10.   Photoelectric emission is the emission of electrons from the surface of a substance — it is caused by photoelectric absorption of u.v. or X-rays.

11. A vacancy occurring in an electron shell as a result of photoelectric absorption is quickly filled by electrons jumping down from higher orbits accompanied by the emission of 'characteristic' radiation, which produces K, L, M, ... 'line' spectra, where the lines are of slightly lower energy than the corresponding absorption edges (see Fig. 25.8). An element is thus 'relatively transparent' to its own characteristic radiation.

26. Radioactivity

The case of radioactive decay as an example of the exponential law is considered in Chapter 5, together with the concepts of half-life and decay constant. The reader is advised to refer to (25.2) for the definitions of terms used in describing nuclear structure. This chapter discusses radioactive decay in more detail and the production of artificial radionuclides.

The term *radioactive* is applied to those nuclei which are unstable. They demonstrate their instability by changing their internal structure to a more stable form, often (but not always) ejecting a charged particle from the nucleus in the process. Each time a nucleus changes its structure it is called a radioactive (or nuclear) *transformation* or *disintegration*, and may result in a change of atomic number (and therefore element), atomic mass number or both.

A pictorial representation of the decay of a particular radionuclide (see examples below) is called a *decay scheme*. In addition, it is possible for a nucleus to undergo more than one type of transformation (e.g. to emit a positron or capture an orbiting electron); this is termed *branching*, examples of which occur in the following sections.

Each nuclear transformation takes place at an unpredictable moment, but the laws of probability may be used to determine the behaviour of a large number of such nuclei (e.g. the 'law of radioactive decay' — 5.2).

The unit of radioactivity (or just 'activity') is the *becquerel* (Bq) where 1 Bq is 1 disintegration/second and therefore has units of s^{-1} (6.2). An earlier unit, which will probably continue for some time, is the curie (Ci) where 1 curie $= 3 \cdot 7 \times 10^{10}$ disintegrations/second. Thus, 1 Ci $= 3 \cdot 7 \times 10^{10}$ Bq. A table relating activities in the two systems of units is shown in Table B at the end of the book.

It is often useful to know the *specific activity* of a radioactive sample. This is the activity of the radionuclide per unit mass of the radioactive sample, so that it is measured in Bq kg^{-1} (or mCi per g etc.), or sub-multiples thereof.

26.1 NUCLIDE CHART

It is useful to draw a graph of the number of neutrons in a nucleus against the number of protons, since all nuclides may be included in such a 'chart of the nuclides'. This is shown in simplified form in Figure 26.1. Note that isotopes (lines of equal Z) are given by any vertical line in the figure.

It is found that there is a broad band of nuclides starting at about 45° to the axes of the graph which are stable, i.e. non- or only weakly radioactive. Thus, for the lighter elements the stable elements have about as many neutrons as protons, while for the heavier elements the nuclei require relatively more neutrons to achieve stability. This is shown in the figure by the increasing slope of the band of stable nuclides as the atomic number increases. The stable heavy nuclei thus contain increased numbers of neutrons compared to protons in order to balance the Coulomb repulsion (9.2) of the protons. This done by the presence of more short-range forces (25.2.1)

Nuclides which are outside the band of stability shown in Figure 26.1 have nuclei possessing higher energies than those within the band. In consequence, such a nucleus is unstable and, on decay, tends to produce a new nucleus of lower energy which is closer to, or within, the stable band. The energy difference between the nuclei before and after decay may be carried by a charged particle or a quantum of electromagnetic radiation emitted from the nucleus. Stability may be achieved either by a single decay (e.g. $^{14}_{6}C$ to $^{14}_{7}N$ by the emission of a beta particle) or by a very circuitous path involving many nuclear

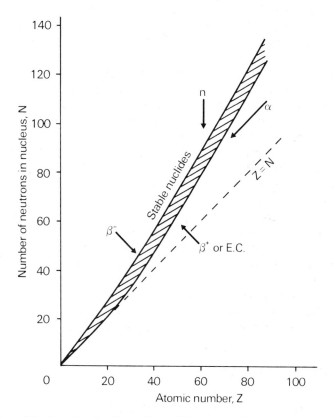

Fig. 26.1 A nuclide chart showing the stable nuclides as a shaded band in the 'N–Z' diagram. As the atomic number increases more neutrons are required to achieve stability. Also shown are the directions which a nucleus takes for various forms of decay (not to scale).

transformations (e.g. $^{238}_{92}U$ to $^{206}_{82}Pb$). In general, the greater the mass number of the nuclide, the more complex will be the decay path to eventual stability.

The effect of different modes of decay is illustrated in Figure 26.1, where the direction of the change of position in the chart is shown for each type of decay. The reader might find it helpful to refer to this while studying the various forms of radioactive decay in more detail in the following sections.

26.2 GAMMA DECAY

A gamma ray (or γ) is a quantum of electromagnetic radiation which may be emitted from the nucleus of an atom when it undergoes radioactive decay. It is important to distinguish this from an X-ray, which is a quantum of electromagnetic radiation emitted either as a result of a change in the *electron shells* of the atom (25.5.3) or in Bremsstrahlung (28.1.3) when a charged particle decelerates in a substance. Thus, both γ-rays and X-rays are part of the electromagnetic spectrum (24.2), but they are distinguished by their *source*, i.e. γ-rays are emitted from nuclei, while X-rays are emitted from electron shells. It is possible, therefore, for a γ-ray to have a lower energy than an X-ray, and *vice versa*. However, γ-rays exceed X-rays in their maximum energies.

If a nucleus has just undergone a transformation whereby it has ejected a β-particle (26.3), for example, the new 'daughter' nucleus may possess excess energy above its minimum possible 'ground state' energy. This situation is depicted in Figure 26.2(a) for $^{60}_{28}Ni$, which is the *daughter product* (i.e. the resulting nucleus) of the decay of $^{60}_{27}Co$. The figure illustrates the energy states of the daughter nucleus by means of the horizontal lines above the thick line, representing the ground state of the nucleus. In this example, after the decay of the $^{60}_{27}Co$, the $^{60}_{28}Ni$ nucleus has an energy of 2·50 MeV above the ground state. This is known as an 'excited state', and decays immediately in two jumps: first

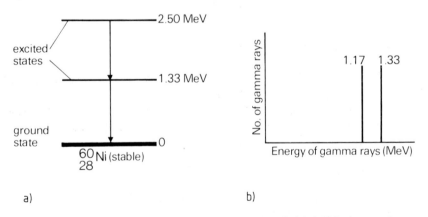

Fig. 26.2 Gamma decay from an 'excited' nucleus. The case of nickel-60 is shown, where the excited states in the nickel nucleus have been caused by the previous decay of cabalt-60. All such gammas are 'monoenergetic' and form a line spectrum as shown in (b).

to 1·33 MeV above the ground state, and then to ground state. *Each of these jumps is accompanied by the emission of a gamma ray from the nucleus.* This is shown in the figure by vertical arrows between the levels, representing the emission of two gamma rays of energies 1·17 MeV and 1·33 MeV (see also Fig. 26.5).

Figure 26.2(b) shows the 'line' spectrum of the gamma radiations emitted from the nucleus, i.e. each gamma ray has a precise (or 'discrete') energy corresponding to the discrete energy transformations within the nucleus.

26.2.1 Metastable states and isomeric transitions

The previous example of $^{60}_{27}\text{Co}$ is a case of so-called 'prompt' gamma decay, where the nucleus stays in the excited state for such a short time as to be incapable of accurate measurement. However, this is not always the case, and those excited states which last sufficiently long for their durations to be measured are called *metastable* states. A transition from a metastable state is an *isomeric* transition. The use of metastable radionuclides is prevalent in nuclear medicine (26.9), owing to the low radiation dose they deliver to patients. Technetium — 99m ($^{99}_{43}\text{Tc}^m$, or $^{99m}_{43}\text{Tc}$ in many texts) is a widely used radionuclide for such purposes, and its simplified decay scheme is shown in Figure 26.3. Obviously, the symbol 'm' stands for 'metastable'. The metastable state of $^{99}_{43}\text{Tc}^m$ has a half-life (5.2.2) of 6 hours and emits a gamma ray of 140 keV

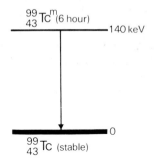

Fig. 26.3 An example of a metastable state.

when it decays to $^{99}_{43}\text{Tc}$. The half-life of $^{99}_{43}\text{Tc}$ is so long ($2\cdot1 \times 10^5 y$) as to be considered stable for all practical purposes.

Nuclear transformations may be written in the form of equations, but with an arrow rather than an equals sign. For example, the simplified decay scheme for $^{99}\text{Tc}^m$ shown in Figure 26.3 may be written as

$$^{99}_{43}\text{Tc}^m \rightarrow ^{99}_{43}\text{Tc} + \gamma\ (140\ \text{keV})$$

Further examples of this form of representing nuclear transformations are given in the rest of this chapter.

The next two sections consider the consequences of gamma emission from the nucleus on the whole atom, rather than on the nucleus only.

26.2.2 Internal conversion

Whenever a nuclide decays by gamma emission there is a competing process known as *internal conversion*, whereby an electron from one of the inner orbits of the *atom* may be ejected from the atom instead. These electrons carry discrete energies, unlike those emitted in beta decay (26.3). This process is a result of the direct interaction between the excited nucleus and the orbiting electron, such that the nucleus is able to jump down to its ground state by giving all its excess energy to the electron. This 'converted' electron escapes from the atom with an energy reduced by its binding energy (25.5.1),

i.e.

KE of converted electron = nuclear energy transition − BE   Equation 26.1

Note the similarity between this and the photoelectric effect (25.5.1), the latter often being described as 'external conversion'.

Insight

The innermost electrons of the atoms have orbits which pass close to, or even through, the nucleus. Thus, it is matter of statistical probability whether the nuclear transformation will result in gamma emission from the nucleus or electron emission from the inner electron shells. Obviously, the K shell is most likely to participate in such internal conversion, followed by the L, M . . . shells. Each mode of decay has its own half-life, both of which combine to form the overall half-life of the radioactive decay of the 'mother' radionuclide.

The *internal conversion coefficient*, α, is defined as the ratio of the number of nuclear transformations which result in internal conversion to the number that result in gamma emission. (α may therefore take a value between zero and infinity, corresponding to no internal conversion and complete internal conversion respectively.) For example, the decay scheme of $^{99}_{43}Tc^m$ as shown in Figure 26.3 is in reality somewhat more complicated. In particular, approximately 9% of the transitions shown in the figure result in internal conversion of electrons from the K shell of the atom, 1·1% from the L shell and about 0·3% from the M shell. The gamma emission of 140 keV from the nucleus therefore appears in about 89·6% of all transitions, and internal conversion for the remainder (10·4%).

Exercise 26.1

From the above figures, show that the internal conversion coefficient (α) for $^{99}Tc^m$ is 0·116.

26.2.3 X-rays and Auger electrons

If a radioactive decay results in a vacancy occurring within one of the electron shells of the atom, then electrons in higher orbits will perform quantum jumps 'downwards' (25.5.3) until there are no inner shell electron vacancies. Each orbital transition will produce an electromagnetic quantum which, for the inner shells of atoms, has an energy within the X-ray region of the electromagnetic spectrum (24.2). This is known as *fluorescence radiation*, whether the wavelength of any such quantum is in the visible band of the spectrum or not.

Note
   In this context 'X-rays', 'characteristic radiation' and 'fluorescence' are the same (see 25.5.3).

Thus, in the process of internal conversion described in the previous section, a K electron (say) has been removed from the atom and a vacancy in the K shell is left. This vacancy is filled by either of the K_a, K_β, ... transitions (25.5.3), followed by L or M transitions, etc., until all of the lowest electron orbits are filled. Each of the quantum jumps results in the emission of electromagnetic radiation, some of which may be sufficiently energetic to be X-rays (i.e. for the inner electron shells of heavy atoms such as tungsten). The atom as a whole stays positively charged until it is able to capture a free electron and place it in its next outermost orbit.

There is one more complication, however, because the fluorescent radiation emitted as a result of changes in the inner electron orbits may be able to interact with electrons in the outer orbits and eject an electron from the atom by the photoelectric effect (25.5.1). Such *Auger electrons* have discrete energies as determined by Equation 25.2. Obviously the ejection of an Auger electron from a shell leaves a vacancy in that shell, and this is filled by electrons jumping down from orbits even further out, with the release of more fluorescent radiation and perhaps more Auger electrons.

Thus, the ejection of an electron from one of the atomic orbits by internal conversion (26.2.2) may result in quite a complicated sequence of orbital quantum jumps, fluorescent radiation and more ejected (Auger) electrons. The term *fluorescent yield* is defined as the fraction of the number of electron orbital transitions which result in fluorescent radiation.

For each decay, the total energies of all the fluorescent radiation and of all the electrons emitted from the shells of the atom are equal to the energy of the nuclear transition. This is because the binding energies of each ejected electron are recovered in the fluorescent radiation emitted in the subsequent cascade of orbital jumps. The whole process thus obeys the law of conservation of energy, as expected (23.2).

To return to the example of the decay of $^{99}Tc^m$, the previous section showed about 11·6% of nuclear transitions were internally converted, i.e. resulted in the removal of one of the inner electrons from the atom. Of the subsequent rearrangement of electron orbits, caused by 'downward' electron jumps between the shells, about 80% of electron transitions result in fluorescent radiations and 20% in Auger electrons (the latter carrying a total energy of about 6·5 keV). The 'fluorescent yield' is thus 0·8, or 80%. Some typical fluorescent radiation energies for $^{99}Tc^m$ are:

$$K_a = 18·4 \text{ keV}, \quad L_a = 2·4 \text{ keV}, \quad M_a = 0·2 \text{ keV}$$

Note that all emitted particles and quanta carry discrete amounts of energy, unlike the case of beta decay considered next.

26.3 BETA DECAY

In the process of beta decay a particle is ejected from the nucleus, the mass of which is equal to that of the electron. The ejected particles, however, may have either a positive or negative charge, and they are known collectively either as beta particles (β-particles) or negatrons and positrons (i.e. *nega*tive or *posi*tive elec*trons*). The negative beta particle (β^-) is in fact exactly the same as an electron. In this chapter, however, the term 'negatron' is used to refer to negative beta particles, and 'positron' to positive beta particles from the nucleus. The term 'electron' is used, as before, for the orbiting electrons of the atom. In either case, the emission of a beta particle from a nucleus results in a change in its atomic number (i.e. the charge on the nucleus) but no change in its mass number, and the daughter nucleus lies closer to or within the band of stable nuclides shown in Figure 26.1. This type of decay is known as an isobaric transition (25.2).

Neither the negatron nor the positron exists as a separate particle within the nucleus (25.2). How then is it possible for either of them to be ejected from the nucleus? The answer to this problem lies in the way in which nucleons are constantly being changed from protons into neutrons (and back) within the nucleus — the so-called 'exchange forces'. For example, a neutron may be thought to consist of a proton and a negatron (i.e. β^-), and a proton as a neutron and a positron (i.e. β^+) as shown by the equation:

$$n \longrightarrow p^+ + \beta^-$$
$$p^+ \longrightarrow n + \beta^+$$

Equation 26.2

There is a finite probability that, during these very rapid changes, the beta particles will be able to escape from some types of nuclei. One of the nucleons has changed, however, since it lost either a negatron or positron. Thus, the atomic number *increases* by 1 for β^- decay, and *decreases* by 1 for β^+ decay. Beta decay therefore results in a new element being formed, with the consequent rearrangement of the electron orbits to suit the new element.

For example, the beta decay of carbon-14 ($^{14}_{6}C$) is well known, and may be represented by the decay scheme shown in Figure 26.4. The emission of the negative beta particle from the nucleus of $^{14}_{6}C$ produces nitrogen-14 ($^{14}_{7}N$), the nucleus of which has a lower ground state. Note that the decay scheme depicts the energy in the 'Y'-direction and atomic number in the 'X'-direction, so that the $^{14}_{7}N$ nuclear state is shown below, and to the right of, the position of $^{14}_{6}C$ nucleus. This simple decay scheme is an example of a 'pure' beta emitter, since no other transformations are involved. This is not the case for the decay of $^{60}_{27}Co$ to $^{60}_{28}Ni$, which decays first by β^--emission (forming the nickel nucleus) and then by gamma emission from the excited states of the $^{60}_{28}Ni$ nucleus as

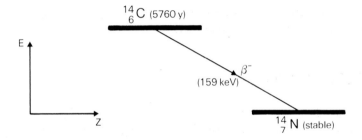

Fig. 26.4 An example of a decay scheme of a pure beta emitter. Increasing energy and atomic number are as shown.

shown in Figure 26.5. This is an extension of the gamma decay considered in Figure 26.2(a), and is sometimes called a 'β-γ' decay.

An example of positron decay is shown in Figure 26.6, where the decay of $^{11}_{6}C$ is shown. Note that, unlike β^--decay schemes, the arrow drops vertically (by 1·02 MeV) and then branches to the left. This is because a positron can only escape from the nucleus if the energy lost by the nucleus is greater than $2mc^2$, where m is the mass of the positron (which is the same as that of an electron), and $2mc^2$ is equivalent to an energy of 1·02 MeV. The decay of $^{11}_{6}C$ is by 'pure' positron emission, and the daughter nucleus of boron ($^{11}_{5}B$) is shown to the left of and below the carbon nucleus since it possesses less energy and has a reduced atomic number. All positron decays produce an atomic number of the daughter nucleus reduced by one, since a positive charge has been removed from the nucleus. As shown above, this is equivalent to changing a proton to a neutron within the nucleus.

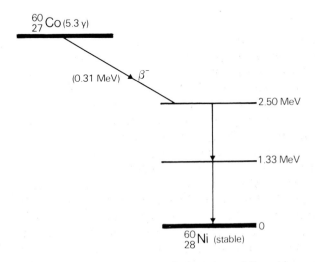

Fig. 26.5 The decay of cobalt-60 as an example of a beta decay followed by a gamma decay of the daughter nucleus.

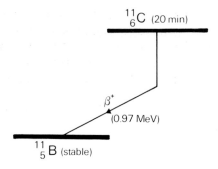

Fig. 26.6 A example of positron decay.

26.3.1 The neutrino

If the relative number of beta particles emitted from the decaying nuclei are plotted on a graph against their energies, then a typical 'spectrum' obtained is shown in Figure 26.7. This spectrum is *continuous* from zero up to the 'end-point' energy, unlike the discrete or 'line' spectra exhibited in gamma decay, internal conversion, fluorescent radiation and Auger electrons as described in the previous sections. However, the transformations within a nucleus are always between discrete energy levels, so there appears to be a problem here concerning the law of conservation of energy (23.2)! This difficulty was resolved by Pauli (in 1933) who postulated that another particle (the *neutrino*) is always ejected with the beta particle. In particular, he postulated that a neutrino (symbol v) is ejected at the same time as a positron, and an antineutrino (symbol $\bar{v}$) with a negatron. The *total* energy of the emitted negatron and the neutrino then corresponds to the energy of transformation within the nucleus, but this total energy may be shared differently between the two

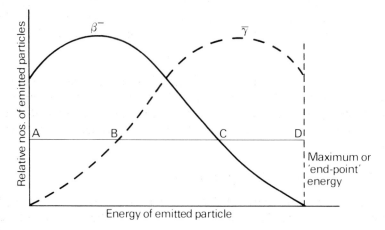

Fig. 26.7 The sharing of energy between the beta particle and the neutrino in beta decay (the case of negatron emission is shown).

particles for each decay of a nucleus. In this way a continuous distribution of energies is obtained both for the β^--particle and the antineutrino, as shown in the figure. For example, if a β^--particle is emitted with an energy of AC, then the antineutrino will have an energy of AB, such that AC + AB = AD (the 'end-point' energy), i.e. the total energy carried by the two particles is constant (Fig. 26.7).

The properties of the neutrino and antineutrino are very unusual, and include the following:

a.   zero rest mass
b.   no charge
c.   extremely small interaction with matter.

It is this last property which made the neutrino so difficult to detect by experiment. The neutrino has a HVT (5.3.1) in lead of many miles!

Insight

A beta particle emitted from the nucleus is influenced by the charge on the nucleus until it has been able to escape from the atom. Thus, the energy of a negative electron is *diminished* by the attractive forces of the nucleus, while the energy of a positron is *increased* by electrostatic repulsion.

As shown above, an *antineutrino* is emitted during β^--decay, and a neutrino is emitted during β^+-decay. The difference between these two particles is the direction in which they are spinning relative to their motion (the neutrino spins anti-clockwise and the antineutrino clockwise).

Equation 26.2 can now be modified to include the emission of the neutrinos:

$$n \longrightarrow p^+ + \beta^- + \bar{v}$$
$$p^+ \longrightarrow n + \beta^+ + v$$

Equation 26.3

Associated with each equation is the release of energy (not shown) which is carried away as the kinetic energy of the β-particle, neutrino and 'recoil' of the atom. Energy and momentum are conserved in this process (23.2 and 23.3).

Exercise 26.2

a.   In what circumstances can a β-decay result in the production of X-rays and Auger electrons? (*Hint:* see Fig. 26.5.) Given that the electron orbits rearrange themselves for the daughter nucleus before any possible gamma emission from the nucleus, are such X-rays characteristic of the parent or daughter nucleus?

26.3.2 The fate of the positron

An energetic positron emitted from a nucleus will move through the surrounding atoms and slow down by collision with them. As its momentum decreases, it is more likely to interact with a free electron in the material. The electron and positron are *'antiparticles'* of each other (i.e. they are alike except for having opposite signs of charge), and when they meet they completely annihilate each other and form two gamma rays. This process is shown diagrammatically in Figure 26.8, where the 'annihilation radiation' consists of two 0·511 MeV γ-photons 'back-to-back'. In this way both energy and *momentum* are conserved (23.3). The mutual annihilation of the electron and the positron is an example of the principle of mass–energy equivalence (23.2.1) as given by Einstein's relationship: $E = mc^2$, and shows that each particle has a mass–energy of 0·511 MeV, in agreement with Table 25.1.

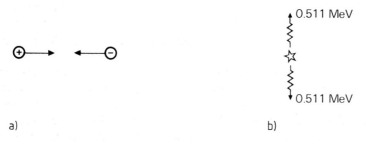

a)   b)

Fig. 26.8 The mutual annihilation of a positron and a negatron (electron).

The annihilation radiation may interact with the neighbouring atoms by the processes of photoelectric absorption, Compton scatter etc. (Ch. 30) and may produce characteristic radiation and Auger electrons.

Insight

A positron and electron may annihilate one another when the positron is still quite energetic, in which case the two quanta of annihilation radiation are not emitted 'back-to-back' and each has a higher energy than 0·511 MeV, as shown in the figure. In either case, energy and momentum are conserved.

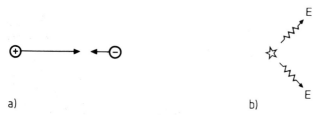

a)   b)

The annihilation of a positron and an electron when the positron is not at rest. *E* is greater than 0·511 MeV.

26.4 ELECTRON CAPTURE

An alternative way by which a nucleus may undergo an isobaric transition (nucleus has same mass number — 25.2) and lose energy is the capture by the nucleus of an orbiting electron. This process is known as *electron-capture* (EC), and the most likely shell to be affected is the K shell. Sometimes the terms 'K

capture', 'L-capture' etc. are used to denote that the captured electron was from the K, L, ... shell. An example of a 'pure' electron capture transition is that of caesium-131 ($^{131}_{55}$Cs) which decays to xenon-131 as shown in Figure 26.9(a).

Electron capture generally takes place in those nuclei which are deficient in neutrons. The capture of an orbiting electron by the nucleus enables it to change a proton to a neutron according to the relationship:

$$p^+ + e^- \rightarrow n + v \qquad \qquad \text{Equation 26.4}$$

Note that a neutrino (26.3.1) is emitted from the nucleus during electron capture.

In those nuclear transformations which result in an energy loss to the nucleus of more than 1·02 MeV, the process of electron capture competes with positron emission. For energy transformation less than this positron emission cannot take place (26.3) and only electron capture will occur. An example of the competing processes of electron capture and positron emission is shown by the decay of $^{58}_{27}$Co into stable $^{58}_{26}$Fe in Figure 26.9(b). Note that both electron capture and positron decay reduce the atomic number by one, but do not affect the mass number. This is because the number of nucleons is unaltered, since a proton is changed to a neutron.

A vacancy in one of the electron shells produced by electron capture will produce the characteristic fluorescent radiation and Auger electrons (26.2.3) of the *daughter* element. This means that the electron orbits for the daughter product are established before the consequent electron transitions occur.

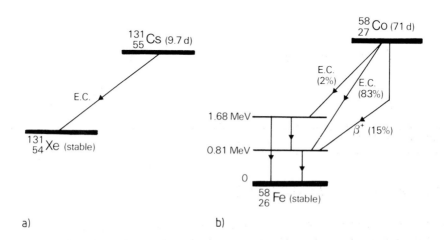

Fig. 26.9 (a) Pure electron-capture decay, (b) electron-capture and positron decay occurring in the same nuclei (85% EC and 15% positron). Also emitted are the X-rays from the iron-58 atoms and the 0·511 MeV gammas from the positron-electron annihilations.

26.5 ALPHA DECAY

The spontaneous emission of an alpha(α) particle from a nucleus occurs in elements of atomic mass numbers greater than about 150. An α-particle consists of two protons and two neutrons tightly bound together (a helium nucleus) and may be considered as a free particle of high kinetic energy which is trapped within the nucleus by a 'potential well' of the general form shown in Figure 26.10. The 'well' is a result of the short-range forces between nucleons

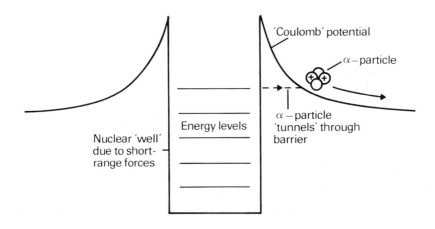

Fig. 26.10 'Alpha decay.' The alpha particle tunnels through the barrier rather than going over the top of it.

(25.2.1), and the downward slope outside the well is the 'Coulomb' potential (9.6) due to electrostatic forces. The α-particle may therefore be visualised as striking, and being reflected, from the vertical sides of the barrier at a very great rate (about 10^{21} times per second).

An example of α-decay is given by the decay of bismuth-212 (thorium C) to thallium-208 (thorium C''), a simplified version of which is shown in Figure 26.11. Also shown is the alternative β^--decay to $^{212}_{84}\text{Po}$ (polonium). This is an example of a 'branched' decay scheme, since there is more than one method by which the nucleus may decay. The emitted α-particles have discrete energies, like gamma emission but unlike beta emission.

The ejection of an α-particle at a high kinetic energy means that, in order to preserve momentum, the nucleus must 'recoil' with an equal and opposite momentum to the α-particle. The energy of the recoiling nucleus is typically about 2% of that of the emitted α-particle. Recoil also exists for β-decay, of course, but is very much smaller owing to the relatively tiny mass of the β-particle.

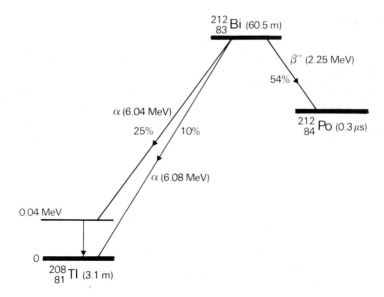

Fig. 26.11 Competing processes of alpha and beta decay for bismuth-212.

Example 26.3

What is the effect on Z and A of α-decay?

Insight

The following Insight attempts to explain the phenomenon of α-decay in terms of modern physics, but may be skipped by the student if found too difficult.

According to the principles of classical physics (Chs. 7 and 23), it would be necessary to 'lift' the α-particle to the top of the barrier in order for it to escape from the nucleus. (It would then be able to 'slide down' the Coulomb curve due to the electrostatic force of repulsion.) However, it is found in practice that α-particles are emitted from a nucleus at an energy which is not sufficient for them to be absorbed by the same nucleus if the direction of the α-particles is reversed. This means that α-particles of a given energy are able to travel 'outwards', but not 'inwards', in violation of classical physics. For example, a uranium-238 nucleus decays by emitting an α-particle of energy 4·2 MeV. However, a beam of α-particles of the same, and much higher, energies is scattered by the repulsion barrier, and do not form heavier nuclei by joining with the uranium-238 nuclei.

Modern physics explains this anomaly by stating that the α-particles do not go *over* the barrier, but *tunnel through* it! The explanation of this is somewhat complicated, and certainly beyond the scope of this book. However, a simple picture may be formed from the use of the Uncertainty Principle (23.5), which states that it is not possible to measure particular quantities concerning the state of a particle simultaneously with absolute accuracy, even when using instruments of infinite precision. Thus it may be shown, for example, that if the particle has an accurately known momentum there is always a relatively high uncertainty as to its precise position. The probability of the true position of the α-particle being within the nucleus is very high and falls to very small (but *not* zero) values outside the barrier (e.g. 1 in 10^{38} particles will be outside the barrier as a result of the Uncertainty Principle). It is the very great number of times that the α-particle tries to escape per second (by colliding with the barrier) and the enormous numbers of such nuclei, even in a very small sample, that produces the observed rate α-particle emissions from such radionuclides. The α-particles reach the other side of the potential barrier at zero kinetic energy and are then repelled by the Coulomb electrostatic field (see Fig. 26.10). Thus, they are emitted with discrete energies, like the γ-rays, so that a line-spectrum is obtained (similar to Fig. 26.2(b)). There is therefore no need to postulate the existence of another particle emitted with the α-particle, unlike the case of β-decay (26.3).

26.6 FISSION

Very heavy elements have large nuclei containing many nucleons. The short-range forces holding the nucleus together exists only between adjacent nucleons (25.2.1), so that the electrostatic forces of repulsion (the 'Coulomb' forces) between distant protons in the nucleus become increasingly important as the nuclear size increases. Such a large nucleus may be pictured as a 'liquid-drop' in which the nucleons are moving about with high energy and continually deforming the shape of the nucleus as they almost (but not quite) manage to escape from the nucleus.

Some nuclei (e.g. thorium 232) break up into two or more large fragments — this is known as *spontaneous fission*. The fragments are the nuclei of elements of lower atomic number and are called *fission products*. In addition , one or more neutrons are emitted, and the whole fission process occurs with the liberation of about 200 MeV of energy (about 10 times greater than α-decay, for example).

A heavy nucleus, on capturing an incoming neutron, may either be stable, or the effect of the energy absorbed by the nucleus due to the binding energy and kinetic energy of the neutron may result in *neutron-activated fission* (or just 'fission'). In the latter case, the nucleus breaks into large fragments as in the case of spontaneous fission.

A pictorial representation of the process of fission is shown in Figure 26.12(a) to (e). The incoming neutron is captured in Figure 26.12(a) and delivers sufficient energy to the nucleus to perturb its shape (Fig. 26.12(b)) into an ellipsoid. If the energy is sufficient, a 'dump-bell' appearance results (Fig. 26.12(c)) in which the eventual break-up of the nucleus into two large fragments is inevitable, because the electrostatic repulsion between the two positively charged volumes is greater than the short-range attraction forces between them. The two fragments fly apart (their kinetic energy taking about 80% of the total disintegration energy) and several neutrons and gamma rays are emitted (momentum and energy being conserved, of course). Thus, nuclear fission has occurred, and the neutrons liberated may cause the fission of other nuclei so that a fission 'chain-reaction' may be set up with a consequent liberation of large amounts of energy (26.6.1).

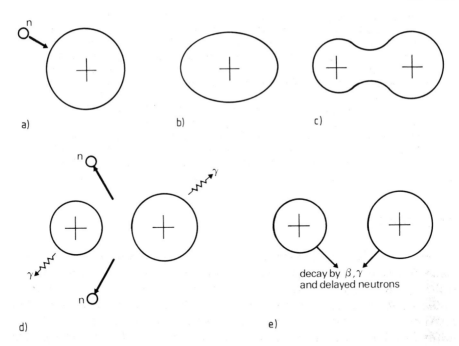

Fig. 26.12 Fission (neutron-activated) — see text.

The fission products from any given type of nucleus are not always the same, i.e. the two (or occasionally three) fragments may have different relative sizes on each disintegration. The fragments themselves are rich in neutrons for their atomic numbers, and do not lie within the stable band shown in Figure 26.1. They thus attempt to become more stable by decreasing the numbers of neutrons with respect to the number of protons. This results in either β-decays (with associated gamma rays) so changing a neutron to a proton within the nucleus of a fragment (26.3), or the ejection of a neutron itself from the fragment if the nucleus is in a highly excited state. These neutrons are known as *delayed neutrons* to distinguish them from the 'prompt' neutrons liberated at the moment of fission. Either type of decay eventually produces a stable element which is within the stable band of nuclides depicted in Figure 26.1.

The obvious example of nuclear fission is that of uranium-235 ($^{235}_{92}U$), which is the 'fuel' used in nuclear reactors (see below). The fission of such nuclei produces many different fission fragments of which $^{140}_{54}Xe$ is an example. This then follows the decay chain:

$$^{140}_{54}Xe \xrightarrow[16\,s]{\beta^-} {}^{140}_{55}Cs \xrightarrow[66\,s]{\beta^-} {}^{140}_{56}Ba \xrightarrow[12\cdot8\,d]{\beta^-} {}^{140}_{57}La \xrightarrow[40\,h]{\beta^-} {}^{140}_{58}Ce \text{ (stable)}$$

Each β^--decay increases the number of protons in the nucleus by one, while unaffecting the mass number (i.e. 140 nucleons in each nucleus). Thus the element changes after each disintegration, and the nuclei are isobars of each other.

A great range of other decay chains are possible from other fission fragments.

Insight

It is possible to initiate fission of a nucleus by using charged particles (e.g. protons) and gamma rays.

$$\text{e.g.} \quad {}^{63}_{29}\text{Cu} + p^+ \left\langle \begin{array}{l} {}^{24}_{11}\text{Na} + n \\[1ex] {}^{39}_{19}\text{K} \end{array} \right.$$

and ${}^{238}_{92}\text{U} + \boldsymbol{h}\nu$ (5·1 Mev) $\longrightarrow$ fission products

The latter example is known as 'photofission'.

26.6.1 The nuclear reactor

The nuclear reactor (or 'pile') produces heat energy by controlled fission. The heat generated within the reactor raises the temperature of a circulating coolant such as pressurised water or carbon dioxide, which in turn is used to produce steam. The steam then drives very powerful electric generators, the electrical power from which may then be transmitted over large distances for use in cities and villages.

The controlled fission in the nuclear reactor is obtained by using the neutrons of fissile-decay to produce fission in other atoms. Thus, for a sustained reaction, at least one neutron released during each fission must produce fission in another nucleus. The 'fuel' used in conventional nuclear reactor is 'enriched' uranium, which is a mixture of ${}^{238}_{92}\text{U}$ and ${}^{235}_{92}\text{U}$. Controlled fission is possible only with ${}^{235}_{92}\text{U}$ because ${}^{238}_{92}\text{U}$ is able to form stable nuclei on the capture of 'fast' neutrons (energies greater than 0·5 MeV). However, ${}^{235}_{92}\text{U}$ is an efficient fissile material for 'thermal' neutrons. The classification of neutron energies into fast, intermediate, slow and thermal is shown in Table 26.1, where it is seen that a thermal neutron has a very low energy, which is necessary for the production of an efficient process of fission with ${}^{235}_{92}\text{U}$. Hence, the energetic neutrons emitted at the moment of fission (see Fig. 26.12(d)) must be slowed down, or *moderated*. A suitable 'moderator' is made from graphite (a form of carbon) which is made into rods and inserted into the nuclear 'pile'. An alternative moderator is 'heavy water' (${}^{2}_{1}\text{H}_2\text{O}$). On average, a neutron takes about 0·1 second to become 'thermal' and to cause another fission.

There is also a requirement to be able to adjust the power generated within the reactor and, in particular, to prevent 'runaway', where the ever-increasing heat produced in the reactor would melt and vaporise the contents to produce a severe radioactive contamination problem in the environment (i.e. 'melt down'). Note that it is not possible for the nuclear reactor to explode in the manner of an atomic bomb! The method by which the number of neutrons present may be altered, so altering the fission rate and hence the amount of heat, is by using adjustable rods containing boron which are inserted in the

Table 26.1 Energy classification of neutrons

Classification	Energy range
Fast	Greater than 0·5 MeV
Intermediate	1 keV to 0·5 MeV
Slow	1 eV to 1 keV
Thermal	0·025 eV

'pile'. Boron is a very good absorber of neutrons — those which are not absorbed are moderated by the graphite and then produce fission in the uranium-235 nuclei.

To start the reactor, the boron rods are almost completely withdrawn and the spontaneous fission (see previous section) of the uranium or the neutrons from cosmic rays are sufficient to release the neutrons necessary for further fission. If there is sufficient uranium in the reactor for a sustained chain reaction to be possible, it is said to have gone 'critical' ('hyper-critical' is an un-controlled fission rate, and therefore dangerous). The increase in the number of neutrons is then quite rapid (e.g. a factor of 10^{12} in about 30 s). The boron rods are progressively reinserted in the pile and adjusted to produce a given number of neutrons in the pile, corresponding to the power level required.

The nuclear reactor may be used to produce artificial radionuclides (described below) by inserting samples in the neutron flux within the reactor.

26.7 SUMMARY OF RADIOACTIVE NUCLEAR TRANSFORMATIONS

Table 26.2 is a summary of all the previous types of radioactive decay described in the above sections and is included at this stage to enable the reader to achieve a clear understanding and comparison of each type of decay and its consequences.

26.8 ARTIFICIALLY PRODUCED RADIONUCLIDES

Radionuclides are produced artificially by bombarding the nuclei of elements with particles, such that the captured particle makes the nucleus unstable. It then decays with a definite half-life (5.2.2) by one or more of the methods described above.

A large proportion of all radionuclides are produced by bombarding a 'target' with neutrons, as produced in a nuclear reactor (see above). The daughter nucleus produced by neutron capture is then, obviously, rich in neutrons, and so is likely to decay by β^--emission. This may be accompanied by γ-emission (26.3). The capture of the neutron is accompanied by the immediate ejection of a γ-ray or particle, and the reaction is written

Table 26.2 Summary of effects of radioactive decay

Type of decay	Symbol	Effect on nucleus Z	N	A	Effect on atom	Comments
Gamma	γ	—	—	—	None, but competing process may be 'internal conversion'	Produced by quantum jump from excited state of nucleus to a lower energy. Excited state of measurable half-life is 'metastable' state, and transition is 'isomeric' (I.T.)
Internal conversion	IC	—	—	—	Characteristic radiation and Auger electrons	Inner orbital electron of atom isteracts directly with the nucleus is ejected from atom — energy of nucleus thereby reduced. Vacancy in shell
Electron capture	EC	$Z-1$	$N+1$	—	Characteristic radiation and Auger electrons of daughter nucleus	Inner orbital electron captured by nucleus and changes proton to neutron. Neutrino emitted carrying energy change of nucleus Nucleus may decay subsequently by gamma emission. Vacancy left in electron orbit
Beta (negatron)	β^-	$Z+1$	$N-1$	—	Electron orbits change to those of daughter nucleus	Proton changed to neutron in nucleus. Negatrons (electrons) emitted with spread of energies, but energy of negatron + antineutrino is constant. Daughter nucleus may decay with prompt or delayed gammas with competing IC
Beta (positron)	β^+	$Z-1$	$N+1$	—	" "	Neutron changed to proton in nucleus. Positron emitted with neutrino (sum of energies is constant). Only occurs if energy lost by nucleus is greater than 1·02 MeV. Positron is annihilated with electron with production of two 0·511 MeV gammas 'back-to-back'. Daughter nucleus may decay by gamma and/or IC
Alpha	α	$Z-2$	$N-2$	$A-4$ "	"	Occurs in heavy elements. Alphas travel through, rather than over, nuclear barrier, and emitted with discrete energies. Daughter nucleus may decay by gamma and /or IC or beta emission
Fission	f	Variable sizes and compositions of fission products			Fragments recoil and break bonds/ionise surrounding atoms	Spontaneous or neutron-activated. Nucleus splits, producing two or more fragments, neutrons (fast), gammas and about 200 MeV of energy. Controlled fission is used in nuclear power stations by 'moderating' the neutrons to thermal energies. Occurs in heavy elements, e.g. uranium-235

symbolically as (n, γ), (n, p) etc. An example of a (n, γ) reaction is the production of $^{99}_{42}Mo$ from $^{98}_{42}Mo$:

i.e. $^{98}_{42}Mo\ (n, \gamma)\ ^{99}_{42}Mo$ Equation 26.5

This is 'shorthand' for:

$$^{98}_{42}Mo + n \longrightarrow {}^{98}_{42}Mo + \gamma$$

Note the increase of atomic mass number due to the capture of a neutron, but no change in the element. The symbolic notation shown in Equation 26.5 will be used for the remainder of this section.

The capture of the neutron by the $^{98}_{42}Mo$ nucleus raises the energy of the resulting $^{99}_{42}Mo$ above its ground state, which it promptly loses by the emission of a γ-photon. The widespread use of a 'technetium generator' in Nuclear Medicine (where the mother $^{99}_{42}Mo$ decays to $^{99}_{43}Tc^m$ by β^--emission, the latter being eluted from a column as sodium pertechnetate) makes this an important example of radionuclide production.

Another useful radionuclide in medicine is $^{131}_{53}I$ which may be used as a 'tracer' (26.9) and for the treatment of thyroid disorders and cancers. It is produced in two stages: first by a (n, γ) reaction and then by the decay of the daughter product ^{131}Te:

$$^{130}_{52}Te\ (n, \gamma)\ ^{131}_{52}Te \xrightarrow[25\ min]{} {}^{131}_{53}I + \beta^-$$

The $^{131}_{52}Te$ produced by the (n, γ) reaction decays rapidly to the longer-lived (8 days half-life) $^{131}_{53}I$.

An example of a (n, p) reaction is in the production of $^{35}_{16}S$:

$$^{35}_{17}Cl\ (n, p)\ ^{35}_{16}S$$

The (n, p) reactions usually require fast neutrons, and have the advantage that, by producing a different element, the product may be chemically separated from the target material, so enabling high specific activities (see beginning of this chapter) to be obtained.

In addition, a cyclotron may be used to produce beams of protons, deuterons* or α-particles to bombard nuclei. The daughter nuclei of such bombardments are usually neutron deficient and decay either by positron emission or electron capture. However, a very wide variety of reactions and subsequent decay schemes are possible.

e.g. $^{60}_{28}Ni\ (p, \alpha)\ ^{57}_{27}Co \xrightarrow[270\ days]{EC} {}^{57}_{26}Fe$ (stable)

Thus, the $^{57}_{27}Co$ produced by the protons in the cyclotron decays by 100% electron capture (26.4) to $^{57}_{26}Fe$.

26.8.1 The growth of activity

If it is imagined that a sample has just been introduced within a nuclear reactor or cyclotron, then the number of daughter nuclei formed by one of the capture

---

* Deuteron — isotope of hydrogen (1 proton and 1 neutron). ^2_1H.

processes increases over a period of time. However, the number of daughter nuclei does not continue indefinitely, for the following reasons (the case of neutron capture is assumed):

a.   as more of the original nuclei continue to capture neutrons, there are fewer left to do the same

b.   daughter nuclei may themselves capture further neutrons and form a different isotope of that element

c.   daughter nuclei undergo natural radioactive decay during the irradiation time.

The relative importance of these processes depends upon many factors such as target material, the half-lives involved and neutron flux and neutron energy spectrum. However, it is usual to irradiate for a time so that only a few per cent of the original nuclei are transformed. The probability of (b) above is often low, so that the amount of radioactivity finally produced in the sample in practice depends only upon the sample itself, the neutron flux, irradiation time and half-life of the daughter product. In these circumstances, the growth of activity is of an exponential form:

$$A_t = kF(1 - e^{-\lambda t})$$ Equation 26.6

where A_t is the radioactivity at time t (in becquerel or curie)
       k is a constant for a given sample and reactor
       F is the neutron flux (number per unit area per second)
       λ is the 'decay constant' of the daughter (5.2.2)

This 'growth-curve', which is similar to that obtained when charging up a capacitor (9.10), is shown in Figure 26.13 for two different neutron fluxes. In both cases, the activity produced in the sample approaches a maximum value after about four half-lives. It is usual, however, to irradiate for only two to three half-lives, as the increased activity obtained for longer exposure times than this is not very great.

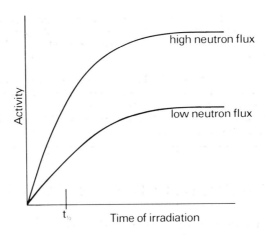

Fig. 26.13 The growth of activity induced by irradiating a sample with neutrons.

A long exposure time of the sample to neutrons (or other particles) compared to the half-life of the product enables the activity curve to reach its maximum value, when there are equal numbers of nuclei being produced and decaying per second. This is known as *radioactive equilibrium*, and may also occur in long decay chains where a nuclide is being produced by decay and is also decaying into another nuclide.

Insight

An example of radioactive equilibrium is the decay $^{99}_{42}\text{Mo}$ into $^{99}_{43}\text{Tc}^m$, as in a 'technetium generator'. 90% of $^{99}_{42}\text{Mo}$ decays to $^{99}\text{Tc}^m$ and the half-lives of each are 67 h and 6 h respectively. If the generator is not 'eluted', then the curve of $^{99}_{43}\text{Tc}^m$ activity 'follows' that of $^{99}_{42}\text{Mo}$ (at 90% of its value) i.e. it is in radioactive equilibrium with it. Elution of the generator removes all

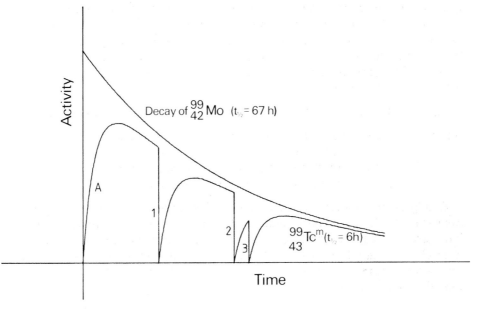

Fig. 26.14 An example of radioactive equilibrium. Molybdenum-99 decays with a half-life of 67 h to technetium-99m (half-life = 6 h). At time = 0, the Tc-99m grows in activity (A in the figure) — this is removed by elution from a 'technetium-generator' (1.2.3), after which the activity grows again.

the $^{99}_{43}\text{Tc}^m$ (1, 2, 3, in Fig. 26.14) which then regrows until it is once more in equilibrium with the ^{99}Mo curve, unless two elutions follow each other too quickly as in 2 and 3. The generator may thus be used as a source of the daughter nuclide over a much longer time than the half-life of the daughter would otherwise permit.

26.9 CLINICALLY USEFUL RADIONUCLIDES

Radionuclides are used to diagnose and treat certain clinical conditions. As a diagnostic aid, they may be 'labelled' to a particular 'radiopharmaceutical' and injected into or ingested by, the patient. Such 'tracers', when detected externally, are divided into two main uses:

   a. to provide information on organ physiology
   b. to produce an 'image' of an organ.

For example, the passage of radioactive iodo-hippurate (or technetium-labelled DTPA*) through a patient's kidneys may be used to determine ureteral obstruction or early kidney transplant rejection. A 'brain scan' using $^{99}_{43}Tc^m$ as pertechnetate may be obtained on a scanner or gamma camera, and the images produced may aid in the detection of abnormalities such as infarcts, abcesses, subdural haematomas and brain tumours.

Of all the decay processes outlined in the previous sections, only that of gamma decay is useful for detection external to the patient, because all the other particles emitted are absorbed very efficiently in the body's tissues. Such absorbed energy within the body governs the quantity of the radiation dose received by the patient, which must be minimised, commensurate with the appropriate 'risk-benefit' of the procedure for that patient (33.1). The radiation dose is reduced by selection of a radionuclide which exhibits a short half-life, a small amount of 'particulate' radiation and a relatively rapid excretion from the body. The radionuclide $^{99}_{43}Tc^m$ decays by 90% gamma emission and 10% internal conversion, X-rays and Auger electrons. The relatively small amounts of 'soft' (i.e. low energy) particulate radiation means that $^{99}_{43}Tc^m$ produces a low radiation dose to the patient. This, together with its half-life of 6 h, gamma energy of 140 keV and wide range of radiopharmaceuticals to which it may be labelled, makes $^{99}_{43}Tc^m$ and almost ideal 'tracer' for many applications. (For example, approximately forty times the activity of $^{99}Tc^m$ may be injected into a patient as ^{131}I — to give the same radiation dose.)

A beta emitter such as tritium (^3_1H) in the form of tritiated water ($^3_1H_2O$), or sulphur-35 as sulphate, may be used to estimate the volumes of various 'compartments' or 'spaces' within the body volume by a technique known as *dilution analysis*. In this procedure, a known activity of tritiated water (say) is injected into the patient and blood or urine samples taken over a period of time. By measuring the activity within such samples and making assumptions about the fate of the tritiated water in the body, it is possible to calculate the total mass of water in the patient. This is important, for example, in some studies in obesity. The detection and measurement of β- and γ-emitters is discussed in Appendix II.

A diagnostic procedure involving radioactivity, but which does not involve any radiation dose to the patient is called *radioimmunoassay*, which is a technique used to measure extremely small amounts of circulating hormone in the patient's blood-stream (e.g. thyroid-stimulating hormone (TSH), growth hormone, human placental lactogen (HPL)). Typically, a known quantity of hormone which is labelled with a suitable radionuclide (e.g. $^{125}_{53}I$ or ^3_1H) is made to compete with an accurately dispensed quantity of the patient's serum for a restricted number of chemical 'binding-sites'. The amount of activity which

---

* DTPA — diethylene triamine penta-acetic acid.

Table 26.3 Medical uses of radionuclides

Application	Radionuclide	$t_{1/2}$	Decay mode	Gamma energies (MeV)	Max beta energy (MeV)	Comments
Diagnostic:						
a. Tracers	$^{3}_{1}H$	12·3 y	β^-	—	0·018	Used in a wide
	$^{14}_{6}C$	5760 y	β^-	—	0·155	variety of chemical forms
	$^{35}_{16}S$	87·2 d	β^-	—	0·167 ⎱	Estimation of
	$^{43}_{19}K$	22 h	β^-	0·37 0·61	0·83 ⎰	cellular volumes
	$^{51}_{24}Cr$	27·8 d	EC	0·32	—	For blood studies
	$^{57}_{27}Co$	270 d	EC	0·122	— ⎱	Investigation of
	$^{58}_{27}Co$	71 d	β^+, EC	0·51, 0·81	0·485 ⎰	pernicious anemia
	$^{59}_{26}Fe$	45 d	β^-	1·10, 1·29	0·46	For blood studies
b. Organ physiology	$^{131}_{53}I$	8·04 d	β^-	0·364	0·61 ⎱	Thyroid uptakes (NaI), kidney function (iodohippurate)
	$^{132}_{53}I$	2·3 h	β^-	0·67, 0·78	2·12 ⎰	
	$^{99}_{43}Tc^{m}$ ⎱	6 h	IT	0·140	—	Kidney function (DTPA)
c. Organ imaging	$^{99}_{43}Tc^{m}$ ⎰					Imaging brain, lung, liver, kidney, spleen,
	$^{113}_{49}In^{m}$	90 m	IT	0·390	—	Brain, liver, kidney
	$^{75}_{34}Se$	121 d	EC	0·14, 0·27	—	Pancreas
	$^{68}_{31}Ga$	68 m	β^+, EC	0·51	1·89	'Tumour-seeking' agent and for inflammatory lesions
	$^{81}_{36}Kr^{m}$	13 s	IT	0·19		Lung 'ventilation' studies
	$^{133}_{54}Xe$	5·3 d	β^-	0·081	0·34	Cerebral blood flow, lung ventilation
Therapy:						
a. By injection	$^{32}_{15}P$	14·3 d	β^-	—	1·71	Treatment of polycythaemia vera (as phosphate)
	$^{90}_{39}Y$	64·2 h	β^-	—	2·27	Arthritis, lymphatic cancer (as colloid)
b. By ingestion	$^{131}_{53}I$	8·04 d	β^-	0·364	0·61	Hyperthyroidism, thyroid cancer

c. Inter- stitial	$^{226}_{88}$Ra	1620 y	(Complex decay)			⎫	Localised treatment of cancer — sources
	$^{182}_{73}$Ta	115 d	(Many βs and γs)			⎬	in form of needles,
	$^{192}_{77}$Ir	74 d	(Many βs and γs)			⎬	tubes, wires etc.
	$^{137}_{55}$Cs ⎱	30 y	β^-	0·662	0·51	⎭	
d. Tele- therapy	$^{137}_{55}$Cs ⎰						External beams of
	$^{60}_{27}$Co	5·3 y	β^-	1·17,	0·31		gamma radiation
				1·33			used to treat cancer

Radioimmunoassay:

	$^{125}_{53}$I	60 d	EC	0·027, 0·035	—	Small quantity of patient's serum added to radioactive compound in solution — used to detect minute quantities of hormones

(Also tritium and carbon-14 — see above)

does not succeed in binding itself to such sites is inversely related to the quantity of hormone in the blood sample. Typically, the activity which remains in solution may be measured in a suitable scintillation counter (see Appendix II), and compared to various 'standards' which form part of the same test batch.

The therapeutical aspects of radionuclides involve internal, interstitial and external sources. An example of an internal source is $^{32}_{15}$P in the form of sodium phosphate which is injected to control polycythaemia vera (a blood disorder). Interstitial sources include tubes, needles and wires of radium, caesium, tantalum, cobalt and iridium and are used in the localised treatment of cancerous growths. External sources used in 'teletherapy' produce intense beams of gamma radiation which may be used to treat various conditions — mainly cancer. The use of such beams of different sizes and at different angles is arranged to produce the greatest radiation dose to the treatment volume while minimising the dose received by the surrounding healthy tissues. Sources of $^{60}_{27}$Co (see decay scheme in Fig. 26.5) and $^{137}_{55}$Cs are commonly used for this purpose (34.2).

The above is a very brief survey of some of the uses of radionuclides in medicine. Table 26.3 summarises many of these points.

Exercise 26.4

(*Note:* Revision of previous chapters may be necessary for some of these questions).

a. What is meant by the term 'radioactivity', and what is the 'law of radioactive decay'? Define the unit (becquerel or curie) used to measure radioactivity.

b. Describe the processes of alpha decay, beta decay and gamma decay in radioactivity. What is the effect on the atomic number, atomic mass number and the number of neutrons in the nucleus for each type of decay?

c. Explain the meaning of the following terms:

(i) metastable state
(ii) isomeric transition
(iii) isobaric transition
(iv) internal conversion
(v) Auger electron
(vi) fluorescent (or 'characteristic') radiation.

d. 'Iron-55 decays to manganese-55 by electron capture with a half-life of 2·7 years'. Describe fully what this statement means.

e. What is meant by the 'decay scheme' of a radioactive decay? Sketch and explain the general appearances of the decay schemes for gamma, beta (both signs), electron capture and alpha decay.

f. Write notes on:

(i) electron shells
(ii) 'characteristic' X-rays
(iii) negatrons and positrons
(iv) the neutrino
(v) 'line' spectra
(vi) annihilation radiation.

g. What is meant by 'mass–energy equivalence'? Discuss this in relation to the fate of a positron emitted in beta decay.

h. Give a brief account of the phenomenon of fission, and describe how fission is used in a nuclear reactor to produce electrical power.

i. What are the methods used to produce 'artificial' radionuclides? Show some different types of nuclear reactions used in this process and list some uses to which artificially produced radionuclides are put in medicine.

j. What factors are important when assessing the radiation dose the patient is likely to receive from the administration of a particular 'radiopharmaceutical'? Hence show why therapeutic doses of $^{131}_{53}I$ are used for thyroid disorders and why organ imaging ('scanning') is undertaken using radionuclides such as technetium-99 m.

SUMMARY

1. Unstable nuclei 'decay' by a variety of mechanisms — this is known as radioactive decay, and results in nuclear transformations, or 'disintegrations'. The unit of activity is the becquerel (1 Bq = 1 disintegration/second) or the curie (1 Ci = 3·7 × 10^{10} disintegrations/second).

2. A nucleus may undergo the following transformations: γ (prompt or metastable), β or α-emission, internal conversion, electron capture or fission.

'Neutron rich' nuclei tend to decay by β^--decay, while 'neutron deficient' nuclei tend to decay by β^+-emission or electron capture.

3.   The effects of all these transformations on the nucleus and on the atom are summarised in Table 26.2.

4.   Transformations occur so as to make the daughter nucleus closer to the band of stability (Figure 26.1). The daughter nucleus is at a lower energy state than the mother.

5.   The laws of conservation of energy and momentum are obeyed in each transformation. The apparent breaking of these in β-decay led to discovery of the neutrino (β-particles show a continuous energy spectrum, unlike the line spectra of the other transformations).

6.   Radionuclides may be artificially produced by the capture of neutrons or charged particles by nuclei, either in a nuclear reactor or cyclotron.

7.   The uses to which radionuclides may be put in medicine are summarised in Table 26.3.

8.   The radiation dose received by a patient from the administration of a 'radiopharmaceutical' is reduced if:

a.   the half-life of the radionuclide is short

b.   there is very little 'particulate' radiation emitted on decay (i.e. beta particles)

c.   the radiopharmaceutical is excreted rapidly from the body, i.e. a short 'biological' half-life.

27. Fluorescence

27.1 FLUORESCENCE, PHOSPHORESCENCE AND CHARACTERISTIC RADIATION

In the previous chapter the term 'fluorescence' was used synonymously with 'characteristic radiation', it being shown that such quanta of electromagnetic radiation are released when electrons drop from outer orbits to inner vacant electron orbits in the atoms. Such radiation is 'characteristic' of the atoms, since each element has a unique arrangement of electron orbits. In general radiographic usage, however, the term 'fluorescence' is usually used to refer to that characteristic radiation which is emitted within the visible part of the electromagnetic spectrum and this corresponds to quantum jumps in the outer electron orbits only (X-rays are produced in the more energetic jumps to the inner electron shells). Thus if a substance emits visible light when irradiated by X-rays or ultraviolet light, it is said to display the phenomenon of *fluorescence* (or 'luminescence'). If it continues to emit visible light after ceasing to be irradiated, then it displays *phosphorescence*, or 'afterglow' (27.3).

Each absorption of energy (whether of X-rays or charged particles) by the fluorescent material (the 'phosphor') which results in a burst of photons of visible light is called a *scintillation*.

The mechanisms of fluorescence may only be explained satisfactorily by the use of the electron band theory of crystalline solids, and the reader is advised to read sections 10.1 and 19.2.

27.2 MECHANISMS OF FLUORESCENCE

All fluorescence is caused by an electron in a high-energy state dropping to a lower-energy state and thereby emitting a quantum of radiation (25.5.3). The electron may be raised to its high-energy state by means of the absorption of a photon (photoelectric absorption — 25.5.1) or by interaction with an energetic beam of charged particles. An efficient *phosphor* (i.e. a substance which fluoresces) contains a small amount of impurity or an excess of one of its constituents (e.g. excess Zn in ZnS, Tl in NaI, excess tungstate in calcium tungstate) which greatly enhances the light output from it. These impurities produce what are known as *luminescent centres*, and they possess discrete electron energy levels which are different from those in the crystal. This is shown in diagrammatic form in Figure 27.1(a) for a crystal with no luminescent centres, and Figure 27.1(b) with the energy levels of a luminescent centre shown relative to the pure crystal.

The importance of the luminescent centres lies in the increased efficiency with which they produce fluorescence. Nevertheless, not all electrons which reach such a centre produce a photon; some electrons are able to work their way 'downwards' from the upper energy level of the fluorescent centre in a series of collisions with the surrounding atoms, so reaching the valence band without performing a quantum jump. These are known as *radiationless transitions*, since no radiation is emitted — the surrounding atoms merely gain a little extra kinetic energy! However, the luminescent centres are more efficient in producing fluorescence than the pure crystal.

The sequence of events leading to a scintillation is as follows (assuming photoelectric absorption):

a. an electron is ejected from an atom with high kinetic energy — it becomes 'free' and travels at high speed in the conduction band

b. the energetic electron, on passing close to other atoms, excites and ionises these atoms, so that more electrons are lifted into the conduction band (leaving positive holes behind)

c. some of these electrons eventually reach the site of luminescent centres (in about a millionth of a second!) and adjust themselves to the electron energy levels of each centre

d. some of the electrons in the luminescent centres are able to perform a quantum jump downwards over an energy difference E_1 (see Fig. 27.1(b)) and emit a photon of electromagnetic radiation of energy $E_1 = \boldsymbol{h}v_1$, where v_1 is the frequency of the photon.

Note that the positive holes (19.1.1) in the valence band must also reach a luminescence centre in order for the electron to be able to fall into an available site in the valence band.

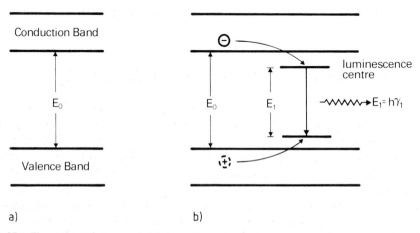

Fig. 27.1 Fluorescence in a crystal. (a) shows the outer electron structure of a pure crystal, and (b) shows the effect of an 'impurity' atom on the electron levels. Such impurities enhance fluorescence and are known as luminescent centres.

Three consequences follow from the above remarks:

    a.   no phosphor is perfectly efficient, because some of the incident energy is converted into heat energy by radiationless transitions (phosphors are typically 2−20% efficient for energy conversion into light)

    b.   the wavelength of the fluorescent light is always longer than any incident wavelength producing the fluorescence, because the energy gap E_1 is less than E_0 (Fig. 27.1(b))

    c.   the number of fluorescent photons is greater than the number of absorbed photons.

Taking these points in turn, the efficiency of the production of fluorescence in a material is described by the 'scintillation efficiency', where:

Definition
> The *scintillation efficiency* is the fraction of the incident energy which is converted into luminescence.

(*Note:* This is also termed the 'absolute' or 'intrinsic' scintillation efficiency.)

    A typical range of scintillation efficiencies of phosphors is 2% for anthracene to 10% for NaI(Tl) and about 18% for oxysulphide intensifying screens ('rare-earth' screens — 27.5.3).

    The energy of the emitted photons is less than that of the total gap between the valence and conduction band of the pure crystal (Fig. 27.1 (b)) so that hv_1 is less than hv_0, i.e. the wavelength of the emitted photon is greater than that of any absorbed incident photons, since the frequency is smaller.

Exercise 27.1
    a.   Why does a photon of lower energy than another have a longer wavelength?

    b.   A 140 keV γ-ray strikes a phosphor and is totally absorbed.
How many light photons are emitted if the scintillation efficiency is 5% and the average energy per fluorescent photon is 3 eV? (3 eV photons correspond to 'blue' light.)

27.3 MECHANISMS OF PHOSPHORESCENCE

Phosphorescence is caused by the presence of *electron traps* within the crystal structure of the phosphor. When an electron falls into one of these traps it is unable to escape down to the valence band — it must be re-energised back into the conduction band, from which it may be able to find a luminescence centre. It is the effect of inter-atomic collisions (i.e. heat) which enables the eventual escape of the electron from some of the higher-lying traps, but this process takes time so that the fluorescence continues when the incident radiation is stopped. This phenomenon is also known as *afterglow*, and may diminish in intensity as a simple exponential decay with time (5.1). Such afterglow would be a great nuisance, of course, in X-ray fluorescent screens, TV sets and image intensifier phosphors since the previous image would be 'remembered' by the phosphor and interfere with the clarity of a later image.

Figure 27.2 illustrates the location of two 'traps' A and B, both of which contain electrons which were previously raised to the conduction band. The electron in trap A is much more likely than that in B to receive sufficient energy from thermal agitation to jump up into the conduction band and stand a chance of producing a photon of luminescence. The statistical probability of a large number of electrons being so energised at any one moment produces the afterglow in phosphorescence.

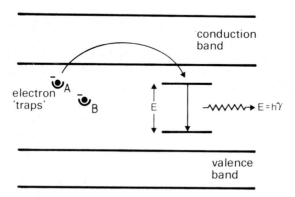

Fig. 27.2 The production of phosphorescence, or 'afterglow'. Electrons in traps A and B are put there by the original absorption event of electromagnetic radiation. They are able to reach the conduction band subsequently as a result of thermal agitation, and hence produce fluorescent photons, as shown.

27.4 THERMOLUMINESCENCE

The 'electron traps' which cause phosphorescence, or afterglow, as outlined in the previous section, may be used to advantage in *thermoluminescent dosimetry*. This is a method of measuring the radiation dose received by a suitable material (e.g. a lithium fluoride 'dosimeter') by the number of electrons captured by the 'deep' traps during irradiation. Such irradiation produces electrons in the conduction band (as described previously), and the numbers which are captured by the 'traps' is proportional to the radiation dose to which the material has been subjected. At normal temperature the electrons which fall into the deeper traps do not manage to receive sufficient energy from thermal agitation of the molecules to jump up to the conduction band. However, if the material is subjected to heating, the kinetic energy of the molecules is increased and some of the electrons reach the conduction band, and subsequently take part in luminescence. This process is called *thermoluminescence*, and the light output of the dosimeter is measured using a photomultiplier (Appendix II), the reading from which is related to the radiation dose received by the dosimeter in a reliable and repeatable manner if such samples are always subjected to the same heating cycle.

The dosimeter is finally raised to an even higher temperature and allowed to cool slowly ('annealing'), thus emptying all the traps and allowing the dosimeter to be re-used.

The practical use of thermoluminescence is discussed in Chapters 32 and 33.

27.5 X-RAY FLUORESCENT SCREENS

27.5.1 Screen factors

The intensity distribution of X-rays obtained after passing through a patient (the 'X-ray image') depends upon the detailed internal structure of the patient's body. If this X-ray image exposes a photographic film by direct action (31.2), a 'density image' is obtained, where the dark areas on the film correspond to the higher X-ray intensities in the incident 'X-ray image'. If, however, the X-ray beam is incident upon a flat fluorescent surface (a 'screen'), then the 'X-ray image' is first converted to an 'optical image' within the screen, being brighter where the X-ray intensity is higher. The 'optical image' may then produce a 'density image' if the light from the screen is allowed to fall on the photographic film.

Fluorescent screens are used in radiography to reduce the radiation dose which the patient would otherwise receive. They do this by significantly reducing the X-ray exposure required to achieve a given photographic density on the X-ray film. The factor by which exposure is reduced is known as the screen intensification factor (or just 'screen factor') and may be formally defined as:

Definition

The *screen intensification factor* (IF) is given by E/E_s where:

E is the exposure without screens and

E_s is the exposure with screens which produces the same photographic density on the radiograph.

Note: In this context, the term *exposure* may be considered to represent the total energy of the X-ray beam incident upon the film per unit area for the total exposure time. It therefore depends upon the kV_p, mAs and the Inverse Square Law (see section 4.7 for a fuller treatment of these points).

If the kV_p and FFD are unchanged between the two exposures (i.e. one with and one without the screen), then the value of the IF is given simply by the ratio of the two values of mAs which produce the same film density. This simplifies even further if the same value of mA is also used, when the IF is just the ratio of the exposure time without the screen to the exposure time with the screen. For example, if an exposure time of 8 s is required to produce a photographic density (31.2.1) of 1·0 without the use of a screen, and an exposure time of 0·5 s is required with the screen, then the intensification factor is just $8/0·5 = 16$ for that screen. A typical value for the IF for calcium tungstate screens is about 50 and about 250 for the newer 'rare-earth' screens (see below). This is equivalent to the statement that each screen contributes about 98% and 99·9% of the light striking the film respectively, the remainder of the film blackening being due to the direct action of X-rays on the photographic emulsion.

Example

If particular settings of kV_p, exposure time and FFD require an exposure of 100 mAs without a screen then the use of a screen with an intensification factor of 50 will enable an exposure setting of 2 mAs for the same photographic density. Further examples are given in section 4.7.

The 'relative screen factor' compares the intensification factors between two or more screens, as indicated by the following definition:

Definition

The *relative screen factors*, $S_1, S_2, S_3, \ldots$ of two or more screens is given by the ratio of their respective intensification factors with respect to any *one* of the screens.

It is assumed that the same type of photographic film is being used in all the screens, of course.

Hence, if the IF of a calcium tungstate screen is 50 and that of a 'rare-earth' screen is 250, the relative screen factor of the latter is 5 when compared to the calcium tungstate screen. Thus the exposures may be taken in one-fifth of the time (using the same FFD, kV_p and mA) when using the 'rare-earth' screen, producing the same photographic density on the same type of film.

27.5.2 Screen construction

A typical fluoroscopic screen is made by gluing tiny fluorescent crystals of a suitable material to a flexible white plastic or cardboard backing and sealing the surface of the crystals with a transparent 'scratch-proof' lacquer to prevent accidental damage. The white surface of the backing material (a thin layer of reflective material such as magnesium oxide paint) ensures that the light emitted by the crystals (in all directions) in reflected towards the film to achieve maximum photographic effect. A screen is usually placed on either side of the film, to achieve a greater photographic effect, and each screen is placed facing the film in close contact with it to ensure good image quality. Even a small air-gap between the film and the screen surface results in significant light spread from each tiny fluorescent crystal before it reaches the film, and hence degrades the image by adding to the geometric unsharpness (3.4). The basic construction of a 'cassette' incorporating the above features is shown in Figure 27.3. The purpose of the metal backing is to absorb those X-rays which manage to pass through both screens and the film. Some of these X-rays would be scattered back from couch, floor etc. and would result only in a generalised 'fogging' of the film.

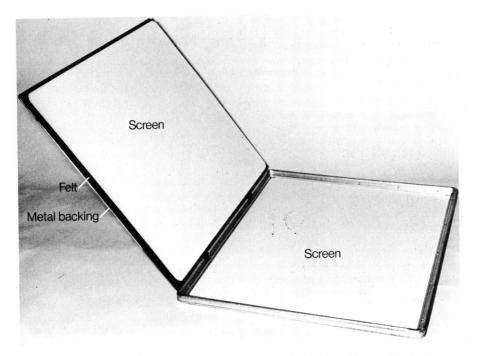

Fig. 27.3 The composition of a radiographic cassette. The film is placed between the two screens.

27.5.3 Calcium tungstate and 'rare-earth' screens

The most common types of crystal used as a phosphor in radiographic screens are those composed of calcium tungstate ($CaWO_4$). These have relatively good absorption of the incident radiation owing to the high atomic number of tungsten, and also show an output spectrum of light which matches the characteristics of conventional X-ray film. These two factors produce intensification factors (27.5.1) between 30 and 90, depending upon the individual screen and the kV_p at which the X-ray tube is operated. Calcium tungstate screens have a proven record of reliability and resistance to ageing effects to which earlier types of screen were subject.

In recent years a more efficient type of screen has appeared which is based upon the 'rare-earth' elements of the Periodic Table (atomic numbers 57 to 71 — see section 25.4) These act as the 'impurities' which produce the luminescent centres (27.2). Two such rare-earth screens are terbium-activated lanthanum oxysulphide ($La_2O_2S:Tb$) and terbium-activated gadolinium oxysulphide ($Gd_2O_2S:Tb$). The rare-earth elements are lanthanum (La) of atomic number 57, gadolinium (Gd) of atomic number 64 and terbium (Tb) of atomic number 65.

These phosphors have an improved performance over calcium tungstate in two important respects: their high atomic number makes them more efficient absorbers of radiation (Ch. 30), and they have a high scintillation efficiency (27.2). Thus, not only do such screens absorb more X-rays (by about a factor of

4), but each X-ray photon that is absorbed produces more light (by about a factor of 4). Thus the overall improvement over calcium tungstate screens is by a factor of about 16, in terms of the light energy emitted during the taking of a radiograph. Alternatively, much finer crystals may be used to reduce the geometric unsharpness. This also has the effect of reducing the amount of light reaching the film owing to self-absorption of light within the smaller crystals. Such a screen, therefore, may be designed to have the same intensification factor as a conventional calcium tungstate screen, but with a superior geometric unsharpness. Obviously, a compromise may be made anywhere between these two extremes.

The spectrum of fluorescent light emitted by rare-earth screens extends beyond the sensitive range of conventional X-ray films, so that 'orthochromatic' films are used, i.e. films sensitive to the whole of the visible spectrum up to the dark red. This colour of light filter is then used in the 'safe' lights in darkrooms to prevent unnecessary fogging of the film.

Figure 27.4 summarises these points in graphical form by showing the simplified emission spectra of both calcium tungstate and a typical rare-earth screen ($Gd_2O_2S:Tb$), together with the responses of the blue-sensitive and green-sensitive films used with either. The advantage of the greater light output of the rare-earth screens is only used to full advantage if a 'green-sensitive' film is used, of course, since the bulk of the emitted light occurs at a wavelength beyond the sensitivity of the blue-sensitive films suitable for calcium tungstate. Thus a relative screen factor for the rare-earth screen over the calcium tungstate may only be 2 or 3 when using conventional film, but may be 10–20 using green-sensitive film. This factor increases with increasing kV_p owing to the increased absorption of X-rays by the rare-earth screen compared to the calcium tungstate screen.

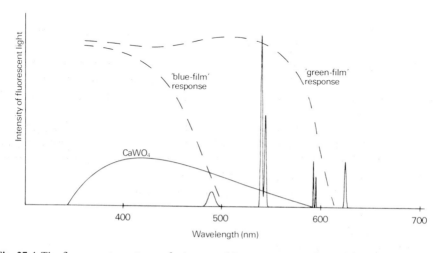

Fig. 27.4 The fluorescent spectrum of a 'rare-earth' screen compared to calcium tungstate (shown magnified). Also shown are the photographic sensitivities of conventional ('blue') and extended ('green') film.

27.6 FURTHER EXAMPLES OF FLUORESCENCE

The screens discussed in the previous sections produce fluorescence by the absorption of X-rays. It is also possible to produce fluorescence using high-speed electrons, as every television owner is aware! The television 'display monitors' used in image intensification also use the same principle as a domestic monitor, i.e. the 'scanning' of an electron beam across a phosphor inside an evacuated tube. The electrons impinging on the phosphor raise electrons into the conduction band within the phosphor (i.e. same effect as X-rays) which then produce fluorescence as they 'drop-back' to the valence band at a luminescent centre (27.2).

An X-ray image amplifier uses the mechanisms of fluorescence at each end: firstly a coating of phosphor (e.g. caesium iodide) to absorb the X-rays, emit light and produce electrons from a photoemissive surface (the 'photocathode') at the cathode end, and secondly a phosphor of reduced size at the anode end of the amplifier which converts the 'electron image' into an optical image by fluorescence. Further information on these devices is to be found in any book specialising in X-ray equipment.

Another example of fluorescence is in the 'fluorescent viewers' used for viewing X-ray films, where an electrical discharge in the gas of the fluorescent tubes emits ultra-violet radiation (24.2). This is absorbed by a suitable phosphor inside the tubes which is chosen to emit a broad band of wavelengths and so appear white. Note, however, that all wavelengths emitted are longer than that of the 'exciting' ultra-violet radiation (27.2).

The final example of fluorescence is that of scintillation counters using sodium iodide crystals and photomultiplier tubes for the detection of very small amounts of X and γ-radiation. These are discussed in Appendix II.

Exercise 27.1

a.   Explain what is meant by the term 'fluorescence', and show how this is put to advantage in an X-ray 'screen'.

b.   Define what is meant by 'screen intensification factor' and 'relative screen factor'. If the intensification factor of one screen/film combination is 30, and another is 120, what is the relative screen factor of the second compared to the first?

c.   If an exposure of 60 mAs is required to produce a photographic density of 2·1 when no screen is used, what value of mAs must be used to produce the same photographic density when using a screen whose intensification factor is 15? (Assume no changes in FFD and kV_p.)

d.   Explain what is meant by the following terms:

  (i)   fluorescence
 (ii)   phosphorescence
(iii)   luminescent centre
 (iv)   radiationless transition
  (v)   scintillation.

e. Describe the mechanism of fluorescence using the 'band' model of electron shells of a crystalline solid. Hence explain why the wavelength of the emitted photon(s) is greater than that of the absorbed photons which produce the fluorescence.

f. What is 'thermoluminescence'? Describe how it is produced and for what practical purpose it may be used.

g. What advantages are to be had when using 'rare-earth' screens compared to calcium tungstate? Explain the reasons for such advantages.

h. List and explain the uses to which fluorescence has been put in radiography.

(See also question (d) in Exercise 4.2 on p. 49.)

SUMMARY

1. In common radiographic usage, the term 'fluorescence' means the emission of visible light when a substance is irradiated by electromagnetic radiation or charged particles. In atomic physics, 'fluorescent' and 'characteristic' radiation are the same, i.e. fluorescence may also include non-visible radiation such as X-rays.

2. 'Phosphorescence' is fluorescence which does not cease within a very short time after the source of 'exciting' radiation is removed.

3. The wavelengths emitted in fluorescence are always longer than that of the electromagnetic radiation causing it. This is the same thing as saying that the emitted photons are less energetic than the incoming photons.

4. The phenomenon of fluorescence may be understood with reference to the band theory of crystalline solids, where electrons are enabled to jump from the valence band to the conduction band by the action of an energetic photoelectron travelling through the crystal after (for example) photoelectric absorption of the incoming quantum. Some of these energetic electrons migrate to a 'luminescence' centre and fall back to the valence band in a quantum jump which releases an electromagnetic quantum. Most of the energy, however, is converted to heat rather than light.

5. Phosphorescence occurs when a substance contains 'electron traps' which release trapped electrons to the conduction band over a long period of time so that the fluorescent radiation is extended. This is known also as 'afterglow' and is to be avoided in radiography.

6. Thermoluminescence uses these electron traps to 'remember' the radiation dose, and measures the dose by heating the sample (lithium fluoride) and recording the light emitted by fluorescence as the traps empty due to thermal agitation.

7. Fluorescent screens are used to reduce the radiation dose to the patient, since they are more efficient at absorbing the X-ray beam than a photographic film. They also release a large number of protons per absorption of an X-ray quantum and hence enhance the photographic effect.

8. The enhancement obtained when using a screen is the intensification

factor, defined as the ratio of the exposures required with no screen to when using a screen.

9. The relative screen factor relates the 'speeds' of different screens relative to each other. They are thus the appropriate ratios of the intensification factors.

10. Rare-earth screens show a marked increase in relative screen factor compared to calcium tungstate because of increased X-ray absorption and increased light output.

11. Other examples of fluorescence include image intensifiers, TV monitors, viewing screens and scintillation counters.

Part E
X-RAYS AND MATTER

28. The production of X-rays

28.1 INTERACTION OF ELECTRONS WITH MATTER

The construction of the X-ray tube is discussed in Chapter 21, together with the functions of the cathode, anode etc. in producing a high-energy focused beam of electrons onto the tungsten target. In that chapter it was stated that the sudden deceleration of the electron beam in the tungsten target produced the X-rays; in this chapter the fate of such electrons is investigated in more detail.

There are several different ways in which an energetic electron may lose its energy to the atoms in the material through which it passes. These all involve 'collisions' with either the orbiting electrons of the atoms or with the nuclei themselves. Further, there are two types of 'collision': *elastic and inelastic* (7.3): there is conservation of *kinetic* energy for the former case only. Thus the four main interactions of the energetic electrons are: inelastic and elastic collisions with nuclei, and inelastic and elastic collisions with the orbiting electrons. The latter is unimportant for electron energies higher than about 100 eV (6.4.3) and so is neglected in this chapter. The other three types of interaction are discussed separately in the following sections. It is important to realise, however, that any one electron may experience very many different interactions (typically about 1000), before being brought to rest within about 0·25 to 0·5 mm of the tungsten surface.

28.1.1 Inelastic collisions with atomic electrons — Characteristic radiation production

The inelastic collision between the incoming electron and the atomic electrons results in the excitation and ionisation (25.5) of the atoms, as shown illustrated in Figure 28.1. The collisions resulting in excitation or ionisation may take place with an electron in any shell, and the cases of excitation from the outer shell and ionisation from the innermost (K) shell are illustrated in the figure. In both cases, the kinetic energy of the electron has been reduced: by the energy difference of the two orbits in Figure 28.1(a), and by the sum of the binding energy (25.5.1) and kinetic energy of the ejected electron in Figure 28.1(b). The ejected electron is also known as a 'delta ray' ('δ-ray') and will also excite and ionise atoms along its path.

The vacancies in the orbits of such excited or ionised atoms are filled by 'downward' transition of electrons, together with the emission of an X-ray of characteristic radiation (25.5.3) as shown by the K_a transition in Figure

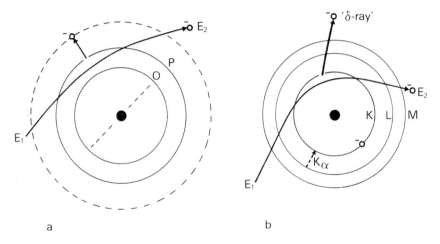

Fig. 28.1 (a) Excitation, and (b) ionisation caused by the passage of an energetic electron close to a tungsten atom. Both processes result in the production of heat, and ionisation produces characteristic radiation (e.g. K_a radiation, as shown). Not all electron orbits are shown, for clarity (E_2 is less than E_1 in both figures).

28.1(b). However, excitation and ionisation both result in the production of heat within the target: *excitation* by the absorption of energy in the target as the electron falls back to its original orbit (see also 27.2), and *ionisation* by the increased kinetic energy received by the tungsten atoms as they slow down the ejected electron by collision.

Inelastic collisions with atomic electrons form the major mechanism by which the energetic electron beam loses its energy when it strikes the tungsten target, producing heat in consequence. It is also the mechanism by which the 'line spectra' of characteristic radiation are produced (28.2).

28.1.2 Elastic collisions with nuclei

The light, negatively charged electron is attracted by the positive charge on the nucleus of a heavy atom such as tungsten. The closer the electron travels to the nucleus, the more it is attracted by it and so the more it is deflected, as shown in Figure 28.2. However, the kinetic energy lost by the electron (i.e. transferred to the nucleus) is very small in these deflections, since the mass of the electron is only 1/334 000 of that of the tungsten nucleus! The number of such events compared to the number of inelastic collisions with electrons (discussed above) increases as the atomic number increases, and so is very frequent in tungsten. The elastic collisions of the electrons with nuclei, then, serve only to produce very tortuous paths of the incoming electrons within the tungsten without absorbing very much energy.

28.1.3 Inelastic collisions with nuclei — Bremsstrahlung production

One of the conclusions of classical physics is that an accelerating or

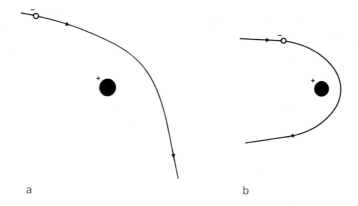

Fig. 28.2 The deflection of an electron by a nucleus — (a) small deflection, and (b) large deflection.

decelerating charged particle *always* produces electromagnetic radiation (e.g. 8.2.3). However, we have seen already that this cannot be the case for an orbiting atomic electron (the Bohr Atom — 25.3). It also is not the case for the elastic collisions of electrons with nuclei, as described above. As shown in Figure 28.2, the electron must accelerate towards the nucleus during its deflection, but despite this acceleration, in only a small percentage of cases is a quantum of electromagnetic radiation emitted. When such a quantum is emitted, the kinetic energy of the electron is reduced by the energy of the electromagnetic quantum, and so is very suddenly slowed down, or 'braked'. This process is described as an *inelastic* interaction, since the total kinetic energy of the electron and the atom is not conserved (because some energy is removed by the emission of the quantum). Note that not every electron passing close to a nucleus produces an X-ray, but only those which are able to undergo a sudden loss of energy by means of an inelastic interaction within it. This is another example of the disparity between classical and modern physics (Ch. 23). The electromagnetic quantum may be in the X-ray region of the electromagnetic spectrum (24.2) and is also known as *Bremsstrahlung* (or 'braking') radiation. It may have any energy up to the total kinetic energy of the electron. In the latter case, the electron is reduced to zero velocity on the emission of the X-ray.

This process is illustrated in Figure 28.3, where the X-ray is emitted at point P and the electron continues with reduced kinetic energy.

Insight

The Bremsstrahlung process may be visualised as an instantaneous change in the energy state of the electron brought about by its interaction with the nucleus — the difference between the energy states producing the quantum of radiation (as in the Bohr model of the atom).

Bremsstrahlung is the reverse process to 'pair-production' (30.6), where electromagnetic radiation produces charged particles in the presence of a nucleus.

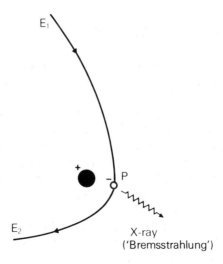

Fig. 28.3 The production of 'Bremsstrahlung' X-rays. An electron at point P suddenly loses energy by the emission of an X-ray. The electron continues with reduced energy.

The probability of Bremsstrahlung radiation being emitted is small (about 1–5%) for diagnostic X-ray units. The remaining 95–99% of the energy of the electron beam is converted into heat. However, the intensity (I) with which Bremsstrahlung radiation is produced increases with atomic number (Z) and energy of electron beam (E), according to the relationship:

$$I \propto ZE^2$$

Equation 28.1

Thus, tungsten is used as a 'target' for the electron beam in an X-ray tube because its high atomic number (74) results in the efficient production of an X-ray beam.

The effect of varying the energy of the electron beam is discussed in section 28.2.2, but it is worth noting here that high-energy beams (4–20 MeV) from linear accelerators used for radiotherapy have much less severe anode cooling requirements than lower-energy therapy machines because of the greater efficiency of X-ray production (because of the E^2 term in equation 28.1)

Lastly, in order to preserve momentum (7.3), the greater the energy of the incident electrons, the more likely is the emitted Bremsstrahlung to be in the same direction as the electrons. Beams of low energies are thus directed almost isotropically (4.2), while high-energy X-ray beams are directed in a 'forward' direction. One result of this is that linear accelerators use 'transmission' targets, i.e. the useful beam is transmitted *through* the anode, in order to take advantage of the higher intensity in this direction. Diagnostic X-ray units utilise X-ray beam produced at 90° to the direction of the electrons (21.2.1).

28.2 THE X-RAY SPECTRUM

The above sections of this chapter have shown that X-rays are produced when (a) inner electron vacancies are filled by the 'dropping down' of electrons from orbits further out (i.e. the 'characteristic radiation') and (b) when the incoming energetic electrons suffer inelastic collisions with the nuclei and are suddenly slowed down (i.e. 'Bremsstrahlung'). In the former case, discrete energies of X-ray quanta are emitted, while the quanta of Bremsstrahlung radiation have a continuous range of energies up to, but not exceeding, the kinetic energy of the electrons striking the target. If the overall X-ray intensity is plotted against the energy of radiation, a summation of these two effects is produced, as shown in Figure 28.4 — this is the X-ray *spectrum*.

[**Note:** All the spectra shown in the ensuing figures of this chapter apply to the emission of X-rays from the anode *without* any subsequent filtration, which is discussed in the next chapter.]

The important features of the spectrum shown in the figure are:

a.   The energy of the Bremsstrahlung radiation expressed in keV lies between zero and a maximum value (the 'end-point') which is numerically equal to the value of kV_p across the X-ray tube. Further, the 'end-point' is the same whatever the *material* of the target. Such a continuous spectrum of radiation is also called 'polychromatic' or 'white'.

b.   The low energy (or 'soft') radiation is decreased in intensity by absorption of such X-ray within the anode itself.

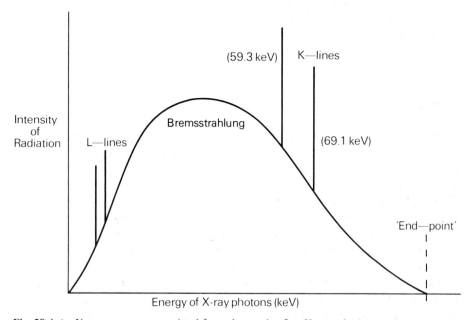

Fig. 28.4 An X-ray spectrum as emitted from the anode of an X-ray tube (see text).

c.   The *average* energy of the X-ray beam is about one-third to one-half of the maximum energy — this is related to X-ray *quality* (29.2).

d.   The line-spectra always occur at the same energies although the *M*, *N*, . . . series are strongly absorbed by the anode and glass of the tube. The discrete energies are also termed 'monochromatic' radiation and '*K*-lines' etc.

e.   The line-spectra will not be produced unless the energy of the electron beam exceeds the binding energy of the appropriate shell of the atom (28.1.1), so that it is possible (for example) to produce the *L*-series of lines without the *K*-series if the electron energy is between 11 keV and 79 keV for a tungsten target.

f.   The total intensity of the X-ray beam is given by the area under the curve.

In Chapter 6 it is shown that the energy of an electron which has been accelerated across a potential difference of *V* volts may be expressed as *V* electron-volts (eV) — see section 6.4.3. The maximum energy of electron which is accelerated across the X-ray tube operating at a given peak kilovoltage (6.4.1) is therefore numerically the same number of kilo-electron-volts (keV). In other words, an X-ray unit operated at (say) 100 kV_p produces electrons of energy 100 keV striking the anode. The maximum energy of an X-ray quantum obtained by the Bremsstrahlung process is thus 100 keV, and it has been shown previously (24.1.2) that the wavelength (λ) corresponding to this maximum energy is given by the simple expression:

$$\lambda = \frac{1 \cdot 24}{kV_p} \text{ nanometers} \qquad \text{Equation 28.2}$$

This corresponds to the *minimum* wavelength of X-ray photon emitted by the X-ray tube.

28.2.1 Effect of rectification

The type of HT rectification (Ch. 20) affects the shape of the X-ray spectrum because of the changing energy of the electron beam striking the anode over each half-cycle. Thus, for full-wave rectification with no smoothing (20.2), the end-point of the spectrum varies from zero to the kV_p value and back to zero for each half-cycle, as shown in Figure 28.5(a), where the instantaneous X-ray spectrum is shown for the kV_p value and for an intermediate value (given by points B and C on the voltage waveform respectively). The time-averaged X-ray spectrum is therefore as shown in Figure 28.5(b), where that due to full-wave rectification has a lower intensity and a lower average energy than a constant-voltage rectification system (20.4). Rectification therefore affects both the intensity and quality of the X-ray beam (29.2). ('Intensity' is defined as the X-ray energy passing through unit area per unit time — see Ch. 4).

28.2.2 Effect of mA and kV$_p$

If the mA is doubled, for example, while all other quantities are kept constant, then there will be twice as many electrons interacting with the target over any given time, so producing twice as many X-rays at each value of wavelength or energy. Hence, the intensity is directly proportional (1.7) to mA:

i.e. $I \propto \text{mA}$	Equation 28.3

If the potential difference across the tube is altered, then the energy (E) of the electrons alters in proportion, since $E = \text{kV}_p$ when the electron energy is

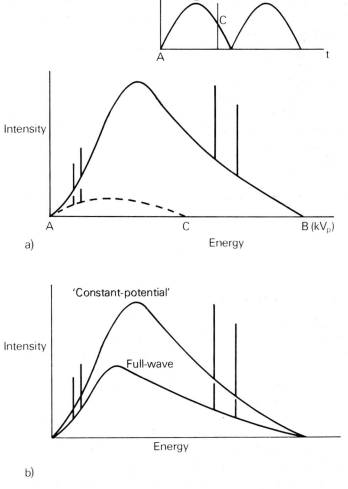

a)

b)

Fig. 28.5 The effect of the type of rectification on the X-ray spectrum. Constant potential circuits give the greatest intensity and quality of the beam.

measured in keV. The efficiency of X-ray production by the Bremsstrahlung process is proportional to E^2 (Equation 28.1), so that:

$$I \propto kV_p^2 \qquad\qquad \text{Equation 28.4}$$

The effect of varying the kV_p on the shape of the X-ray spectrum is shown in Figure 28.6. As shown in the figure, an increasing kV_p produces a higher end-point energy of the spectrum (equal to the new kV_p value,) increases the height of the spectrum at all energies and moves the peak of the spectrum to a higher energy. The average energy of the X-ray beam of higher kV_p is thus greater, resulting in a more penetrating beam of higher quality (Ch. 29). The positions of the characteristic line-spectra are unaltered, of course.

The total intensity of each spectrum is given by the area under each curve (28.2), and it is this area which is proportional to the kV_p^2, as given by equation 28.4.

If all the foregoing factors are combined, we have finally:

$$I \propto Z . mA . kV_p^2 \times F \qquad\qquad \text{Equation 28.5}$$

where F is a factor depending upon the rectification (unity for constant-voltage rectification, and less than unity for other types).

In this equation, I is the intensity of the X-rays at a particular point in the beam. We have seen previously (Ch. 4) that the intensity also depends upon

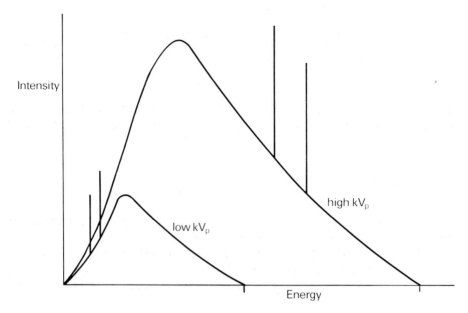

Fig. 28.6 The effect of kV_p on the X-ray spectrum. The overall intensity (given by the area under such curves) is proportional to kV_p^2. Note that the lower of the two curves is not able to produce the K lines.

the distance from the source of radiation in a manner determined by the Inverse Square law. It is shown in the following chapter that the amount of *filtration* is an additional factor which affects the intensity of the X-ray beam.

Exercise 28.1

a. Describe the processes whereby X-rays are produced in the target of an X-ray tube. Draw and describe the X-ray spectrum emitted from the tube.

b. What is meant by 'Bremsstrahlung' radiation? What are the similarities and differences between this radiation and 'characteristic' radiation?

c. Sketch graphs of the spectrum of X-rays emitted by an X-ray tube

  (i) with energy, and
  (ii) with wavelength on the X-axis of the graph.

A beam of electrons is accelerated by a potential difference of 80 kV$_p$ across an X-ray tube. What is

  (i) the maximum energy of X-rays emitted
  (ii) the wavelength corresponding to the maximum energy?

d. Explain how the following factors affect the intensity of X-rays emitted from the anode of an X-ray tube:

  (i) the potential difference across the tube
  (ii) the current flowing through the tube
  (iii) the atomic number of the 'target' material
  (iv) the type of high-tension rectification
  (v) the amount of beam filtration.

e. Why is tungsten used as a 'target' in X-rays tubes?

f. What practical consequences in the taking of radiographs on thick patients follow from the relationship:

'X-ray intensity is proportional to mA $\times$ kV$_p^2$'?

(*Hint:* It is more effective to change the kV$_p$ rather than the mA when radiographing such patients — use this relationship to explain why this should be so.)

SUMMARY

1. Electrons are slowed down in the tungsten target of an X-ray tube by many collisions with the atomic electrons and nuclei.

2. The majority of the energy of the electrons is transformed into heat energy within the target and only 1–5% into X-rays.

3. X-rays are produced by two processes — characteristic radiation and Bremsstrahlung.

4. Characteristic radiation is a result of the inelastic collisions between the incoming energetic electrons and the inner electron shells, producing a vacancy in one of them. This is subsequently filled by the outer electrons

'dropping down' with the emission of electromagnetic radiation, i.e. X-rays. The discrete energies of such characteristic radiation may be called 'line-spectra' or 'monochromatic radiation'.

5.   The Bremsstrahlung process occurs for a small percentage of electrons which suffer an inelastic collision with the nuclei of the target. In this process, the energy of the electron is suddenly decreased and the difference in energy appears as a quantum of radiation, i.e. X-rays. The X-rays produced in this process may have any energy up to the maximum energy of the electron (corresponding to only one collision in the target).

6.   The X-ray spectrum is therefore composed of a continuous curve, caused by Bremsstrahlung, upon which is superimposed the characteristic 'lines' (see Fig. 28.4).

7.   The total intensity of X-radiation varies with atomic number, mA and kV_p i.e. $I \propto Z \cdot mA \cdot kV_p^2$.

8.   Unsmoothed rectification reduces the intensity of the X-ray beam by reducing the energy of the electron beam below the kV_p value. A 'constant voltage' supply produces the highest possible intensity (all other factors being constant).

29. Quality and filtration

29.1 FILTRATION AND THE X-RAY SPECTRUM

The X-rays emitted by the anode of the X-ray tube form a continuous spectrum up to the maximum energy given by the kV_p (28.2). The very low energies ('soft' X-rays) are, however, not suitable for the formation of radiographic images, since they are so rapidly absorbed within the patient's tissues that they contribute nothing to the blackening of the film. However, they do contribute significantly to the radiation dose which the patient receives. It is the function of the *filter* placed in the path of the X-ray beam (see Fig. 2.1) to preferentially absorb the low-energy radiation *before* it reaches the patient. In this way a lower radiation dose is received by the patient and all the X-rays are involved in the production of the radiograph. The procedure of using filters to modify the shape of the X-ray spectrum is called *filtration*.

Spectrum A in Figure 29.1 shows the distribution of X-ray energies emitted

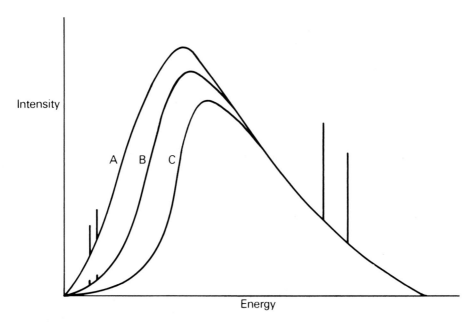

Fig. 29.1 The effect of inherent filtration (B) and total filtration (C) on the X-ray spectrum emitted by the anode of an X-ray tube (A). As shown, progressive amounts of 'soft' radiation are removed from the beam.

from the anode itself, i.e. as measured *inside* the vacuum of the X-ray tube insert (21.1 and 21.2). The passage of such a beam through the glass envelope of the insert, the cooling oil and the exit window of the shield results in the absorption of some of the 'soft' X-rays, so that B is the spectrum of the X-ray beam which emerges from the X-ray unit. There are fewer 'soft' X-rays in spectrum B than spectrum A, since the low energies have been absorbed, while the high-energy radiation is virtually unaffected. This absorption of the X-ray beam by the glass of the insert and the shield is termed *inherent filtration*. However, inherent filtration alone does not remove a sufficient quantity of the 'soft' radiation to reduce the radiation dose to the patient to a minimum. For this reason, a thin sheet of aluminium is placed in the beam to perform *additional filtration*, as shown by curve C in Figure 29.1. The amount of the low-energy radiation has been substantially reduced, which makes the average energy of the beam higher; the filtered beam is said to have become *harder*. Note that the overall intensity of the beam has been reduced by the filter.

The material used for the filtration of diagnostic X-ray tubes is usually aluminium of about 1.5 mm to 2 mm thickness (copper is sometimes used for the higher kV_p's). No significant change in the exposure time required to produce a satisfactory radiograph is experienced when these filters are used, reflecting the almost complete absorption of the soft X-rays which occurs in the body when an unfiltered beam is used.

The inherent filtration may be expressed in terms of the 'equivalent thickness of aluminium' and is usually between about 0.5 mm to 1 mm of aluminium. This means that the effect of the glass, oil and exit window of the X-ray unit on the X-ray beam is the same as if it had passed through that thickness of aluminium instead.

The *total filtration* is the sum of the inherent and additional filtrations and is usually chosen to be between 1.5 and 2.5 mm of aluminium, depending upon the maximum kV_p at which the unit is designed to operate.

Insight

Aluminium has a low atomic number (13) and so is only able to absorb strongly at low energies by photoelectric absorption (30.4). High energies of X-ray quanta have a low probability of being either photoelectrically absorbed or Compton scattered in the thin aluminium and so are relatively unaffected. This makes aluminium an ideal filter for diagnostic X-ray beams.

A certain amount of low-energy characteristic radiation is produced in the aluminium as a result of photoelectric absorption, but this is of very low intensity and may be ignored.

29.2 QUALITY

The term *intensity* has previously been used to describe the quantity of radiation emitted by an X-ray tube (Ch. 28). By itself, the intensity does not indicate the penetrating power of a beam, since it could be composed of a large proportion of either low or high-energy photons. An X-ray beam with a preponderance of high-energy photons is more penetrating, of course. The *quality* of an X-ray beam is a measure of its penetrating power, and is dependent upon several factors as outlined in the following sections.

29.2.1 Quality in radiography

In order to be able to predict the behaviour of an X-ray beam as it passes through an absorbing medium it is necessary to know the exact spectrum of the beam. The absorption of each energy in the medium may be considered in turn and the spectrum of the transmitted beam determined. However, this method represents a sophistication which is not necessary for practical radiography. It is the usual practice to quote the kV_p value as a direct measure of quality. Obviously, the higher the kV_p, the greater the penetrating power, or quality. However, if it is desired to obtain an accurate estimate of quality (or to check the kV_p calibration), a more accurate estimate of the quality of the beam may be made by measuring the Half-Value Thickness (HVT) in aluminium, for example.

A measurement of the HVT plus a statement of the kV_p then defines the quality of an X-ray beam. HVT is always quoted for therapy beams of higher energy. The measurement of HVT is discussed in (5.3.1) as an example of the exponential law. Aluminium is used for the measurement of quality of diagnostic X-ray beams, while copper and lead are used for the more penetrating therapy beams of higher energies.

An alternative, quicker, method of comparing the quality of the output of one X-ray unit to another is to use an aluminium 'step-wedge' consisting of an aluminium block whose thickness increases in a series of steps form one end to the other. The photographic density of a series of equivalent exposures taken through the wedge is measured on each unit and the kV_p of one unit is calibrated against the other.

Insight

If the X-ray beam contains a significant fraction of 'soft' radiation, the HVT value is not constant since the average energy of the beam becomes greater as the soft radiation is absorbed. However, once the soft radiation has been removed, the average energy of the X-ray spectrum is approximately constant and the absorption follows the usual exponential law as shown in Figure 29.2. Strictly speaking, the exponential law of absorption applies to a *homogeneous* beam (i.e. all of the same energy) rather than the *heterogeneous* beam (a distribution of energies) produced by an X-ray unit because of the changes in spectral shape caused by an absorber.

29.3 FACTORS AFFECTING QUALITY

Any quantity which affects the *spectral shape* of the emitted beam of X-radiation will also affect the *quality* of that beam. Such quantities are:

a. kV_p, since a higher kV_p produces a beam of higher average energy;

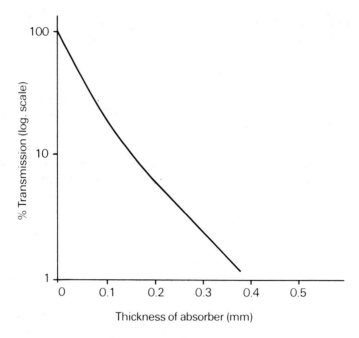

Fig. 29.2 The absorption of a heterogeneous X-ray beam departs from the exponential law —
soft radiation is more rapidly absorbed than hard radiation in the same beam.

b. filtration, since a filter is used to 'harden' the beam;
c. rectification.

The effect of rectification on the X-ray *intensity* was discussed in 28.2.1 —
see Figure 28.5, where it was shown that full-wave rectification produced an
X-ray spectrum containing a larger fraction of low-energy X-rays compared to
a 'constant voltage' rectification system. The quality of the beam produced
from a constant potential unit is therefore of higher average energy and
consequently of higher quality than other rectifier circuits (Ch. 20).

Exercise 29.1
a.   What is meant by 'inherent', 'additional' and 'total' filtration? Show
the effect of filtration on an X-ray beam.
b.   Why is it necessary to *filter* an X-ray beam? By what means does a
filter modify the spectral shape of the beam?
c.   Explain what is meant by:

(i) the intensity
(ii) the quality of an X-ray beam.

d.   Explain how (if at all) the following quantities affect the intensity or
quality of an X-ray beam:

(i) mA
(ii) kV_p

(iii) atomic number of target
(iv) rectification
 (v) filtration
(vi) distance from the anode.

29.4 SUMMARY OF FACTORS AFFECTING QUALITY AND INTENSITY

The factors discussed in this, and the previous, chapter which affect either the intensity or quality of an X-ray beam are summarised in Table 29.1.

Table 29.1 Summary of factors effecting quality or intensity of an X-ray beam

Factor	Intensity	Quality	Comments
mA	$I \propto$ mA	Unaffected	Shape of spectrum unaltered
kV_p	$I \propto kV_p{}^2$	Increases with kV_p	
Z	$I \propto Z$	Unaffected	
Rectification	Maximum for 'constant potential'		Pulsating waveforms on kV alter shape of spectrum over each half-cycle, towards lower energies
Filtration	Decreases with filtration	Increase with filtration	Filtration removes soft radiation by absorption
Distance from focus (d)	$I \propto 1/d^2$	Unaffected	Inverse Square Law for intensity (Ch. 4)

SUMMARY

1.   Filtration of an X-ray beam is necessary to remove the low-energy (soft) radiation, since the latter produces an unnecessary radiation dose to the patient while contributing nothing to the radiograph.
2.   The filtration consists of (a) the 'inherent' filtration of the tube and shield and (b) the 'added' filtration due to a thin sheet of aluminium — the sum of these two is the 'total' filtration and should be equivalent to between 1·5–2·5 mm of aluminium.
3.   'Quality' is a measure of the penetrating power of an X-ray beam. It may be measured by the HVT of the beam in aluminium, but it is usual to state just the kV_p for radiographic units.
4.   Whatever factors affect the shape of the X-ray spectrum will also affect the quality of the beam. These are summarised in Table 29.1, which also shows the factors which affect intensity.

30. X-ray interaction with matter

30.1 THE ATOM AS A TARGET

Consider a parallel beam of X-rays passing through a solid substance. The atoms of that substance are able to interact with the X-rays via the processes described below. Each of the possible types of interactions affects individual X-ray quanta, either by completely removing them from the original, or 'primary', beam ('absorption') or by deflecting (i.e. 'scattering') them from their original direction. Either type of interaction is an example of *attenuation*. The interactions considered involve mainly the orbiting electrons rather than the nuclei of the atoms in the substance. Thus, for an interaction to occur, an X-ray quantum must pass very close to those electron orbits with which it is capable of interacting.

Hence, the atoms within the solid may be viewed as 'targets' which, if hit, will remove an X-ray quantum from the primary beam.

30.1.1 Probability and cross-sections

The probability of an X-ray interacting with any one atom is low, but the very large number of atoms in even a very small volume of a solid substance makes the probability of an interaction *happening at all* very much greater. In Figure 30.1 a beam of X-rays of area A is incident upon a medium whose atoms appear to the beam to have an area a. This area is called the *cross-section* of the atom to a particular radiation, a typical value being 1.5×10^{-28} m².* If a quantum 'hits' one of these tiny atomic targets, then it is removed from the primary beam. (The area a is not the true size of the atom, but is its apparent size from the point of view of the X-ray quanta — it therefore depends upon many factors including atomic number and energy of quantum.)

The probability of any interaction occurring is just the total area of all the atoms within the irradiated volume divided by the total area A, since this is a measure of how much of the available area A is 'occupied' by the atoms. The number of atoms within the irradiated volume is obtained by multiplying the number of atoms per unit volume (N) by the volume, i.e. $N \times Ax$ (see Fig. 30.1). Thus, the total atomic area presented to the X-ray beam is $aNAx$ and the probability of an interaction occurring is obtained by dividing this quantity by A. Thus,

* 10^{-28} m² is an area called a 'barn'.

$$\text{probability of interaction} = aNx \qquad\qquad \text{Equation 30.1}$$

30.1.2 The total linear attenuation coefficient (μ)

The value of aN Equation 30.1 is the total atomic area presented to the X-ray beam for a unit volume of the substance, and is given the symbol μ. It may be shown (see Insight below) that equation 30.1 may be written as:

$$I_x = I_0 e^{-\mu x} \qquad\qquad \text{Equation 30.2}$$

This equation was first introduced in (5.3), where the attenuation of X-rays was given as an example of the exponential law. The reader is referred to that section for a general discussion of the exponential law applied to X-rays where, in particular, μ is defined as the total linear attenuation coefficient, where:

Definition

The *total linear attenuation coefficient*, μ, is the fraction of X-rays removed from the beam per unit thickness of a medium.

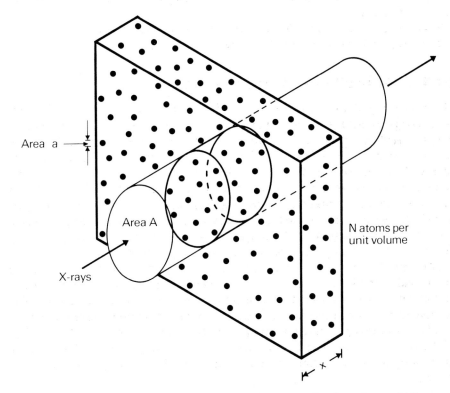

Fig. 30.1 The atom as a target. If any of the X-ray photons passing through area A hits an atom (area a), it is removed from the beam. The beam is said to have been attenuated.

Insight

For a small thickness, dx, of absorber equation 30.1 may be rewritten:

$$-\frac{dI}{I} = aN\,dx$$

since the probability of an interaction is the same as the fraction of X-rays removed from the beam.

i.e. $\dfrac{dI}{dx} = -aNI = -\mu I$ since $\mu = aN$ (see above)

Integrating, we have:

$$I = I_0 e^{-\mu x}$$

which is the expected exponential attenuation formula for X-rays (5.3).

30.1.3 The total mass attenuation coefficient (μ/ρ)

Section 30.1 above has shown that the probability of an interaction between an X-ray quantum and a medium containing N atoms per unit volume is proportional to N (Equation 30.1). However, the *density* (ρ) of a substance is defined as the mass of a unit volume of that substance, and is therefore also proportional to the number of atoms per unit volume. The total mass attenuation coefficient is the value of μ/ρ and may be defined as:

Definition

The *total mass attenuation coefficient*, μ/ρ, is the fraction of the X-rays removed from an X-ray beam of unit cross-sectional area in a medium of unit mass.

It may be useful to compare the units of the two attenuation coefficients μ and μ/ρ. μ has units of m^{-1} (or cm^{-1}) whereas μ/ρ has units of m^2 kg^{-1} (or cm^2 g^{-1}). For example, the value of μ for 100 keV X-rays passing through lead is approximately 567·5m^{-1} so that the value of μ/ρ is obtained by dividing by the density of lead (11 350 kgm^{-3}), i.e. 0·05 m^2 kg^{-1}.

The total *mass* attenuation coefficient is a more fundamental measure of the attenuation of X-rays in matter than the total *linear* attenuation coefficient, since it is independent of the state of the absorber, i.e. it can be a solid, liquid or gas and μ/ρ has the same value. This is because μ is proportional to the density of the absorber, while μ/ρ is independent of the density and so does not depend upon the particular physical state of the absorber.

It is the purpose of the following sections to consider the effects of the different *types* of X-ray interactions on the values of μ (or μ/ρ) for different materials and energies of X-ray beam. This is fundamental to an understanding of the formation of the radiograph (Ch. 31).

30.2 ATTENUATION AND ABSORPTION

The four processes of X-ray interaction with matter described below all involve *attenuation*, since the intensity of the X-ray beam is reduced (or 'attenuated') as a result of each process. Some of these processes result in complete *absorption* of an X-ray quantum, and some in partial or no absorption. Used in this sense, the term 'absorption' implies that energy is transferred to the atoms of the absorber from the X-rays.

As shown in the following sections, coherent scattering (30.3) shows attenuation but no absorption (since the X-rays are deflected with no loss of energy); photoelectric absorption (30.4) shows both attenuation and usually complete absorption; Compton scatter (30.5) produces attenuation and partial absorption, and pair production (30.6) produces attenuation and partial or complete absorption.

In the same way that the total mass attenuation coefficient is applied to the overall *attenuation* of X-rays, each process has its own *mass attenuation coefficient* and *mass absorption coefficient*. The first coefficient describes the probability of a particular event occurring at all (e.g. photoelectric absorption) and, if it has occurred, the mass absorption coefficient determines the fraction of the energy (on average) absorbed per unit mass and may be defined as:

Definition
> The *mass absorption coefficient* is the fraction of energy contained in the X-ray beam which is absorbed per unit mass of the medium through which it passes when unit area is irradiated.

This difference between attenuation and absorption should be borne in mind when such terms are used in the following sections.

30.3 ELASTIC ('COHERENT') SCATTERING

When the energy of a photon of electromagnetic radiation is considerably less than the binding energies (25.5.1) of the electrons orbiting the atoms of the absorber, the photon may be deflected from its path with no loss of energy after interaction with one of the electrons. This process is known by any of the terms 'classical', 'coherent', 'elastic' or 'Rayleigh' scattering.

The sinusoidally changing electric field of incoming electromagnetic radiation (24.1.1) causes the negatively charged orbiting electron to oscillate at the same frequency, provided that it does not gain sufficient energy to become excited or ionised (25.5). However, an oscillating charge radiates electromagnetic radiation (8.2.4) so that the electron both absorbs and emits electromagnetic radiation at the same frequency (thus 'elastic', since no energy is lost) and in-phase (15.4.1) with each other — hence the term 'coherent'. The photon is scattered predominantly in the forward direction, because the recoil experienced by the atom as a whole during the scattering process must not be sufficient to produce excitation or ionisation, or the coherent scattering cannot take place. Thus, there is *no absorption*, since no energy has been lost by the photon, and the attenuation, though present, is small since the majority of the scattered photons are deflected only slightly from their original direction. This is particularly so for materials of low atomic number and for X-ray energies above about 100 eV, since it may be shown that:

$$\frac{\sigma_{coh}}{\rho} \propto \frac{Z^2}{E}$$ Equation 30.3

where σ_{coh}/ρ is the mass attenuation coefficient (30.2) for elastic scattering, Z is the atomic number of the absorber and E is the energy of the photon. Thus, the probability of elastic scattering is much reduced for low values of Z and also as E is increased.

In radiography, the effect of elastic scattering may be ignored since the average value of the atomic number of tissue is low (approximately 7·4) and the small proportion of the incident X-rays which are scattered elastically contribute nothing to the radiation dose received by the patient and have a negligible effect on the radiograph.

Elastic scattering may also occur from the nuclei of atoms as well as from the orbiting electrons ('Thomson scattering'), but this has even less effect than 'Rayleigh' scattering and may safely be ignored.

Insight

For those familiar with X-ray diffraction studies on crystals, it is the Rayleigh scattering which is responsible for the coherent 'reflections' from the various atomic planes within the crystal lattice. Monoenergetic X-rays of low energy are used, only a small percentage of which is able to take part in the scattering process.

30.4 PHOTOELECTRIC ABSORPTION

The previous section has shown that elastic scattering is significant only for low energies of X-ray quanta. However, even at these low energies the process of photoelectric absorption is more important. This process (discussed briefly in 25.5.1) is a result of an *inelastic* interaction between the X-ray and an orbiting electron, since kinetic energy is not conserved (7.3).

In photoelectric absorption, the X-ray interacts with a bound electron by giving to it the whole of its energy. The X-ray quantum thus disappears and the electron is ejected from the atom. This process is only possible, of course, if the quantum has sufficient energy to overcome the binding energy of the electron to the atom (25.5.2). Otherwise, the electron cannot be ejected.

The process of photoelectric absorption is shown schematically in Figure 30.2, where it is assumed that an X-ray quantum of energy $h\nu$ ejects an electron from the innermost (or K) shell of the atom, which has a binding energy of B. The kinetic energy of the ejected electron is thus $(h\nu - B)$. The vacancy left in the K shell is filled very soon afterwards by electrons in higher orbits performing a series of 'quantum jumps' downwards, producing the characteristic fluorescent radiation of that atom (25.5.3), with the possible emission of Auger electrons (26.2.3) from orbits further out.

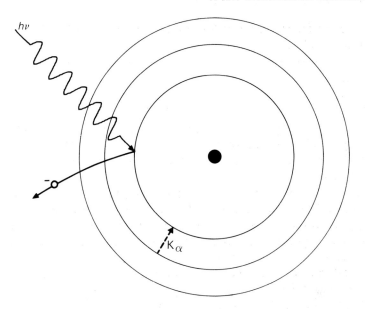

Fig. 30.2 The process of photoelectric absorption and the subsequent emission of a 'characteristic' quantum.

The probability of a photoelectric interaction occurring at a particular electron shell is zero when the energy of the X-ray photon is less than the binding energy, is greatest when the photon energy is equal to the binding energy, and decreases rapidly thereafter with increasing photon energy. A graph of the mass absorption coefficient for photoelectric absorption in lead is shown in Figure 30.3 to illustrate these points. The outer orbits are affected at the lower photon energies, only to have a reducing absorption as the energy increases. One by one, the inner orbits are able to absorb photoelectrically when the quantum energy reaches the binding energy of each orbit, producing a sudden increase in the mass absorption coefficient since more X-rays are absorbed. The K 'edge' of absorption is shown in the figure. Between 'edges', the mass attenuation coefficient is reduced by approximately $1/E^3$ as the energy E increases, i.e. it varies rapidly with the energy of the X-rays.

The mass attenuation coefficient for photoelectric absorption (τ/ρ) varies in a somewhat complicated manner with Z and E. As a very approximate guide, we may use the relationship:

$$\frac{\tau}{\rho} \propto \frac{Z^3}{E^3} \qquad \text{Equation 30.4}$$

This equation applies to X-ray energies up to about 200 keV. At higher energies, the E^3 term approximates to E^2 and eventually to E. The mass attenuation coefficient for this process is thus strongly dependent upon both the atomic number, Z, and the energy of the X-ray photons, E, because each is raised to the power 3.

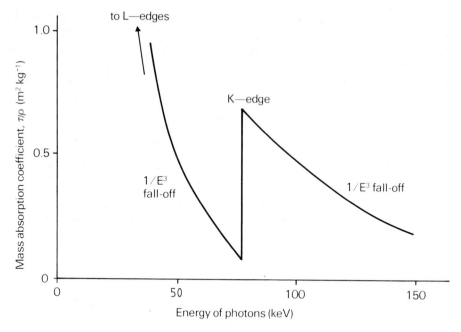

Fig. 30.3 The mass absorption coefficient for the photoelectric effect in lead and its variation with energy.

The X-ray beam is both *attenuated* and *absorbed* since the individual X-ray photons are eliminated from the beam ('attenuation') and energy is imparted to the medium ('absorption'). The absorbed energy is composed of the following parts:

a. energy of the ejected electron
b. energy of recoil of the atom
c. energy of characteristic radiation and Auger electrons.

The ejected electron is quickly brought to rest by the surrounding atoms and delivers its energy to them in the process, as do any Auger electrons. It is possible, however, for the characteristic radiation to escape from the absorber, particularly if the energy of such photons is high and the original absorption occurred near the surface of the absorber. In this case, the mass *absorption* coefficient is somewhat less than the mass *attenuation* coefficient, since not all of the energy of the original X-ray photon has been absorbed by the medium. This effect is of importance only in materials of high atomic number, since the energy of the characteristic radiation is high for such materials. In radiography, therefore, it may be assumed that the characteristic radiation emitted is of a sufficiently low energy to be completely absorbed within the tissues, in which case a photoelectric event results in the whole of the energy of the X-ray photon being absorbed in the body. Thus, the mass attenuation coefficient and the mass absorption coefficient (30.2) are approximately equal for photoelectric absorption in practical radiography.

The dependence of photoelectric absorption on the atomic number of the medium, as shown in the above equation, is the major reason for the clear contrast between bones and other tissues in radiographs, since the calcium and phosphorus in the bones provides a higher average atomic number than in the muscles and fat, which are mainly water. The bones thus absorb considerably more X-rays than the same thickness of tissue and are therefore clearly seen on the radiograph as regions of reduced optical density.

Insight

Why does the photoelectric effect have to take place between an X-ray quantum and a *bound* electron, i.e. why cannot it give a 'free' electron all its energy?

If we assume that it is possible for this to happen, and that T and p are the kinetic energy and momentum of the electron subsequent to the interaction, then

$$\textbf{\textit{hv}} = T \quad \text{(Conservation of Energy)}$$

and $\quad \dfrac{\textbf{\textit{hv}}}{c} = p \quad \text{(Conservation of Momentum)}$

giving $T = cp$ $\hspace{6cm}$ Equation (A)

If m is the mass of the electron moving at velocity v, then

$$T = mc^2(1 - \sqrt{(1 - v^2/c^2)}) \quad \text{(see 23.2.1)}$$

and $\quad p = mv$

Substituting into equation (A), and cancelling as appropriate, we obtain finally:

$$1 - \frac{v}{c} = \sqrt{\left(1 - \frac{v^2}{c^2}\right)} \hspace{4cm} \text{Equation (B)}$$

Equation (B) has two solutions: $v = 0$ and $v = c$. The first solution states that the interaction has not taken place, and the second solution states that the velocity of the electron is the same as that of light after the interaction. This is impossible, since both the mass and energy of the electron then become infinite (by Einstein's Relativity Theory).

Thus, it is not possible for a photon to give all its energy to a free electron since the process is not able to conserve both energy and momentum simultaneously. The process of photoelectric absorption is with the whole atom and the recoil of the atom ensures the conservation of momentum. This is also the case for pair production (30.6).

30.5 COMPTON SCATTER

Photoelectric absorption predominates at low energies since the X-ray quanta interact most efficiently with bound electrons when the energy of the quanta are close to the binding energies of the electrons (see previous section). As the energy of the X-rays increases, the binding energies become progressively less significant, until the X-ray quanta may be considered to be interacting with individual 'free' electrons. This type of interaction is known as *Compton scatter*, and results in partial absorption of the energy of any X-ray which undergoes such scatter. The 'electron density' (number of electrons per unit mass of absorber) is an important factor in determining the probability of a Compton scatter, and hence in determining the attenuation and absorption coefficients (30.5.1).

The process of Compton scattering by a 'free' electron is shown in Figure 30.4.

The incident photon of energy $E_1 (= \boldsymbol{h}\nu_1)$ and momentum $p_1 \left(= \dfrac{\boldsymbol{h}\nu_1}{c} \right)$ 'collides' with the electron, which recoils and takes some of the energy of the photon with it. The energy left is taken by the 'scattered' photon of energy $E_2 (= \boldsymbol{h}\nu_2)$. Since E_2 must be less than E_1, ν_2 is less than ν_1 and so the wavelength of the scattered photon is longer, as shown in Figure 30.4. Such Compton scattering interactions are thus termed 'inelastic', since the energy of the photon is not conserved, although the *total* energy is conserved, of course.

After a Compton scatter process, the scattered photon may travel in any direction whatever, but the electron can only travel in the 'forward' direction. This means that θ (Fig. 30.4) may take any value, while ϕ lies between $+90°$ and $-90°$. The way in which the energy of the original X-ray photon is shared between the electron and the scattered photon depends upon the values of the energy of the original photon (E_1) and the angle through which it is scattered. In particular, it may be shown that, in order to preserve both energy and momentum, the following equation must be obeyed:

$$\lambda_2 - \lambda_1 = \frac{h}{mc}(1 - \cos\theta) \qquad\qquad \text{Equation 30.5}$$

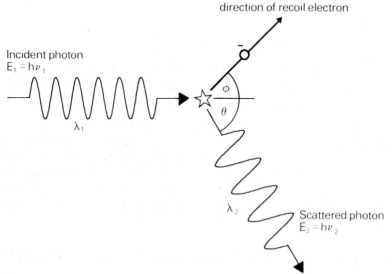

Fig. 30.4 The process of Compton scattering. The scattered photon has a smaller energy than the incident photon and may be scattered at any angle — the electron is always scattered 'forwards'.

where the quantity $\lambda_2 - \lambda_1$ is called the 'Compton wavelength shift'. (As before, h is Planck's constant, m is the mass of the electron and c is the velocity of light.)

This is an important equation, from which several conclusions may be drawn:

a. $\lambda_2 - \lambda_1$ depends upon only h, m, c and θ, and not upon the wavelength of the incident photon, or the type of absorbing material.

b.   For a given angle of photon scatter (θ in Figure 30.4), the value of $\lambda_2 - \lambda_1$ is constant. Now, low-energy photons have long wavelengths, so that the wavelength change corresponds to a small *fractional* change in λ, and hence only a slight reduction in the energy of scattered photons. However, high-energy photons have a small wavelength so that a given wavelength change (specified by the value of θ) implies a considerable relative change in both wavelength and energy.

An alternative way of writing equation 30.5 is to use the energies of the photons rather than their wavelengths, and is:

$$\frac{1}{E_2} - \frac{1}{E_1} = \frac{1}{511}(1 - \cos\theta) \qquad\qquad \text{Equation 30.6}$$

where E_1 and E_2 are in keV.

Example

Consider the case where (i) a 100 keV photon and (ii) a 1 MeV photon are both completely 'backscattered' in Compton events, so that $\theta = 180°$ in each case. Equation 30.6 then simplifies to:

$$\frac{1}{E_2} - \frac{1}{E_1} = \frac{2}{511}, \quad \text{since } \cos 180° = -1$$
$$\therefore \quad E_2 = 511\, E_1/(2E_1 + 511)$$

giving values of 71·9 keV and 203·5 keV for the back-scattered photons respectively. Note that the lower-energy photon has lost much less energy than the high-energy photon in agreement with point (b) above.

Equation 30.5 shows what happens to the photon wavelength when scattered by an angle θ; it does not give any information of the relative probability of actually being scattered by θ. Mathematical treatment based on quantum mechanics, and practical measurement, have shown that low-energy photons (up to about 100 keV) are scattered in all directions with almost equal probability, while high-energy photons (greater than 1 MeV) are scattered predominantly in the forward direction (34.2.1).

30.5.1 Attenuation, absorption and scatter coefficients

The mass attenuation coefficient, σ/ρ, for Compton scattering is given approximately by:

$$\frac{\sigma}{\rho} \propto \frac{\text{Electron density}}{E} \qquad\qquad \text{Equation 30.6}$$

The value of σ/ρ is the probability of a Compton event occurring in unit mass and unit area of the absorber when an X-ray beam of a particular energy is incident upon it. As shown in the above equation, σ/ρ is inversely proportional (1.7.2) to energy and so decreases as E increases.

In order to calculate the 'electron density' of a material we must be able to estimate the number of atoms per unit mass of the substance, and hence the number of electrons per unit mass may be obtained if the number of electrons per atom is known. Now the number of atoms per 'mole' of an element is given by Avogadro's number N_A (7.5) and is $6 \times 10^{23}\,\text{mol}^{-1}$. If each atom has a 'mass number' (25.2) of A, then the number of atoms per unit mass is just N_A/A. The number of electrons per atom is the same as the number of protons per atom, and this is determined by the atomic number Z (25.2). Thus, the number of electrons per unit mass (i.e. the 'electron density') is given by the simple expression $N_A \times Z/A$. As we have seen previously (26.1) the value of Z/A is approximately 0·5 for all elements, as this situation corresponds to equal numbers of protons and neutrons in the nucleus. However, the exception to this is hydrogen, which contains no neutrons so that Z/A is 1·0 in this case. Hydrogen thus contains 6×10^{23} electrons per gram (or 6×10^{26} electrons per kg), while all other elements and compounds contain about half of this value in the range 2·5 to 3·5 $\times 10^{23}$ electrons per gram. The higher values in this range are due to the presence of hydrogen in the compound (e.g. water has about

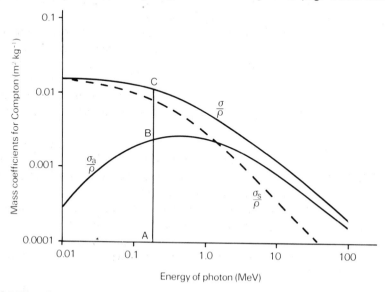

Fig. 30.5 The mass attenuation, absorption, and scattering coefficients for Compton scattering. As the energy increases, the absorbed energy (σ_a/ρ) becomes an increasing proportion of the total energy of the interaction (σ/ρ).

3.3×10^{23} electrons per gram), and the lower values are for the heavier elements (e.g. lead has about 2.4×10^{23}) which have more neutrons in their nuclei than protons so that the value of $(N_A Z)/A$ decreases.

The mass attenuation coefficient in equation 30.6 is therefore very similar for all materials except for hydrogen, where it is twice as large. The same equation shows that the probability of a Compton scatter decreases with increasing energy of X-ray photon.

The mass *absorption* coefficient for Compton scattering, σ_a/ρ, represents the average energy transferred to the electrons (and hence to the medium itself) as a fraction of the total energy of the beam. As shown in the previous section, the higher the energy of the photon the greater is the average energy loss by that photon as a result of Compton scatter. This means that the electron takes more and more energy in the recoil process as the energy increases. Figure 30.5 shows a graph of both the mass attenuation and the mass absorption coefficients against photon energy for the Compton scattering process. It is usual on such graphs to use a logarithmic scale (1.8.1) for both axes in order to accommodate the large variations in the values encountered.

The mass attenuation coefficient is seen to decrease with photon energy, as expected from Equation 30.6. As shown, the mass absorption coefficient increases with energy and then decreases again after about 1 MeV. However, the *fraction* of absorbed energy increases with energy although the absolute amount of that energy decreases after 1 MeV. Thus, the value of AB/AC increases in the figure, so that the two curves approach each other at high energies, even though the value of AB reaches a peak. For example, AB/AC is about 0.10 at 100 keV and 0.9 at 100 MeV, reflecting the greater fraction of absorption by the medium as the energy increases.

Also shown dotted in the figure is the mass *scattering* coefficient (σ_s/ρ) which represents the average fraction of the total beam energy left to the photons after a Compton scatter. The point at which the scattered photon and recoil electron show equal amounts of energy is where the curves cross, i.e. at 1.5 MeV. Below this energy, the scattered photon carries away more energy (on average) and above this energy the electron carries away more energy after the interaction.

The mass attenuation coefficient is a measure of the *total* removal of energy from the primary beam, whereas the corresponding absorption and scattering coefficients are a measure of the proportions of energy removed from the beam by the electron and scattered photon respectively.

Since the sum of the energies of the recoil electron and the scattered photon must be equal to the energy of the original photon, we have:

$$\sigma = \sigma_a + \sigma_s$$

and $$\frac{\sigma}{\rho} = \frac{\sigma_a}{\rho} + \frac{\sigma_s}{\rho}$$

Equation 30.7

30.6 PAIR PRODUCTION

Pair production is the formation of a pair of electrons (one positive and one negative) from an energetic photon. This process occurs in the proximity of the nucleus of an atom, and only for photons of energy greater than 1·02 MeV. Pair production is illustrated in Figure 30.6(a), where the photon is shown reaching

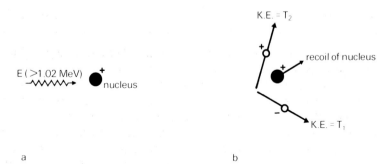

Fig. 30.6 Pair production. A photon of energy greater than 1·02 MeV is able to produce a positron and an electron in the presence of a nucleus.

a point close to the nucleus of an atom. Here it may interact with the electric field of the nucleus and completely disappear by giving all its energy (apart from a small recoil energy of the atom) to the formation of a positron (Table 25.1) and an electron. The recoil of the atom serves to conserve the momentum of the interaction (Figure 30.6(b)). This process is an elegant example of 'mass–energy equivalence' (23.2.1), since mass has been created from energy. Using the principle of the Conservation of Energy (23.2), we have:

$$E = \underbrace{(m_0c^2 + T_1)}_{\substack{\text{total energy of} \\ \text{electron}}} + \underbrace{(m_0c^2 + T_2)}_{\substack{\text{total energy of} \\ \text{positron}}}$$

Here, the total energies of both the positron and the electron are the sum of their 'rest–mass' energies given by Einstein's '$E = mc^2$' plus their kinetic energies T_2 and T_1. The sum of these is equal to the energy of the original X-ray, E.

Simplifying, we have:

$$E = 2m_0c^2 + T_1 + T_2$$

If we express the energies in MeV, $2m_0c^2$ has the value of 1·02 MeV, so that, in order for pair production to take place,

$E(\text{MeV}) = 1·02 + T_1 + T_2$	Equation 30.8

Hence, the energy of the photon must be at least 1·02 MeV in order to create the two particles, and any energy above this value produces kinetic energy of the two particles.

30.6.1 Attenuation, absorption and scatter coefficients

The linear attenuation coefficient is usually given the symbol π, so that the mass attenuation coefficient is π/ρ, and depends upon both atomic number and photon energy as follows:

$$\frac{\pi}{\rho} \propto (E - 1{\cdot}02) \,.\, Z \qquad\qquad \text{Equation 30.9}$$

Thus, pair production increases with atomic number and energy. (Note that all the other processes *decrease* with increasing energy.)

The kinetic energies given to the positron–electron pair are absorbed by the medium as the particles slow down in it. Thus, the energy absorbed by the medium is *less* than the energy of the original photon, and is given by $(E - 1{\cdot}02)$ MeV, from equation 30.8. However, the positron eventually meets an electron and both are annihilated with the emission of two photons of $0{\cdot}51$ MeV (26.3.2). Matter is thus transformed into energy — the reverse of pair production. If these two photons are completely absorbed in the medium, then the total energy absorbed is $(E - 1{\cdot}02) + 2 \times 0{\cdot}51 = E$, i.e. the whole of the energy of the original photon causing the pair production. There is no certainty that this will happen, however, in which case the absorption coefficient (π_a) is less than the attenuation coefficient (π), by a fraction $(E - 1{\cdot}02)/E$, i.e. $1 - (1{\cdot}02/E)$. Thus,

$$\pi_a = \pi\left(1 - \frac{1{\cdot}02}{E}\right)$$

By analogy to the 'absorption' and 'scatter' coefficients in Compton scattering, (Equation 30.7) we may write:

$$\pi = \pi_a + \pi_s$$
$$\frac{\pi}{\rho} = \frac{\pi_a}{\rho} + \frac{\pi_s}{\rho} \qquad\qquad \text{Equation 30.10}$$

Here, π_s is the fraction of the energy carried away by the two 'annihilation' photons of $0{\cdot}511$ MeV, so that $\pi_s = 1{\cdot}02/E$.

However, in all but the most accurate work, it is usual to ignore the scattering coefficient, π_s, since it is a very small contribution to the total scatter at energies just above $1{\cdot}02$ MeV (where the Compton process predominates), and is a reducing fraction of the total pair production coefficient, π, as the energy increases. The exact equation 30.10 may therefore be replaced by the *approximate* relationships:

$$\pi_a = \pi$$
$$\pi_s = 0 \qquad\qquad \text{Equation 30.11}$$

30.7 RELATIVE IMPORTANCE OF ATTENUATION PROCESSES

At any particular photon energy, some or all of the above processes of attenuation will be competing in the removal of photons from the X-ray beam. As mentioned earlier (30.2) the *total* linear coefficient, μ, is composed of the contributions from all processes. For example, for photoelectric absorption alone we may write $I_1 = I_0 e^{-\tau x}$, where τ is the linear attenuation coefficient for the photoelectric effect (30.4). Similarly, for Compton scattering and pair production alone,

$$I_2 = I_0 e^{-\sigma x} \quad \text{and} \quad I_3 = I_0 e^{-\pi x}$$

The fractions of transmitted intensities in each case are $\dfrac{I_1}{I_0}$, $\dfrac{I_2}{I_0}$, $\dfrac{I_3}{I_0}$ respectively.

If now all three processes are present, then the overall fraction transmitted is

$$\frac{I_1}{I_0} \cdot \frac{I_2}{I_0} \cdot \frac{I_3}{I_0}$$

i.e. $e^{-\tau x} \cdot e^{-\sigma x} \cdot e^{-\pi x} = e^{-(\tau + \sigma + \pi)x}$ (see 1.5.1)

This quantity is also equal to $e^{-\mu x}$, from the definition of μ. Therefore,

---

$$\mu = \tau + \sigma + \pi$$

and $\quad \dfrac{\mu}{\rho} = \dfrac{\tau}{\rho} + \dfrac{\sigma}{\rho} + \dfrac{\pi}{\rho}$

Equation 30.12

By applying the same argument to *absorption*, we arrive at very similar equations:

$$\mu_a = \tau + \sigma_a + \pi$$

and $\quad \dfrac{\mu_a}{\rho} = \dfrac{\tau}{\rho} + \dfrac{\sigma_a}{\rho} + \dfrac{\pi}{\rho}$

Equation 30.13

Also, for scatter:

$$\mu_s = \sigma_s$$

and $\quad \dfrac{\mu_s}{\rho} = \dfrac{\sigma_s}{\rho}$

Equation 30.14

---

where the contribution from pair production to scatter is ignored (30.6.1). Note that photoelectric absorption contributes to energy absorption (Equation 30.13), but not to scatter (Equation 30.14).

Some of these points are illustrated in Figures 30.7 and 30.8, where the mass attenuation coefficients for the photoelectric effect (τ/ρ), the Compton effect (σ/ρ) and pair production (π/ρ) are shown for air and lead. The total mass

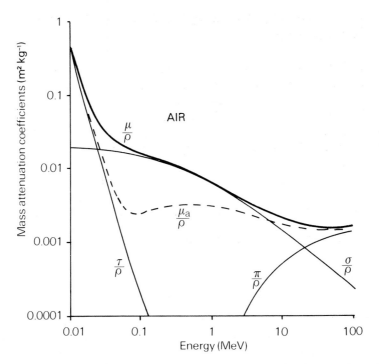

Fig. 30.7 Mass attenuation coefficients for air. Also shown (dotted line) is mass absorption coefficient.

attenuation coefficients (thick lines) and the total mass absorption coefficients (dotted lines) are also shown in the figures.

The following important points emerge from these, and similar graphs:

a.   photoelectric absorption dominates at low energies (up to 50–500 keV depending upon the Z of the absorber).

b.   The absorption 'edges' are more pronounced as the atomic number increases.

c.   The Compton effect dominates over a wide range of energies in all materials (about 500 keV to 5 MeV).

d.   The Compton region is almost identical in all absorbing materials (except those containing hydrogen) because of the similarity of the electron densities (30.5). The shape of the curve is independent of the nature of the absorbing material.

e.   Pair production is only significant for very high energies and materials of high Z. For these materials, increasing the energy of the photons results in a *less* penetrating beam, which is the opposite way round to practical radiography (where no pair production takes place, of course).

In conclusion, the attenuation of the X-ray beam as it passes through the patient's tissues depends in a somewhat complicated manner on the density, thickness and atomic number of the tissues through which the beam passes,

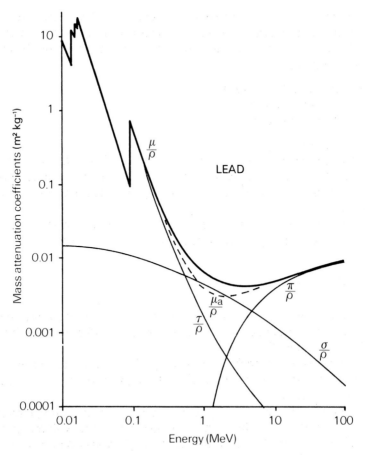

Fig. 30.8 Mass attenuation coefficients for lead. Dotted line is total mass absorption coefficient.

together with the energy of the X-ray quanta. It is possible only to alter the latter, of course, and this forms an important aspect of practical radiography, as discussed in the next chapter. The choice of absorbing materials for use in radiation protection is influenced by graphs of the type shown in Figures 30.7 and 30.8, as explained in Chapter 33.

Exercise 30.1
   a.   Explain what is meant by the 'exponential attenuation of X-rays through matter'. Hence define half-value thickness (HVT) (see Ch. 5).
   b.   What is meant by the following terms:

   (i)   the total *linear* attenuation coefficient (μ)
   (ii)   the total *mass* attenuation coefficient (μ/ρ)
as applied to a beam of X-rays?

   c.   What is the difference between the 'attenuation' and 'absorption' of X-rays?

d.   What are the four processes by which X-rays interact with matter? Which of these processes is relevant to practical radiography and why?

e.   Explain how the following processes depend upon atomic number and energy of X-ray quanta:

(i)   photoelectric absorption
(ii)   Compton scatter
(iii) Pair production

Draw graphs as appropriate.

f.   Sketch the general appearance of a graph of the total *attenuation* coefficient of lead with energy of X-ray quanta. Use this graph to illustrate the ranges of energies over which each of the attenuation processes is most important.

g.   On the above graph, superimpose the total mass *absorption* coefficient of lead, and explain any differences between the two curves.

SUMMARY

1.   All electromagnetic radiation (of which X-rays are a part) is attenuated in matter according to the exponential law: $I = I_0 e^{-\mu x}$, where μ is the 'total linear attenuation coefficient'.

2.   The atoms of the absorber act as 'targets' which, if hit, remove a photon from the beam, either by the absorption of energy, or deflection ('scatter'), or a combination of both.

3. μ varies with energy of X-ray beam and with the absorbing material, such that $\mu = Na$, where N is the number of atoms per unit volume and a is the 'target area' which each atom presents to the photons (known as the 'atomic cross-section').

4.   The density (ρ) of a material is also proportional to N, so that a more fundamental measure of the attenuation of an X-ray beam is μ/ρ, which is the 'total *mass* attenuation coefficient'. μ/ρ is the same value for a particular substance, whether it be in the form of a solid, liquid or gas.

5.   The four main processes of X-ray interaction with matter are: elastic (coherent) scattering, photoelectric absorption, Compton scatter and pair production. Each of these processes has its own linear (and mass) attenuation coefficients which sum to form the total coefficient,

i.e. $\mu = \tau + \sigma + \pi$

(The effect of elastic scattering is usually very small, and is ignored in this equation.)

6.   The *absorption* coefficients for each process (τ_a, σ_a, π_a) are the fractions of the energy which is given up as kinetic energy to the electrons and therefore absorbed in the medium. The *scattering* coefficients (σ_s, π_s) of each process are the fractions of the energy which are taken away by the scattered photon.

7.   Since the absorbed energy plus the scattered energy must be equal to the energy of the original photon removed from the beam, we have:

$\tau = \tau_a$ (no scatter for photoelectric absorption)

$\sigma = \sigma_a + \sigma_s$

$\pi = \pi_a$ (π_s makes only a small contribution to μ)

8. The factors which affect the amounts of the various processes of interaction are shown in the following table.

Summary of X-ray Interaction Processes

Process	Description of Interaction	Effect of Z, E	Comments
Elastic	Photon interacts with bound atomic electron, and is re-radiated with no energy loss	$\dfrac{\mu_e}{\rho} \propto \dfrac{Z^2}{E}$	No absorption in medium. Photon scattered in 'forward' direction. Negligible in biological tissues (low Z)
Photoelectric	Photon ejects electron from shell, leaving vacancy. K. E. of electron = E − binding energy Atom recoils, conserving momentum	$\dfrac{\tau}{\rho} \propto \dfrac{Z^3}{E^3}$	Ejected electron is slowed down by surrounding atoms, giving its energy to them i.e. absorption takes place. Electron vacancy filled, and characteristic radiation emitted.
Compton	Photon behaves like a particle, and collides with electrons (considered 'free'). Energy is shared between electron and scattered photon.	$\dfrac{\sigma}{\rho} \propto \dfrac{\text{electron density}}{E}$	Electron energy absorbed in medium, so Compton process produces attenuation and partial absorption. Electron densities of all materials very similar (except hydrogen) so that σ/ρ values are largely independent of type of absorber.
Pair Production	Photons of energy greater than 1·02 MeV may spontaneously disappear and produce a positron and an electron in the vicinity of a nucleus. Atom recoils, and preserves momentum. Positron eventually annihilated with an electron, to form two 0·511 MeV photons.	$\dfrac{\pi}{\rho} \propto (E - 1\cdot02)Z$	Probability of Pair Production *increases* with E, above 1·02 MeV. Contribution of π_s is always small compared to μ and is often ignored.

31. The radiograph

The geometrical factors which contribute to the quality of the radiograph include focal spot size, focus-to-film distance (FFD) and the position of the patient's internal structures relative to the film. Such factors determine film magnification and geometric unsharpness (penumbra), and the reader is referred to Chapter 3 for a fuller discussion of the interrelationships between these quantities.

The photographic quality of the radiograph depends upon more than geometrical considerations, however, and it is the purpose of this chapter to outline the way in which *physical* quantities affect the radiograph. What this means, in practice, is that we must investigate the behaviour of the X-ray beam as it passes through the body, and how the transmitted part of the X-ray beam is used to form the radiographic image. An understanding of photoelectric absorption (30.4), the Compton effect (30.5) and the 'total linear attenuation coefficient, μ' (30.1.2) is therefore crucial to this chapter.

It is convenient to consider the formation of the radiograph in two stages: firstly, the production of an 'X-ray image' composed of the intensity pattern of X-rays transmitted through the body and, secondly, the consequent production of a 'film density image' whether by direct action of the X-rays on the photographic emulsion, or by the use of fluorescent screens (27.5). These processes are considered separately in the following sections.

31.1 THE 'X-RAY IMAGE'

31.1.1 Attenuation through the body

It is assumed, for simplicity, that an X-ray beam of uniform intensity is incident upon a patient of constant thickness so that the intensity pattern of the transmitted beam depends only upon the attenuation caused by the intervening structures within the body. It is therefore the *differences* in the attenuations caused by bone, muscle and fat which are responsible for the visualisation of anatomical structure on the radiograph. (Obviously, if the attenuation was the same in all tissues, then the transmitted intensity would be uniform and a radiograph would result having constant photographic density and therefore be of no diagnostic value whatever.)

A simple example of the effect of such 'differential' attenuation is shown in Figure 31.1, where two separate blocks of bone and soft tissue are shown

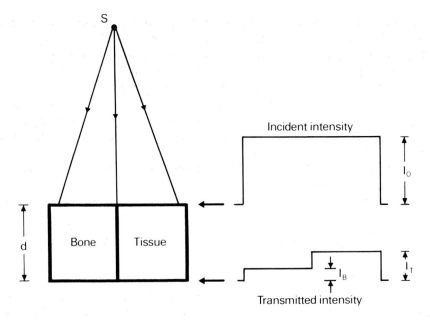

Fig. 31.1 The increased attenuation of X-rays in bone compared to tissue.

irradiated. The profiles of incident and transmitted intensities are also shown, and it is clear that the exponential attenuation of X-rays by matter (5.3) produces the following simple relationships:

$$I_B = I_0 e^{-\mu_B d}$$
$$I_T = I_0 e^{-\mu_T d}$$

Equations 31.1

where I_0 is the X-ray intensity which would have occurred in the absence of the samples, μ_B and μ_T are the total linear attenuation coefficients of bone and soft tissue respectively, and all other quantities are as defined in the figure. It is seen that the X-ray intensity transmitted through the bone is less than that transmitted through the tissue, and this is simply because μ_B is greater than μ_T. There are two physical reasons for this:

a. The average atomic number of bone ($Z_B = 14$) is greater than that of soft tissue ($Z_T = 7·5$).

b. The density of bone is greater than that of tissue ($\rho_B = 1·8 : \rho_T = 1·0$).

Exercise 31.1

How do the above two statements explain the increased attenuation of bone compared to soft tissue?

It was shown in the last chapter (30.1.1) that all linear attenuation and absorption coefficients are proportional to the number of atoms present in a given volume, and hence proportional to the density of the medium. Thus μ_B

is proportional to ρ_B, and μ_T is proportional to ρ_T, so that, all other things being equal, bone will show a greater attenuation than soft tissue owing to the difference in densities. However, the difference in *atomic numbers* produces a much more profound effect on X-ray attenuation owing to its effect on *photoelectric absorption*, particularly at the lower energies.

There are only two processes of attenuation of any significance in radiography: photoelectric absorption and Compton scatter. Coherent scattering (30.3) may be ignored, and pair production (30.6) does not take place below $1\cdot02$ MeV.

To summarise the results of the last chapter for our present purposes, we have (see summary of Ch. 30):

$$\tau \propto \rho \, \frac{Z^3}{E^3}$$

$$\sigma \propto \rho \cdot \frac{\text{electron density}}{E} \qquad \qquad \text{Equations 31.2}$$

where τ, σ are the attenuation coefficients for the photoelectric effect and Compton scatter, respectively. The strong dependence of τ on Z (i.e. Z^3) shown in the first of these equations is thus the major reason for the greater attenuation of the X-rays when passing through bone.

We may summarise these very important findings by reference to Table 31.1.

Table 31.1 Comparison of X-ray attenuations of bone and soft tissue

	Photoelectric $\left(\tau \propto \rho \dfrac{Z^3}{E^3}\right)$	Compton scatter $\left(\sigma \propto \rho \dfrac{\text{electron density}}{E}\right)$	Total attenuation $(\mu = \tau + \sigma)$
Bone ($Z=14$; $\rho=1\cdot8$)	Large at low energies — about 12 times greater than tissue	Predominates at high energies (500 keV to 5 MeV)	Mainly photoelectric at 'diagnostic' energies
Soft tissue ($Z=7\cdot5$; $\rho=1\cdot0$)	Significant at low energies only (50 kV$_p$ and below)	Main attenuation process	Compton scatter predominates for kV$_p$s greater than about 60

Average atomic numbers are shown
Density is in g ml^{-1} (multiply by 1000 to obtain kg m^{-3})

The essential point is that the relatively high atomic number of bone results in photoelectric absorption being the main process of attenuation in bone, whereas the lower atomic number of soft tissue results in Compton interactions being the main process of attenuation in tissue.

A further example of attenuation is given in Figure 31.2, which simulates the presence of a bone within surrounding soft tissue. The profile of transmitted intensity is also shown, and is at a minimum corresponding to the maximum thickness of the bone (point A in the figure).

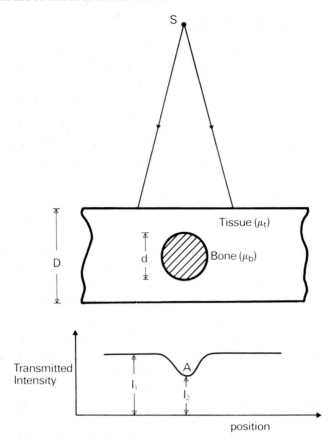

Fig. 31.2 A profile of transmitted X-ray intensity obtained from a bone embedded in soft tissue.

The fraction of X-rays transmitted through a thickness, d, of bone is just $e^{-\mu_B d}$, and the fraction transmitted through a thickness, $D-d$, of soft tissue is $e^{-\mu_T(D-d)}$. The overall transmitted fraction obtained by *multiplying* these two factors, so that:

$$\frac{I_2}{I_0} = e^{-\mu_B d} \cdot e^{-\mu_T(D-d)}$$

$$\text{so that } I_2 = I_0 e^{-\mu_T D - (\mu_B - \mu_T)d}$$

$$\text{and } I_1 = I_0 e^{-\mu_T D}$$

Equations 31.3

Note that if $\mu_B = \mu_T$ (i.e. the bone is replaced by soft tissue) then the first of these equations simplifies to $I_2 = I_0 e^{-\mu_T D}$, which is the same as I_1. In this case, there would be no difference in the attenuations, as expected. The difference between the transmitted intensities I_1 and I_2 is thus determined by the *difference* between the attenuation coefficients (i.e. $\mu_B - \mu_T$).

31.1.2 Scatter and 'grids'

The previous section was somewhat idealised in the sense that the radiation emerging through the patient was assumed to be composed of the transmitted primary beam only. This is true for photoelectric absorption, where an X-ray is completely removed from the beam by total absorption (30.4). However, it is definitely not the case for Compton scatter, where only partial absorption occurs (30.5). The scattered X-ray may well escape from the patient and reach the photographic film. Unfortunately, the contribution of such scattered X-rays to the radiograph is by no means negligible and, unless reduced, leads to a serious loss in image quality.

The amount of scattered radiation escaping from the patient depends upon:

a. the volume of the patient irradiated (the smallest practicable field size is used in order to reduce this effect)

b. the average energy of the X-ray beam. The greater the energy of the X-ray beam, the fewer the fraction of scattered photons but the greater is their penetration in tissue. This point is discussed further in the next section, where the effect on the radiograph of altering the kV_p is considered.

Approximately 80–90% of scattered X-rays are removed by the use of a *grid*, which is composed of alternating strips of a strong and a weak absorber, as shown in Figure 31.3. The principle of the grid is that the scattered X-rays deflected away from the original direction of the primary beam may be preferentially absorbed in the grid by making them pass through a relatively long path length in lead (or other suitable absorber). For example, rays 1 and 2 are primary rays, both of which should ideally be used to help form the final image. However, ray 1 is absorbed, and so is a fraction $d/(D + d)$ of the primary beam, since this is the fraction of the image area covered by lead. The scattered X-rays are much more strongly absorbed, however, because the angled rays 'see' a greater surface area of lead, e.g. ray 3. A slightly scattered ray, such as 4, passes through the grid, but such rays do not contribute so much to image degradation as the X-rays scattered through larger angles. The latter are strongly absorbed by the grid, however, and do not therefore reach the film.

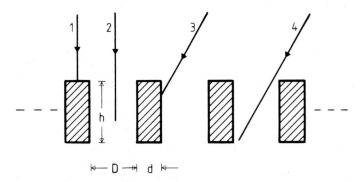

Fig. 31.3 The principle of action of a grid — scattered X-rays are absorbed more than the primary beam.

Various factors of grid design may be chosen to optimise its performance for a particular application (e.g. for skull radiographs). Such factors include:

a.   the separation (D) and width (d) of absorbers
b.   the *grid ratio, r*, where $r = h/D$.

The smaller D and the greater r, the more scattered X-rays are removed from the primary beam. Unfortunately, the primary beam is also absorbed to a greater extent, so that some optimum values of these, and other, factors are determined by the manufacturers for a given X-ray application. The use of focused, pseudo-focused, crossed and moving grids is not considered in this book. However, the physical principle of all such grids is the same, namely to absorb more scattered radiation than primary beam, and hence to improve the appearance of radiographs.

The radiographic exposure required to produce a given photographic density (31.2.1) is greater when using a grid than without the grid, owing to the absorption of both primary and scattered beam within the grid. The 'grid factor' expresses this increased exposure as a ratio, and is defined as:

Definition
   The *grid factor* is the ratio: *exposure with grid/exposure without grid* when each exposure produces the same photographic density.

The grid factor is typically in the range from 2 to 6, and is determined from two exposures usually taken at the same value of kV_p. Under these circumstances, the grid factor as defined above simplifies to the ratio of the *mAs values* with and without the grid. For example, if 20 mAs produces a photographic density of 0·5 at a potential difference of 75 kV_p when no grid is used, and 70 mAs is required to produce the same photographic density using the same kV_p, then the grid factor is just $70/20 = 3·5$. Increasing the kV_p alters both the intensity and quality of the X-ray beam (28.2.2 and 29.2) and adds an extra complication in calculating the mAs value to select when using a grid subsequent to a change in the kV_p. These points are discussed in more detail in section 4.7.

31.1.3 Effect of kV_p

The X-ray specturm varies with the kV_p as described in section 28.2.2 and illustrated by Figure 28.6, where it is shown that the average energy of the X-ray spectrum is one-third to one-half of the kV_p value. The average energy of a beam generated at, say, 90 kV_p is therefore about 40 keV. The attenuation, absorption and scatter coefficients of the various interaction processes between X-rays and matter (Ch. 30) are therefore those which apply for 40 keV radiation. (It is assumed that the spectrum of radiation is unaltered as it passes through the body, which is ony approximately true.) The effect of increasing the kV_p is therefore to increase the average energy of the radiation in proportion, and this *reduces* the values of the total linear attenuation coefficients in bone and tissue, reflecting the increased penetration of the higher average energy X-rays.

From equations 31.2, it is clear that increasing the average energy, E, of the X-ray beam will reduce the photoelectric process (τ) to a much greater extent than the Compton process (σ). For example, doubling the value of E reduces τ by a factor of 2^3 (i.e. 8), while σ is merely reduced by a factor of 2. The total linear attenuation coefficient, μ, is given by $\tau + \sigma$ and is also reduced in value. Thus, the X-ray beam is *more penetrating* as the kV_p increases, both in bone and soft tissue. However, μ_B is reduced to a much greater extent than μ_T, because of the very strong variation of the photoelectric effect with energy. Hence, $\mu_B - \mu_T$ is reduced, so that the 'X-ray image' will show less variation of transmitted intensity between bone and soft tissue as the kV_p is increased (see end of 31.1.1) The 'contrast' is said to have been reduced, as explained in the next section.

As far as the effect of the kV_p on the scattered X-rays reaching the film is concerned, the important quantity to be considered is the intensity of scattered radiation compared to the intensity of the primary beam at the film. If we denote these two quantities by I_s and I_p respectively, then it is desirable to have as small a value of I_s/I_p as possible, since in this case a relatively small amount of scatter contributes to the radiograph. Now an increased kV_p also increases the average energy of the beam, and we have already seen that this reduces the amount of Compton scatter (since σ decreases). However, those X-rays that are scattered are more penetrating, since they have a higher energy. This means that the reduction in the number of Compton events *reduces I_s/I_p*, as we would wish, but the increasing penetration of the scattered X-rays *increases I_s/I_p*. The overall situation is consequently rather complicated, but in the 'diagnostic range of kV_p's, it is the increased penetration of the scattered X-rays which predominates, so that *an increasing kV_p increases the proportion of scatter reaching the film*. This is true whether or not grids are used.

Increasing the kV_p therefore degrades the 'X-ray image' in two ways: by reducing the variations in the intensity pattern of the transmitted primary beam, and increasing the proportion of scattered radiation contributing to the image. However, the practical advantages of using a relatively high kV_p are that there is a greater intensity of transmitted beam so that a shorter exposure may be made, and that the patient receives a lower radiation dose owing to the reduction of the 'soft' X-rays. This is discussed further in section 31.3.

Insight

To simplify, the 'best' radiograph is obtained when the most absorbing structure is just perceived on the film. Obviously, the whole point of the radiograph is to see detailed structure within the body, not just to be able to see the gross difference between bone and soft tissue, for example. A sufficiently high kV_p is therefore chosen to allow adequate penetration of the structures being investigated in order that 'fine detail' may be seen. Too low a kVp setting will only lead to the conclusion that the patient has bones, which was known already! On the other hand, a low kV_p is used for 'soft-tissue' investigations, since the small differences in density and atomic number between (say) fat and muscle show up better at low energies, owing to the significant photoelectric effect at these energies (see Equations 31.2)

31.1.4 'Subject' and 'perceived' contrast

The greater the difference in the intensity of the 'X-ray image' between two points, the greater the 'subject contrast' is said to be. The subject contrast partly determines the difference in the visual appearance of the two points when the final image is formed (on film or fluorescent screen). The differences in the *perceived* intensity pattern (i.e. as seen by the eye) of the image is called 'perceived contrast', or just *contrast*. Visual contrast and subject contrast are not the same, however, owing to the behaviour of the human eye to variations in intensity, as described below.

The difference between the X-ray intensities shown in Figure 31.1. (for example) is simply $I_T - I_B$, and the difference in the intensities of light emitted from a fluorescent screen placed in the path of the transmitted beam is proportional to this value. This is because the light emitted from such a screen is proportional to the quantity of energy absorbed in it as determined by the scintillation efficiency of the screen (27.2). However, the response of the human eye to brightness is not linear, but *logarithmic*. Thus, in order to calculate the *perceived* contrast C between two intensities of light I_1 and I_2 we must take the logarithms of each and then subtract:

---

i.e. $C = \log I_1 - \log I_2$ Equation 31.4

In particular if $I_1 = I_0 e^{-\mu_1 x}$, then it may be shown (see Insight below) that $\log I_1 = \log I_0 - 0.434 \mu_1 x$. In the simple system between pure bone and soft tissue depicted in Figure 31.1, we may substitute $I_1 = I_0 e^{-\mu_T d}$ for tissue, and $I_2 = I_0 e^{-\mu_B d}$ for bone, so that, if the eye were sensitive to X-rays, the perceived contrast would be:

$$C = \log I_0 - 0.434 \mu_T d - \log I_0 + 0.434 \mu_B d$$
i.e. $C = 0.434 d (\mu_B - \mu_T)$ Equation 31.5

The use of a *fluorescent screen* would result in light intensities (L_1, L_2) from the two areas being proportional to the X-ray intensities I_1 and I_2,

i.e. $L_1 = K I_1$ and $L_2 = K I_2$

where K is a 'constant of proportionality' (1.7). The contrast is then:
$$\log L_1 - \log L_2 = \log K + \log I_1 - \log K - \log I_2$$
i.e. $\log L_1 - \log L_2 = \log I_1 - \log I_2$

This is the same as equation 31.4, and therefore leads directly to a perceived contrast as given by equation 31.5 i.e. the scintillation effciency (27.2) of the screen, given by K, does not affect the perceived contrast.

The perceived contrast in this simple system is thus seen (by Equation 31.5) to increase as d increases (i.e. as more attenuation takes places) and as $\mu_B - \mu_T$ increases. Obviously, if the attenuation coefficients of bone and soft tissue were identical, then we would not expect there to be any difference in attenuation, and so the contrast would be zero.

Insight

We have seen (1.10.2) that to obtain the logarithm of two numbers multiplied together, we need only add the logarithms separately. In the equations above, however, we need to obtain the logarithm of the term $I = I_0 e^{-\mu d}$.

Now $\log_{10} I = \log_{10} (I_0 \cdot e^{-\mu d})$

$$= \log_{10} I_0 + \log_{10} e^{-\mu d}, \text{ by the above.}$$

Also $e = 10^c$ or $c = \log_{10} e$ (by definition of a logarithm),

so that $e^{-\mu d} = (10^c)^{-\mu d} = 10^{-\mu dc} = y$, say.

$\therefore \log_e y = -\mu d$

and $\log_{10} y = -\mu dc$ from the definition of a logarithm,

so that $\log_{10} y = c \log_e y = \log_{10} e \cdot \log_e y$

Combining all these equations, we obtain finally:

$$\log_{10} I = \log_{10} I_0 - 0 \cdot 434 \mu d \quad (\text{since } \log_{10} e = 0 \cdot 434)$$

as stated above.

31.2 THE 'FILM DENSITY IMAGE'

The 'X-ray image' discussed in the previous sections may be used to form a visible image using fluorescent screens (with or without image intensification) or a 'density' image on photographic film. The visible image formed by a fluorescent screen is 'linear', in that the intensity of light emitted from any point is proportional to the X-ray intensity incident upon that point. Such an image has the same contrast as the 'X-ray image' (31.2.4). The photographic density image (i.e. the radiograph) is non-linear, however, since the optical density varies in a complicated manner with the film exposure — the so-called 'film characteristic' (31.2.1). As shown later, this non-linearity may be used to advantage by improving the contrast of the radiograph compared to that of the 'X-ray image'.

The formation of the 'latent' image and its chemical development and fixing are not considered here, as this topic is adequately covered in many readily available specialist textbooks on radiographic photography. For the purpose of this chapter, we need only appreciate that electromagnetic radiation (light, X-rays) produces a pattern of silver atoms within the photographic emulsion, and that the number of these silver atoms is greatly increased by chemical 'developing'. The number of silver atoms increases with the total number of photons striking the film, and so a silver pattern is produced which is related to the X-ray image itself. The silver pattern shows up as semi-opaque areas on the film; the more opaque, the greater the 'optical density'. The purpose of 'fixing' is to produce a stable photographic image which is no longer sensitive to light.

31.2.1 The film characteristic

The 'film characteristic' is usually shown as a graph of optical density, D, against 'relative exposure', E. Optical density (or just 'density') expresses the fractional amount of absorption of light as it passes through the film, and is expressed mathematically as:

$$D = \log_{10}\left(\frac{I_0}{I_t}\right) \qquad \text{Equation 31.6}$$

where I_0 is the intensity of light incident upon the film at a given point (e.g. from a fluorescent viewing screen), and I_t is the intensity of light which is transmitted at the point. The value of I_0/I_t increases as more light is absorbed (since I_t becomes less) and the density therefore increases. The *logarithm* of I_0/I_t is used for two reasons: it reduces the scale of D over a useful range of 0 to 4 (it would otherwise be 1 to 10 000), and it matches the way the eye responds to different levels of brightness. This is because the eye also has a logarithmic response to intensity (31.1.4) in that large variations of true intensity are *perceived* as much smaller intensity changes, for only by this type of response is the eye able to cope with the vast range of light intensities it experiences (e.g. from a moonlit night to that of the noon-day sun). Defining density in this manner (Equation 31.6) means that the 'density' image is the same as the 'intensity' image as perceived by the eye.

Insight

If we assume that the perceived intensity, I_p, is related simply to the true intensity, I_t, reaching the eye by an equation of the type:

$I_p = \log_{10} kI_t$ where k is a constant,

then $D = \log_{10}(I_0/I_t) = \log_{10} I_0 - \log_{10}I_t$

to give:

$I_p = \log_{10} k + \log_{10} I_0 - D$

The difference between the perceived intensities from two areas of an X-ray film is thus:

$I_{p_1} - I_{p_2} = -(D_1 - D_2)$

since $\log k$ and $\log I_0$ cancel when subtracted. Hence, the difference in perceived intensities of light transmitted through the radiograph is the same as the differences in densities of the two areas. Obviously, the minus sign indicates that the 'density' image is just the reverse of the 'intensity' image, since high density means low transmission, and vice versa.

The 'film characteristic' is shown graphically by plotting the densities which result from a known photographic series of 'relative photographic exposures'. The use of 'relative', rather than 'absolute', exposures simplifies the practical measurements of the characteristic, an example of which is shown in Figure

31.4 (absolute measurements of exposure may also be used, of course). The photographic exposure may be due either to the direct absorption of X-rays by the photographic emulsion or of light from fluorescent screens. The characteristic curve is slightly different in each case, but both have the same basic shaped as shown in the figure. The density is plotted against the *logarithm* of the relative exposure, as shown, in order to accommodate the wide range of possible exposures (a typical factor of approximately 1000 between the smallest and the largest exposures).

Even an unexposed film will have a measurable density after development. This is called the 'fog level' and has a density value of about 0·2, corresponding to about a 60% transmission of light when used on a 'viewer' (from equation 31.6). At the 'threshold' exposure, a developed film will show a density just above the fog level. Increased exposure above this threshold value are on the 'toe' region and result in an increasing density change up to about $D=0·5$, The 'linear' region of the film characteristic then follows, where the density changes are proportional to the changes in log E. The quantity *gamma* (γ) is defined in this region by:

$$y = \frac{D_2 - D_1}{\log E_2 - \log E_1} \qquad \text{Equation 31.7}$$

The quantity γ is thus the maximum slope of the characteristic curve, and approximates to the slope over the whole of the linear region (which is not

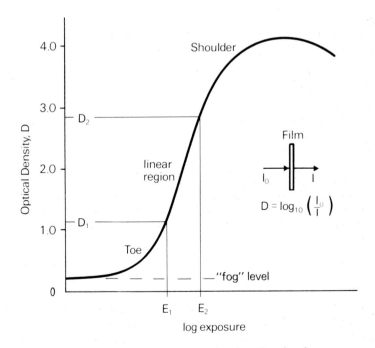

Fig. 31.4 A film characteristic, showing optical density plotted against log exposure.

perfectly straight) over a density range of about 1 to 3, depending upon the type of film and the details of its chemical development.

Increasing photographic exposures above the linear region produce less change in the photographic density, so that the characteristic curve is reduced in slope in the 'shoulder' region. For very large exposures, the density actually decreases, but this region is not important in radiography since the radiographic exposure (i.e. combination of mAs, kV_p etc.) would have to be too high by a factor of about 1000 to reach this part of the curve.

The gamma of the film, is in fact, a special case of the 'film contrast', which is defined as the slope of the characteristic curve at a particular value of D. The gamma is thus the maximum value of the film contrast, and applies only to the linear region. The film contrast is not to be confused with the perceived contrast between different areas on the film as seen by the eye (31.1.4). This is because the film contrast is just the slope of a graph, while the more general term 'contrast', C, is concerned with the visual perception of the radiographic image, and is the difference between the densities of two regions.

$$C = D_2 - D_1 \qquad\qquad \text{Equation 31.8}$$

As show in the previous Insight, the difference between two photographic densities is the same as the differences in the transmitted light as perceived by the eye (i.e. including the eye's logarithmic response to brightness).

Rearranging equation 31.7, we have

$$C = D_2 - D_1 = \gamma \, (\log E_2 - \log E_1) \qquad\qquad \text{Equation 31.9}$$

The photographic exposures E_1 and E_2 were obtained over the same time, t, from X-ray intensities I_1 and I_2.

$$\therefore \quad \log E_1 = \log I_1 t = \log I_1 + \log t \quad \text{and} \quad \log E_2 = \log I_2 + \log t$$
$$\text{Thus} \quad \log E_2 - \log E_1 = \log I_2 - \log I_1$$

and equation 31.9 becomes

$$C = \gamma \, (\log I_2 - \log I_1) \qquad\qquad \text{Equation 31.10}$$

This equation may be compared to equation 31.4, where the 'perceived' contrast is shown to be equal to $(\log I_2 - \log I_1)$. The contrast of the film image is therefore a factor γ greater than this. γ has a typical value of 3, so that the improved, contrast of the film over the fluorescent screen enables more detail to be seen. This point is discussed further in 31.3.

The characteristics of two films of different speeds are shown in Figure 31.5. Film A is said to be 'faster' than film B because the same density is reached for lower values of $\log E$, and therefore E. For example, and exposure E_1 is required to produce a density of 1·0 on film A, while E_2 is required to produce the same density on film 2. The *relative speed* of film 1 over film 2 is then given by the ratio E_2/E_1. Different values of the density chosen for comparison purposes will produce different values of the relative speeds between the two

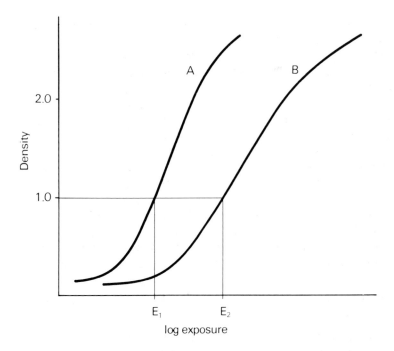

Fig 31.5 The film characteristics of a 'fast' (A) and 'slow' (B) film.

films, so it is necessary to state the density or densities chosen. The speed of the film is increased if screens are used, of course, since the same 'X-ray exposure' then produces a much greater effect.

The *latitude* of a film is the exposure range over which the film will produce a visually acceptable photographic image. Basically, therefore, the latitude refers to the exposure range of the linear part of the characteristic. Figure 31.6 shows the characteristic of a film with a small latitude (curve A) and also one with a 'wide' latitude (curve B). It is possible to produce an acceptable image over the range L_A for film A, whereas film B is usable over the much larger exposure range L_B. However, the film contrast (equation 31.7) is much higher for A over its narrow working range than that of B, and so produces images of greater visual contrast over that range. However, the selection of the exposure is more critical in that a small error in the mAs or kV_p produces a great difference in the appearance of the film (too light or too dark). Thus, a film is used which has sufficient latitude to encompass the exposure ranges produced by a typical 'X-ray image' (31.1), while retaining an acceptable gamma (and therefore visual contrast) over the linear region of its characteristic.

31.2.2 Reciprocity

If an X-ray beam of intensity I is incident upon a photographic film for a time t, then the photographic 'exposure', as given by the total energy absorbed

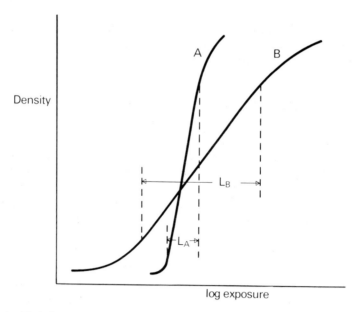

Fig. 31.6 A wide latitude (B) and narrow latitude (A) film.

during t, is proportional to $I \times t$. A series of radiographic exposures may be made where both I and t are changed, but where the value of $I \times t$ is kept constant. Thus, we may double I and halve t (say) to achieve the same photographic exposure. Thus, all such exposures obey the relationship:

$$I \cdot t = K \text{ where } K \text{ is constant,}$$

i.e. $$I \propto \frac{1}{t}$$

Equation 31.11

This is a relationship of *reciprocity* between the intensity of radiation upon the film and the time of irradiation, such that equal photographic densities should be produced (since the same value of photographic exposure should produce the same density, according to the characteristic curve). This is found to be to the case when X-rays impinge directly on the film, but not when fluorescent screens are used. In the former case, each absorbed X-ray photon produces a latent image in the film which is developed, whereas the more numerous but less energetic light photons emitted from the screens do not produce a developable image for low intensities and short exposure times. This is known as *reciprocity failure*, since equation 31.11 is not rigorously obeyed over the whole of the possible combinations of I and t. Its effect is only significant for the short or long exposure times, however.

For a given kV_p, FFD and patient geometry, the intensity of the X-ray beam is proportional to the mA (28.2.2), so that equation 31.11 may be rewritten as

$$mA \propto \frac{1}{t}$$

or,   mAs = constant   Equation 31.12

since mAs = mA × time of exposure in seconds. Modern X-ray units correct automatically for reciprocity failure (i.e. when equation 31.12 does not hold exactly) by increasing the mA values for the shorter exposure times.

31.3 PRACTICAL CONSIDERATIONS

The mastery of the complex interrelationships between the factors which affect the quality of the 'X-ray image' and those that affect the 'density image' on the radiographic film provide much of the 'job satisfaction' experienced by most radiographers. Since there is a strong subjective element involved in the decision as to which of two radiographs is the superior (the personal preferences of the radiologist is also a factor), no absolute rules can be laid down as to which focal spot size or kV_p (for example) is to be used under particular circumstances. In any case, the wide variability in the shapes and sizes of the patients themselves, together with other practical difficulties (e.g. restless patients) would provide so many exceptions as to make the strict adherence to any such rules a nonsense. The experience of the radiographer is therefore one of the most crucial factors in the production of radiographs of a consistently high standard under all conditions. The following sections should therefore be considered with these general comments in mind.

The kV_p value is the crucial factor in determining the 'subject' contrast, i.e. the range of the intensity pattern of the primary X-ray beam transmitted through the patient. This is because the linear attenuation coefficients of the different bodily structures vary with the average energy of the beam (31.1.1). The constraints on the choice of kV_p are therefore governed at the higher values of kV_p by the decreasing subject contrast and increasing contribution of scatter (31.1.4), and at the lower values of kV_p by the loss of detail in the denser structures and by the increasing radiation dose given to the patient. The proportion of scatter in the 'X-ray image' may be reduced by the selection of the smallest practicable *field size*, and by the use of a suitable *grid* (31.1.2).

The subject contrast (31.1.4) is proportional to the *mA* since the intensity of X-rays which are transmitted through a patient at a given point is proportional to the incident intensity, and hence to the mA. The perceived contrast is relatively independent of the mA because of the logarithmic response of the eye to brightness of light (31.1.4). However, the ability of the eye to distinguish between levels of brightness is somewhat poorer than this idealised logarithmic response would suggest when *low* light levels are being visualised. In practice, therefore, there must be a period of 'dark adaption' by the radiologist prior to screening investigations in order to optimise the eye's performance. In this way, the radiation dose to the patient is minimised, for the mA value required to produce a clinically diagnostic image on the screen is also minimised.

The combination of kV_p and *mAs* determines the optical density (31.2.1) on the radiograph. As shown previously (31.2.1), the perceived contrast from a radiographic film is the same as, but opposite in sign to, the density differences on the film. A film of sufficient *latitude* is used to reduce the deleterious effects of an inappropriate setting of mA or kV_p, although somewhat at the expense of contrast. A film *gamma* (31.2.1) of about 3 is normally chosen, as this has been found by experience to optimise the contrast over the wide range of photographic exposures on the radiograph. Fine detail is obscured if the contrast is either too high or too low.

Good *film detail* enables small structures to be seen as distinct areas of different density on the radiograph. This is determined by a combination of the *unsharpness* (geometrical, movement and screen/film — see 3.4) and the overall contrast ('subject' and 'film'). The former is reduced by the use of a smaller focal spot, patient immobilisation and screens using small fluorescent crystals, and the latter is varied by the choice of kV_p, mAs, grid and screen/film combination.

The range of densities normally encountered on a radiograph usually lies between 0·2 and 2·0. This means that the lighter areas on the film, corresponding to a density of 0·2, allow about 60 times (antilog of 1·8) more light to be transmitted compared to the most dense areas. Conventional viewing screens are sufficiently bright to enable adequate optical transmission through the densest areas without dazzling the eye by the transmission through the lightly exposed areas. Obviously, it is important that the light from the viewing screen is uniformly bright, or difficulties of correct interpretation will arise. Masking the bright areas reduces dazzle.

The use of a fluorescent screen/film combination worsens the geometric unsharpness (3.4) although greatly reducing the mAs required to achieve the same density — the Intensification Factor (27.5.1). The overall contrast is better when using such screens because light is used rather than X-rays to expose the film, and the more energetic X-rays absorbed in the phosphor produce more light than the low-energy X-rays, and hence produce a greater photographic density. The lower-energy X-rays are therefore partially discriminated against, which has the effect of reducing the scatter contribution to the radiographic image.

An image intensifier/TV system may be used to provide an image on the TV monitor which is much brighter than that viewed on a fluorescent screeen alone. As mentioned previously, the eye is better able to distinguish between levels of brightness when those levels are higher. Thus, the TV monitors enable the eye to be used more effectively than a conventional fluorescent screen. In addition, the electronic controls on the monitors enable an optimum brightness and contrast to be set for a given image. The contrast may also be adjusted to show different areas within the image to advantage, e.g. areas of low or high illumination (brightness).

Exercise 31.2

a. Upon what factors does the photoelectric absorption of X-rays depend? Hence explain the greater absorption of X-rays by bone compared to soft tissue. Why is this greater absorption not so marked at X-ray energies of about 1 MeV?

b. What is meant by the term 'subject contrast' as applied to an X-ray beam transmitted through a patient? In what way does the subject contrast depend upon:

  (i) kV_p
  (ii) mA
  (iii) atomic number
  (iv) density of absorber
  (v) thickness of absorber

  c. What is the purpose of using 'contrast media' in radiography? Make a list of all those used in your department, together with the investigations for which they are employed. Explain how they influence the appearance of a radiograph from the basic principles of X-ray attenuation through matter.
  d. What is meant by the 'characteristic' of a photographic film? Draw the appearance of such a characteristic in graphical form and explain what is meant by 'optical density' and 'exposure'.
  e. From the graph of the previous question, define what is meant by the terms: film contrast, gamma and latitude.
  f. 'A radiograph gives a greater perceived contrast than a fluorescent screen.' Explain what is meant by 'perceived contrast', and why the use of a photographic film should improve it.
  g. How does a grid improve the appearance of a radiograph?
  h. What practical factors dictate the choice of kV_p, mAs, focal spot size, type of grid and screen/film combination for a radiograph of (a) a lateral skull and (b) an abdomen?

SUMMARY

1. The 'X-ray image' formed by the transmission of X-rays through the patient is composed of the attenuated primary beam and scattered X-rays. The contrast in this image (the 'subject' contrast) is due to the differences in the thicknesses and linear attenuation coefficients (μ) of different structures within the body. Scatter adds a general level of intensity but without structural detail, thus reducing subject contrast.
2. The differences between the values of μ of the bodily structures are due to the difference in their average atomic numbers and densities, and also depends upon the average energy of the X-ray beam ($\tau \propto \rho\,(Z^3/E^3)$; $\sigma \propto \rho \times$ electron density/E). The lower the average energy, E, the greater are the differences in μ, so that the subject contrast is also greater.
3. The higher the kV_p (mean energy E is one-third to one-half of kV_p) the greater the effect of scatter because, although the probability of scatter decreases, this is outweighed by the increasing penetration of those photons that are scattered. The fraction of scattered X-rays to the primary beam which reach the film therefore increases, and has a deleterious effect on the radiograph by reducing contrast (see 1 above).
4. The majority (80–90%) of scattered X-rays are removed by use of a grid, which presents a larger surface area of an absorber (e.g. lead) to deflected X-

rays than to the undeflected primary beam. Approximately 10–15% of the primary beam is also absorbed in the grid, so that there is an overall reduction of the scatter/primary ratio of about a factor of 6 to 10. This enhances the 'subject' contrast markedly.

5.   Photographic film when 'developed' and 'fixed' shows an optical density, D, which varies with the 'photographic exposure', E. The relationship between D and E is known as the film 'characteristic' and is usually plotted as D against log E to accommodate the large possible variations of E . E is just the total energy absorbed by the film, and is proportional to intensity $\times$ time. It is also possible to use 'relative' rather than 'absolute' exposures when the precise measurement of exposure is unnecessary.

6. D is defined as $\log_{10}(I_0/I_t)$, which is mathematically the same as $\log_{10} I_0 - \log_{10} I_t$, where I_0 is the intensity of the light on the film and I_t the intensity of the light transmitted by the film when it is being viewed (e.g. on an 'X-ray viewer'). 'Fog levels' have a density of about 0·2, and the typical range of densities on a radiograph are from 0·2 to 2·0.

7.   Over the 'linear' part of the film characteristic the density changes are proportional to the logarithm of the film exposure changes, where the constant of proportionality is the 'gamma' of the film:

$$D_2 - D_1 = \gamma (\log E_2 - E_1)$$

γ has a typical value of 3, and corresponds to the region of maximum film contrast. Hence it is desirable to produce the radiograph in the 'linear' range.

8.   The eye has a logarithmic response to light intensity, and 'sees' the same as the 'density image' on the film. The *contrast* between two areas, as defined by $D_2 - D_1$, is thus proportional to the film γ (see 7), and is thus greater than the 'subject' contrast of the X-ray image incident upon the film.

9.   The greater the exposure range over which D vs log E is linear, the greater the 'latitude' of the film. This is always at the expense of contrast, however, but is important in relaxing the stringent requirements on the value of E, and hence allows some 'latitude' in the selection of mAs etc.

10.   The 'relative speed' of two films is defined by the ratio of the exposures needed to produce the same density on both films. This is normally measured by the ratio of the mAs values, all other qualities being kept constant (kV_p, FFD, grid, screen type). The choice of density value also affects the value of the relative speed. If the comparison is between the same film used with and without screen, the ratio of the exposures is the Intensification Factor (27.5.1).

11.   Experience is an important contribution to the production of good radiographs, as there is a significant subjective element involved. It is usual to select a given kV_p to ensure a 'known' subject contrast, and a known grid, film and screen combination in the interests of standardisation. The mAs and focal spot sizes may then be selected to determine the best total unsharpness and the correct photographic exposure (i.e. within the 'linear' region of the film characteristic).

Part F
DOSIMETRY AND RADIATION PROTECTION

32. Radiation dosimetry

We live in an environment in which we are continually subjected to ionising radiation from natural causes, such as cosmic rays and naturally occurring radionuclides. Man-made contributions to the total amount of radiation received by the population are a result of radioactive 'fall-out' from atomic weapons testing, leakage from nuclear power plants, manufactured radionuclides and radiological procedures, both diagnostic and therapeutic. All such radiations, whether 'natural' or man-made, constitute a hazard to a greater or lesser extent, and the accurate measurement of the radiation dosage received by members of the population is an essential step in being able to assess those hazards. The second greatest single contribution to the radiation dose received by the population as a whole is that due to irradiation during medical procedures, so that it is important to employ careful techniques which minimise both the radiation doses received by patients, and the number of repeat investigations due to operator error. However, the hazards associated with the medical uses of X-rays and radionuclides must be considered along with the benefits likely to be received by individual patients. This is the so-called 'risk/benefit' relationship, and is discussed further in the next chapter (33.3).

The first part of this chapter considers the physical principles leading to the concepts of Exposure and absorbed dose, while the remainder is concerned with a simplified treatment of the various practical methods by which radiation doses may be measured. The SI system of units is used throughout this and the following chapter. The earlier units of the roentgen, rad and the rem will be used concurrently with the SI units for some years, and are described briefly in Appendix VI.

32.1 UNITS OF EXPOSURE AND DOSE

32.1.1 Exposure

Any X-ray beam passing through air produces excitation and ionisation of the air molecules (25.5). The electron ejected in the first (or 'primary') interaction (e.g. by photoelectric absorption) produces other electrons by ionisation — the 'delta' rays. Such delta rays are responsible for the great majority of ionisations, which are also called 'secondary ionisations'. The net effect on the air is thus:

a. the formation of electric charges by ionisation

b. the absorption of energy by the air as the electric charges are slowed down by collision (producing further ionisation), and

c. the consequent production of heat energy (i.e. increased kinetic energy of the air molecules — 8.1).

'Exposure' concerns the first of these effects only, and is a measure of the total electric charge formed by ionisation, when considering a unit mass of air.

Definition

The *Exposure* at a particular point in a beam of X- or γ-radiation is the ratio Q/m, where Q is the total electric charge produced (of one sign) in a small volume of air of mass m.

The Exposure is thus normalised to a unit mass, and has units of coulomb per kilogram (C kg^{-1}). Note that Exposure only applies to air, and no other medium.

Equal numbers of positive and negative charges are produced in the ionisation processes, of course, since each electron ejected from one atom leaves that atom with a net positive charge. Only the total charge of *one* sign is considered (e.g. electrons) in this definition.

The Exposure *rate* (C kg^{-1}s^{-1}) is a measure of the Intensity of an X-ray beam of a given quality (29.2), since the greater the number and energy of X-ray photons passing through a unit area (4.1) the greater the ionisation of the air.

In air, the *proportions* of ionisation, excitation and heat produced by the absorption of radiation are approximately constant and therefore do not depend upon the energy of the radiation. The total amount of ionisation produced in air is thus proportional to the energy absorbed from the beam. For example, the average energy required to produce an ionisation in air is about 33 eV, so that an X-ray photon of 33 keV which is fully absorbed in air produces about 1000 ionisations (a total charge of about 1.6×10^{-16} coulomb). The remainder of the energy of the absorbed photon produces excitation and heat.

The average atomic number of air is 7.64 and is close to that of muscle at 7.42, so that the mass attenuation and absorption coefficients (30.2) of air and muscle are very similar. This means that the energy absorbed from an X-ray beam by a given mass of air is almost identical to that absorbed by the same mass of muscle. The Exposure measured in air is thus proportional to the energy absorbed both in air and muscle, which is the main reason for the importance of air as a medium for radiation dosimetry, since the absorbed dose (see below) in tissue may be calculated simply from a knowledge of the air Exposure.*

However, the term 'Exposure' is expected to gradually fall out of common usage and to be replaced by the term 'absorbed dose in air', as explained in the next section.

*In the earlier units, this is known as the 'Roentgen to rad conversion factor', which is always close to unity for tissue (reflecting the closeness of the average atomic numbers) and is much greater than unity for bone for low energies of radiation owing to the increase of the photoelectric effect due to the higher atomic number of bone (30.4) — see Fig. 32.3(b).

32.1.2 Absorbed dose and kerma

The measurement of the quantity of electric *charge* produced by ionisation when X-rays are absorbed in a medium is not the same as the measurement of the *energy* actually absorbed by that medium, although the quantities are proportional to each other.

The energy absorbed by the medium is the 'absorbed dose' and is defined as follows:

Definition

The *absorbed dose* in a medium is the ratio E/m, where E is the energy absorbed by the medium due to a beam of ionising radiation in a small mass m.

The unit of absorbed dose is the *gray* (Gy), where 1 gray $= 1$ joule per kg (1 Gy $= 1$ J kg^{-1}) and is 100 times bigger than the earlier unit of absorbed dose, the rad (Appendix VI), i.e. 1 Gy $= 100$ rad.

Note that the Exposure is defined for X and γ-radiation only (charged particle beams produce different proportions of ionisation, excitation and heat within the air), while the absorbed dose is defined for any 'ionising' radiation, i.e. any radiation which is capable of ionising the medium through which it passes. Thus, the energies absorbed in the medium due to α-particles, protons, β-particles and neutrons are all measured in gray. However, visible and ultra-violet light (for example) are capable only of the excitation rather than the ionisation of the atoms and molecules of the medium, and so are outside the scope of this definition of absorbed dose.

If all the electrons produced by primary and secondary ionisation within the medium are stopped within it, then it is clear that the energy *removed* from the beam of ionising radiation is the same as the energy *absorbed* by the medium. (It is assumed here that all fluorescene radiation is absorbed, as is the case for biological tissues.) However, this does not necessarily apply for a particular small volume within the medium, i.e. such a volume may be removing energy from the beam, but the absorbed dose may be deposited mainly *outside* the volume, owing to the distance travelled by the electrons in coming to rest. This effect is more marked for electrons of the higher energies, since such electrons travel an appreciable distance before coming to rest (about 5 mm for 1 MeV electrons in tissue, for example). This effect is illustrated in Figure 32.1, where an incoming X-ray beam of high energy interacts with a volume element V within the medium. All the electrons produced by Compton scatter (30.5) are scattered in the 'forward' direction so that much of the absorption of the energy of the electrons occurs outside V. The secondary ionisations resulting in the production of the 'delta' rays are not shown in the figure.

In general, if the secondary electrons produced *within* the volume deposit a total energy E within the medium, and E_{IN}, E_{OUT} are the total energies of the electrons entering and escaping from the volume, then the absorbed dose in gray is given by:

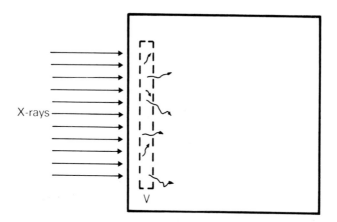

Fig. 32.1 X-rays interacting with atoms in volume V produce electrons which may travel outside V.

$$\text{absorbed dose} = \frac{E + E_{IN} - E_{OUT}}{m} \qquad \text{Equation 32.1}$$

where m is the mass of the particular small volume considered. If a larger volume is considered, then this formula expresses the *average* absorbed dose in that volume.

Electronic equilibrium is said to occur if $E_{IN} = E_{OUT}$, i.e. if there is no net loss or gain of electrons over the small volume considered. If $E_{IN} - E_{OUT}$ is a constant not equal to zero, there is said to be 'quasi-electronic' equilibrium. Obviously, when the irradiation varies in intensity, the net loss or gain of electrons to a given small volume varies in proportion. An example of electronic equilibrium is the 'free-air' ionisation chamber, as described below (33.2.2).

The absorbed dose expresses the quantity of energy absorbed in the medium due to a beam of ionising radiation passing through the medium. However, as stated in the beginning of this section, the site of an attenuation event (e.g. photoelectric absorption) may be at some distance from the subsequent absorption processes because of the distance travelled by the ejected electron in coming to rest. The quantity which measures the amount of attenuation in a small volume is called the **kerma**, the initials of which stand for '**K**inetic **E**nergy **R**eleased per unit **M**ass'. Kerma is also measured in gray (i.e. joule kg^{-1}), and may differ significantly from the 'absorbed dose' at any particular position within the medium. The absorbed dose and kerma along the axis of a beam of X-radiation are shown in Figure 32.2. Figure 32.2(a) shows the case for radiography, where a beam of 100 kV$_p$ X-rays is incident upon soft tissue. The electrons released in primary and secondary ionisations are of relatively low energy and so are absorbed close to the site of each photoelectric or Compton interaction. Hence the kerma and absorbed dose at any particular point are essentially identical (the curves are coincident in the figure). This is

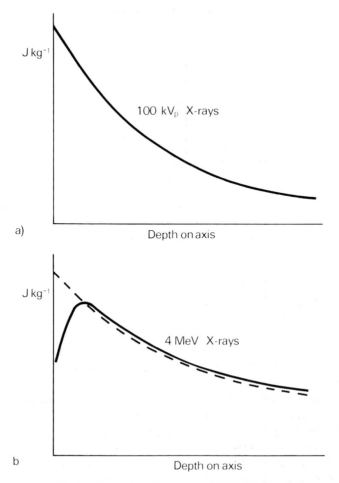

Fig. 32.2 Kerma (dotted line) and absorbed dose for (a) 100 kV$_p$ 'diagnostic' beam and (b) 4 MeV therapy beam. In (a) the two curves are coincident, but are different in (b) because of the increased range of the energetic electrons.

not the case for X-ray beams of high energy, however, since the electrons produced by ionisation have considerable energy and hence deposit the majority of their energy at some distance from the original attenuation process. Thus, the kerma and the absorbed dose due to 4 meV X-rays in a medium are not the same, as shown in Figure 32.2(b). These curves may be understood if it is remembered that the kerma is a measure of the *attenuation* (i.e. the number of photoelectric and Compton events) while the absorbed dose is a measure of the *energy deposited* in the medium caused by the primary and secondary electrons being brought to rest.

32.1.3 Effect of different media

Instruments which are used to measure absorbed dose or absorbed dose rate are called 'dosemeters' and 'dose-rate meters' respectively. Some of these instruments are described in more detail below (32.3). It is the usual practice to calibrate such meters in terms of the absorbed dose (or dose rate) received by the *air* through which the X or γ-radiation is passing. Such a dosemeter may read (for example) 0·5 mGy (50 mrad) as the total absorbed dose at a point within an X-ray beam. It must *not* be inferred, however, that this is the absorbed dose which would have been received by any other medium (such as bone) if it were placed in the same position. For two media to receive the same absorbed dose, they must both absorb the same total energy from the beam per unit mass (since the absorbed dose is defined 'per unit mass'). This is exactly the same as saying that the mass absorption coefficients of the two media must be equal, since the definition of the mass absorption coefficient (30.2), μ_a/ρ, may be paraphrased as the 'fraction of energy absorbed per unit mass.' Hence, if D_{air} is the absorbed dose at a point in air due to a beam of X-rays, and D_m is the absorbed dose in a medium (due to the same X-ray beam), then it follows that in the general case when the mass absorption coefficients are not equal:

$$\frac{D_m}{D_{air}} = \frac{(\mu_a/\rho)_m}{(\mu_a/\rho)_{air}}$$

i.e.

$$D_m = D_{air} \times \frac{(\mu_a/\rho)_m}{(\mu_a/\rho)_{air}}$$
                                                           Equation 32.2

Thus, if the mass absorption coefficients of air and the medium are known at a particular energy of X-ray quanta, the absorbed dose in the medium may be calculated using the above equation. This is very convenient, in practice, since it is not always possible to measure the absorbed dose *in situ* for biological materials without subjecting the patient to an unwarranted degree of discomfort.

The variation of the mass absorption coefficients of air and bone with energy and the ratio of the two coefficients are shown in Figure 23.3(a) and (b) respectively. Firstly, at low energies (e.g. 50 keV, as shown) the higher atomic number of bone ($Z = 13·8$) is responsible for a greater absorption of the incident quanta in the bone compared to the air owing to the importance of the photoelectric effect at such energies ($\tau/\rho \propto Z^3/E^3$ — see 30·4). As shown in Chapter 31, this is responsible for the radiographic contrast between bone and soft tissue on the film. At energies of about 1 MeV, however, both mass absorption curves are very close, and the ratio of the two coefficients is thus close to unity. This situation reflects the dominance of the Compton process in this region ($\sigma/\rho \propto$ electron density, which is approximately the same for all materials except hydrogen — 30.5). The two curves diverge again at the higher energies owing to the greater amount of pair production in the bone compared to air ($\pi/\rho \propto Z$ — 30.6). Thus, it is clear that the scale of an instrument calibrated to read absorbed, dose in air cannot be used directly to measure the absorbed dose in bone or any other medium because there is no simple relationship between the mass absorption coefficients. This is particularly the

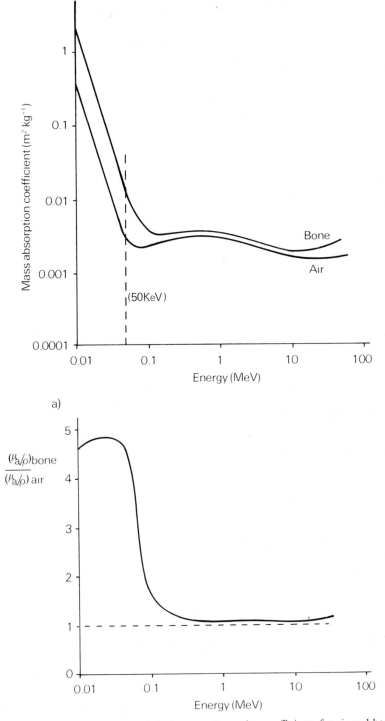

Fig. 32.3 The variation with energy of (a) the mass absorption coefficients for air and bone, and (b) the ratio of the two coefficients.

case in the 'diagnostic' range of X-ray energies, where the photoelectric effect is very sensitive to both atomic number and energy.

Insight

Equation 32.2 may be derived more formally as follows:

$I_x = I_0 e^{-\mu x}$ from the exponential law of attenuation (5.3).

Differentiating with respect to x and simplifying:

$$\mu = \frac{-dI_x/I_x}{dx} = \frac{-dI_x/I_0}{dx} \text{ at } x = 0$$

μ is composed of absorption and scatter components (30.2) such that $\mu = \mu_a + \mu_s$, and the corresponding absorbed and scattered intensities are dI_a and dI_s, where $dI_x = dI_a + dI_s$. Considering only the absorbed component, we have

$$\mu_a = \frac{-dI_a/I_0}{dx}$$

Dividing by the density, ρ, to produce the *mass* absorption coefficient, we have

$$\frac{\mu_a}{\rho} = \frac{dI_a/I_0}{\rho dx}$$

Now, ρdx is just the mass, dm, in a block of material of unit cross-sectional area and depth dx, so that we obtain:

$$\frac{\mu_a}{\rho} = \frac{dI_a/I_0}{dm}$$

or, in words: 'the mass absorption coefficient of a medium is the normalisation to unit mass of the fractional absorption of the electromagnetic energy when incident upon a unit cross section and very small mass.'

Now, $-dI_a/dm$ is just the absorbed dose rate, D/t, in the medium, so that we may set up two equations:

$$\left(\frac{\mu_a}{\rho}\right)_{air} = \frac{D_{air}}{I_0 t}; \quad \left(\frac{\mu_a}{\rho}\right)_m = \frac{D_m}{I_0 t}$$

Divide one equation by the other and simplifying, we obtain:

$$D_m = D_{air} \times \frac{(\mu_a/\rho)_m}{(\mu_a/\rho)_{air}}$$

in agreement with our more intuitive derivation of Equation 32.2

32.1.4 Quality factor and dose equivalent

As described in the previous section, the 'absorbed dose' measures the amount of energy absorbed in a medium per unit mass when it is subjected to ionising radiations of whatever kind (i.e. X-rays, gamma rays, electrons, alpha particles, neutrons, π^--mesons or protons). However, the effects on a biological sample do not depend solely upon the absorbed dose, but also upon the type of ionising radiation and the absorbed dose *rate*. It is found that α-

particles have a greater biological effect than X-rays when both deliver the same absorbed dose to a sample, and the effect of any ionising radiation is greater if the same absorbed dose occurs over a shorter time.

The differences in the biological effects of different types of ionising radiations are due to the differing density of ionisations (ionisations per unit length of track) which they produce in the sample. Electrons (whether primary, or produced by X and gamma rays) do not produce as many ion-pairs* so close together as are caused by the more massive protons and α-particles of the same energy. Thus α-particles and protons are brought to rest within the medium quickly by losing their kinetic energy in the production of many ions over a short distance — their biological effect is therefore greater because the disruption of chemical bonds (33.2) so close together reduces the chances of complete repair. The distance travelled by a 1 MeV α-particle in tissue is about five-thousandths of a millimetre (5×10^{-3} mm), whereas the corresponding values of protons and electrons are three-hundredths (3×10^{-2} mm) and 5 millimetres respectively.

Neutrons also produce dense ionisation caused by the ejection of protons from nuclei and by nuclear recoils, and π^{-}-mesons produce dense ionisation by nuclear disintegrations caused by nuclear capture of the mesons.

The absorbed dose in gray is thus not an accurate measure of the *biological* effects of all these different types of ionising radiations owing to the very different patterns of ionisation produced. The unit used to measure the overall biological effect of different ionising radiations is called the *dose equivalent* and is measured in sievert (Sv) — the earlier *rem* unit is discussed in Appendix VI. The absorbed dose in gray and the dose equivalent in sievert are proportional to each other and are related by a constant of proportionality (1.7) Q, where:

---

dose equivalent (Sv) = $Q \times$ absorbed dose (Gy) $\times N$ Equation 32.3

Q is known as the *quality factor*, and depends upon the type of ionising radiation and, to some extent, upon its energy. N includes '*other factors*' which may have an effect, such as the effect of the dose *rate*. The value of N is usually put to 1, so that Equation 32.3 is frequently quoted without the factor N appearing.

Table 32.1 shows the value of the quality factor for different types of radiation. Note that Q is unity for X and γ-radiation so that the absorbed dose is the same as the dose equivalent for them. The biological effect of particulate radiations is therefore compared to that of X and γ-radiation by means of the value of Q. As shown in the table, electrons have a Q of 1 which is to be expected since X and γ-photons produce secondary electrons within the medium with exactly the same ionisation density along their tracks as are produced by an external beams of electrons. However, α-particles have a Q of 20, indicating that the same absorbed dose produces 20 times the biological effect as X-rays.

---

* *Ion-pairs* — the ejection of an electron from an atom (i.e. ionisation) results in a net (positive) charge on the atom as well as the electron — thus 'ion-pair'.

Table 32.1 Quality factors for different ionising radiations

Type of ionising radiation	Quality factor (Q)
X or γ	1
Electrons	1
Thermal neutrons	2·3
Fast neutrons (or of unknown energy)	10
Protons	10
Alpha particles	20
Recoil nuclei (e.g. in α-decay	20
Fission fragments	20

Since Q is just a number and contains no units, the sievert has the same units as the gray, i.e. J kg^{-1} — 'energy absorbed per unit mass'. The quality factor may thus be considered as a 'scaling' factor relating the absorbed dose to the biological effect of all ionising radiations when compared to X and γ-rays.

It is mentioned briefly here that the dose equivalent is too crude a unit for use in radiobiology, which is the study of the detailed effects of ionising radiations on biological tissues. Here, the relationships between the different ionising radiations to produce the same biological effect depends upon the precise effect being considered (e.g. 50% death of all cells, impairment of cell reproduction etc.), and (by analogy to the quality factor) the more precise 'scaling' factor in this case is the *relative biological effectiveness* (RBE). The RBE compares the absorbed doses of different ionising radiations required to produce the same biological effect. These doses are compared either to each other, or, more usually, to X and γ-radiation.

However, the dose equivalent in sievert has a vital role to play in radiation protection, where it is required to sum the effects of exposure to different ionising radiations (33.2).

The remainder of this chapter is concerned with a brief review of some of the methods used to measure Exposure and absorbed doses.

32.2 ABSOLUTE MEASUREMENT OF ABSORBED DOSE

The absolute measurement of the absorbed dose in air due to a beam of X-rays requires very careful techniques and specialised equipment, and is therefore more suited to a specialised laboratory rather than a hospital environment. Such laboratories (National Physical Laboratory in the UK, and National Bureau of Standards in the USA) calibrate and check their specialised dosemeters (termed 'absolute standards') under carefully controlled conditions. Dosemeters used in hospitals are sent to such centres on a regular basis to be calibrated against their absolute standards — they are therefore known as 'secondary standards' and, while not being as accurate as those in the specialised laboratory, are adequate for their purpose. Further dosemeters in the hospital (or group of hospitals) may be calibrated against the secondary standard and known as 'sub-standards'. This section considers briefly the manner in which an absolute assessment of the absorbed dose in a medium may be made, while the following section (32.3) considers the more numerous *relative* methods (i.e. methods which need to be calibrated against an absolute method). Only X and γ-radiation will be considered.

32.2.1 Calorimetry

X and γ-rays are absorbed in a medium by the processes discussed in Chapter 30, each of which produces many ionisations within the medium. The kinetic energy of the electrons so ejected from their atoms is eventually completely absorbed by the atoms of that medium, thereby giving them increased kinetic energy, and therefore heat (Ch. 8). The medium thus experiences a rise of temperature which is proportional to the heat energy absorbed by the medium and therefore to the absorbed dose. In (8.1.2) it is shown that:

$$Q = mc(T_2 - T_1)$$

where c is the 'specific heat capacity' of the medium. Also the absorbed dose D is the 'energy per unit mass' (see above),

i.e. $D = Q/m$

Thus

$$D = c(T_2 - T_1) \hspace{4cm} \text{Equation 32.4}$$

so that the absorbed dose may be calculated directly from a knowledge of the specific heat capacity and by a measurement of the increase of temperature experienced by the medium after being irradiated. This is known as the *calorimetric* method of absorbed dose measurement.

However, the rise in temperature is very small (e.g. 1 Gy produces a temperature rise of about 2×10^{-4} °C) and needs very careful measurement in controlled conditions, so that this is definitely a specialised technique! However, the calorimetric method is a useful adjunct to the more sensitive method of charge collection in an air ionisation chamber, as described below.

32.2.2 Free-air ionisation chamber

The ion-pairs produced by the absorption of an X-ray beam in air, or other gas, may be collected by oppositely charged plates situated in the air. The electrons are attracted towards the positive plate and the positive ions are attracted towards the negatively charged plate so that a current flows whose magnitude is proportional to both the Exposure in coulomb per kilogram and the absorbed dose in gray (32.1.1 and 32.1.2). Precautions are necessary, however, in order to achieve accurate results. Firstly, and as shown in Figure 32.4, one of the collecting plates is separated into two sections: a central disc and a

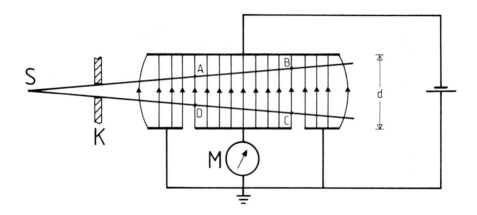

Fig. 32.4 The 'free-air' ionisation chamber.

surrounding annulus which are at 'earth' potential, or 'zero volts'. This construction enables an accurate estimation of the volume of air from which the ion-pairs are to be collected, and it is therefore essential that the lines of electric force (9.4) should be directed at right-angles to both collecting plates. Note that this is not the case at the edges of the plates, where the electric lines of force are 'bowed' outwards and so include an unknown quantity of air beyond the edge of the plates. The volume of air from which the ion-pairs are collected may therefore be calculated (because the area ABCD is known). Ion-pairs produced outside this known volume are still collected by the plates, but do not pass through the meter M (or its associated electronic amplifier) and so do not contribute to the current it indicates.

Some electrons escape from region ABCD and produce ionisations over the annulus of the bottom plate rather than the central disc. It might be thought from this that the current measured by meter M would be too low, but this is not the case because, on average, an equal number of electrons is gained and lost by any given volume in the air so that there is no *net* loss of electrons from the volume under consideration. This is a case of 'electronic equilibrium' (32.1.2).

The potential difference across the plates must be sufficiently high to collect all the ion-pairs produced by ionisation in the air. The current flowing through the meter M varies with the applied potential difference, V, as indicated in Figure 32.5. Below the 'saturation' voltage, some of the positive and negative ions are able to recombine by mutual attraction. At or above the saturation level, however, the electric field intensity (9.4) between the plates overcomes this attractive force and compels the ions to permanently separate and move towards the appropriate plate. The value of the potential difference chosen in practice depends upon the separation of the plates, but is typically of the order of a few hundred volts.

The separation of the plates, d, shown in Figure 32.4 must be sufficiently large so as to enable the production of *all* the secondary ionisations in the air, i.e. no electron produced during the ionising processes must reach the plates

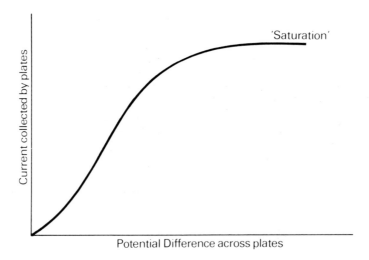

Fig. 32.5 The variation of the current flowing through the meter in Fig. 32.4 with the applied PD.

before producing all the ion-pairs of which it is capable. If d is too small, then a low current is measured by the meter M, since there are fewer ion-pairs produced in the available air volume. Hence the estimates of the Exposure and absorbed dose will be too low. The required plate separation depends upon the energy of the X or γ-ray beam, since high photon energies produce correspondingly energetic electrons which travel further in the air. Typical values vary between about 20 cm for photon energies up to about 250 keV, and several metres for photon energies beyond 1 MeV. The greater the energy of the beam, the more cumbersome is this method owing to the very large plate separations which become necessary.

Insight

It is not necessary for the ions to actually strike the collecting plates in order for a current to flow, because the separation of the positive and negative charges in the gas immediately induces a charge on the plates by *electrostatic induction* (9.5.1). The greater the separation of the ion-pair, the greater the induced charge due to that ion-pair

---

The total charge in coulomb measured by the free-air ionisation chamber is a direct measure of the Exposure in $C\ kg^{-1}$ and is proportional to the absorbed dose in $J\ kg^{-1}$ (i.e. in gray). The mass of the air being irradiated depends upon the temperature and pressure of the air and must therefore be corrected for the effect of their variations. If ρ_0 is the density of air at a known temperature and pressure (e.g. 760 mm of mercury and 293 K), then the mass of air m_0 in the irradiated volume, v, is just ρ_0 v. At a new temperature and pressure (T_1 and p_1), the density changes to $\rho_0 T_0 p_1 / T_1 p_0$ so that the mass of air, m', being irradiated is given by:

$$m' = m_0 . \frac{T_0}{T_1} . \frac{p_1}{p_0}$$ Equation 32.5

The Exposure in $C\,kg^{-1}$ is therefore the ratio of the total charge collected to the value of m', and the absorbed dose is calculated from the energy absorbed divided by m'. (The energy absorbed is known from the charge collected, since it takes a fixed average quantity of energy — about 33 eV — to produce one ion-pair in air.)

The ionisation chamber is not suitable for use with liquids owing to the rapid recombination of the ions produced by radiation and the relatively high current through many liquids, even when no radiation is present. A semiconductor may, however, be used to collect the ion-pairs produced by radiation (32.3.6).

In summary, therefore, the 'free-air' ionisation chamber is suitable for the absolute measurement of Exposure and absorbed dose in air up to an energy of approximately 3 MeV. The absorbed dose which would have occurred in another medium placed in the beam of X-radiation is calculated from the mass absorption coefficients, as explained above (32.1.3).

32.2.3 Chemical methods

Radiation affects the chemical bonding between the atoms of a material through which it passes, both by ionisation and excitation of the atomic electrons. In particular, it is able to transform a dilute solution of ferrous sulphate, $FeSO_4$, to ferric sulphate, $Fe_2(SO_4)_3$, by rearrangement of the chemical bonds. The number of ferric ions so produced is proportional to the absorbed dose (about 15 ferric ions for every 100 eV of absorbed dose), and hence a chemical measurement of the concentration of such ions may be used to estimate the radiation dose absorbed.

Such a 'chemical' dosemeter may be calibrated against either of the two preceding methods of absorbed dose measurement, and is included in this present section on 'absolute' methods of dose measurement because once the conversion factor between absorbed dose and quantity of ferric ions is known, no subsequent calibration is necessary. This is similar to the calculation of the absorbed dose in the free-air ionisation chamber from a knowledge of the energy required to produce an ion-pair in air.

This method of dose measurement is termed the 'Fricke' dosemeter, but is only suitable for the estimation of very large absorbed doses, in excess of about 20 gray (2000 rad), because of the relatively insensitive method of determining the quantity of ferric ions and the effect of chemical impurities. It is, however, particularly suitable for use with high-energy beams of radiation and specialised shapes of irradiated volumes.

32.3 TYPES OF DETECTORS AND DOSEMETERS

The previous section considered the measurement of absorbed dose by 'absolute' methods, which form a standard against which measurements on other types of dosemeters are compared. These 'relative' methods of absorbed dose measurement are therefore calibrated directly or indirectly against a known standard. There are many ways by which a beam of X or γ-rays may be detected and an estimate of the absorbed dose made, each of which has its own particular advantages and disadvantages. Some of these are outlined briefly below.

32.3.1   'Thimble' ionisation chamber

The 'free-air' ionisation chamber discussed in the previous section is necessary for the absolute standardisation of radiation doses, but would be highly impracticable as a method of routine dose measurement in a hospital environment. It would be useless, for example, in the estimation of the absorbed dose rate at the surface of the patient's skin to a beam of ^{60}Co radiation (emitting gamma rays of 1·17 MeV and 1·33 MeV), since the plates would need to be separated by at least 5 metres to collect all the secondary electrons produced in the air.

The 'thimble' ionisation chamber circumvents these difficulties by, as it were, 'condensing' the air to a solid medium surrounding a central electrode, as shown in Figure 32.6. The cap of the thimble chamber is made of a material which has approximately the same atomic number as air (e.g. graphite, bakelite, plastic) and so behaves as the same *mass* of air, because the mass absorption coefficients (30.2) will be almost identical. Some of the energetic electrons produced in the cap by the radiation are able to penetrate into the air surrounding the central aluminium wire electrode and are attracted towards it because of the positive charge upon it supplied by an external electrical supply. The inside surface of the cap is coated with conducting material and may be 'earthed'. Thus, a potential difference exists between the cap and the central electrode enabling the electrons to experience a force due to the electric field.

By suitable choice of materials and size of caps the thimble chamber behaves as if it were 'air equivalent', i.e. as though it were made of the same mass of air. Such a device is calibrated over several photon energy ranges against a radiation 'standard' as described in the previous section, and a correction factor is used to convert the indicated reading of current or total charge to a true absorbed dose. The choice of wall thickness of the cap is one of the factors which influences the applied correction, since a thin cap may not produce

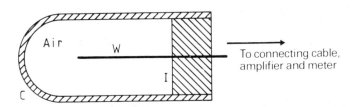

Fig. 32.6 Construction of the thimble chamber. Key: C — cap; W — central wire; I — insulator.

sufficient electrons entering the chamber and a cap which is thicker than optimum absorbs more radiation than it needs to. Notice that the vast majority of the electrons contributing to the electrical current are produced in the *cap*, and not in the air cavity inside the chamber, but it is the passage of such electrons into the air cavity which enables a current to be measured. Corrections for variations in temperature and pressure are made as in the case of the 'free-air' chamber.

The thimble chamber forms the basis of much of the radiation dosimetry measurements both in radiography and radiotherapy. To take an example from radiotherapy, the calibration of the radiation outputs of teletherapy machines such as cobalt-60 units and linear accelerators (34.2) is usually accomplished by the use of a thimble chamber connected to an electronic amplification system which measures and displays the electric charge produced within the chamber during irradiation. A suitable unit is the *Baldwin-Farmer* system using a 0.6 cc chamber connected by a long screened cable. However, in order to relate the reading obtained as a result of a given exposure to the radiation output of the machine (usually expressed in cGy/min), various *correction factors* need to be applied. These include the following:

(i) temperature and pressure correction (end of 32.2.2)
(ii) a calibration factor relating the reading of this sub-standard to a 'secondary standard' unit (32.2) calibrated by a national body (NRPB) — this factor depends upon the energy ('quality') of the radiation
(iii) the factor required to be applied to the secondary standard to obtain the Exposure (32.1.1) — this is also quality dependent
(iv) a factor to convert Exposure to *absorbed dose* (32.1.2) at the appropriate radiation quality.

In addition, there may be some machine-dependent correction factors, such as correcting for a reading at a depth (e.g. 50mm) in a water tank to obtain the 'surface' value, and correcting for switch-on and switch-off errors (6.5.5).

32.3.2 Geiger–Muller counter

The thimble chamber described in the previous section is an example of an 'ionisation chamber', where the charge collected by the electrodes is proportional to the energy absorbed from the X-ray beam. The Geiger–Muller counter works in the 'avalanche' or 'gas multiplication' region (18.5) and always gives the same magnitude of electrical pulse per absorption event whatever the magnitude of the absorbed energy. The structure of the Geiger tube is shown in Figure 32.7(a). A glass envelope contains an inert gas (argon) at low pressure and two electrodes: a positively charged central wire and a cylindrical negatively charged mesh. Ions caused by X-rays or charged particles (when a 'thin' window is used to allow the particles to penetrate into the gas) are attracted to the appropriate electrode as they pass through the gas. Ionisation may occur in the gas itself, or electrons may be ejected into the gas by the interaction of the X-rays with the wall of the chamber.

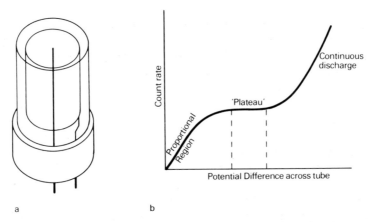

Fig. 32.7 (a) Basic construction of Geiger tube (see text), and (b) its operating characteristic. The Geiger tube is operated on its 'plateau'.

If the potential difference between the electrodes is sufficiently great, the electrons achieve the necessary kinetic energy on their passage to the central wire to ionise the gas atoms in their path — the additional electrons so produced continue this process, and rapid gas multiplication takes place, especially close to the central wire, since the field strength is greatest in that region. The effect of the gas multiplication is to produce well in excess of a million ions collected by the electrodes for every single ion produced in the primary absorption process.

The presence of a small quantity of alcohol vapour in the gas helps to 'quench' the gas multiplication process so that it does not become continuous. It does this by absorbing the kinetic energy of the positive ions in the gas, so that they are prevented from striking the wall with sufficient energy to release further electrons and thereby keep the whole process continuing indefinitely. Alternatively, the potential difference applied across the Geiger tube may be momentarily reduced after the arrival of an electrical pulse, thus terminating the gas multiplication. In either event, there is a 'dead time' after each pulse during which another absorption event (if present) is not recorded. (See Appendix V for a discussion of the effect of dead times etc. on the observed counting rate.)

The correct potential difference to be applied to a particular Geiger tube is determined in practice by plotting a graph of the count rate against the applied voltage obtained when (for example) a small radioactive source is placed near the tube as shown in Figure 32.7(b). Three distinct regions are obtained:

a. the 'proportional' region where some gas multiplication takes place and the electrical pulses are proportional to the energy deposited in the gas

b. the working region, or 'plateau' where the maximum possible gas multiplication takes place and all electrical pulses are the same magnitude

c. the 'continuous discharge' region where the electric field intensity is sufficient to ionise the gas atoms and so produce continuous unwanted gas multiplication.

The 'plateau' is usually between 100 V and 1500V, depending upon the size of the Geiger tube.

The Geiger tube is therefore suitable mainly for the *detection* of radiation rather than the accurate estimation of absorbed doses, since the pulses of constant magnitude bear no relationship to the energy of the radiation causing them. It is therefore usually used as a 'contamination monitor' for radioactive spillage and for other general-purpose uses in radiation protection.

32.3.3 Scintillation detectors

The operation of a scintillation detector employing a sodium iodide crystal and a photomultiplier tube is described in Appendix II. Any suitable scintillating material may be used, whether solid or liquid, and the principle of operation is that the electrical pulse produced by the photomultiplier is proportional to the energy deposited in the scintillator.

Scintillating plastics which have an atomic number close to that of air, and are therefore 'air-equivalent', have a similar variation of absorption with energy of photon, so that they are useful for estimating the absorbed dose in air. A scintillator of high atomic number (such as sodium iodide) will show a marked variation of absorption with energy at and near their 'absorption edges' (25.5.2), requiring correction factors for different energy ranges if an accurate estimate of the absorbed dose in air is to be made. This is particularly so for thin crystals, which show a more marked variation of total absorption with energy than thick crystals.

Scintillation counters are very sensitive devices, and are used in many applications, from the detection of radioactive contamination, the estimation of *in-vivo* radioactivity, to dosemeters and 'gamma cameras' (Appendix II).

32.3.4 Thermoluminescent dosimetry (TLD)

The principle of thermoluminescence has been described previously (27.4) as part of the fluorescence phenomenon. Thermoluminescence may be used to estimate radiation doses by means of lithium fluoride powder or lithium fluoride impregnated teflon discs and rods. The impurities in the lithium fluoride generate the electron 'traps' (27.3), and the number of electrons in those traps is proportional to the absorbed dose in the lithium fluoride. The average atomic number of lithium fluoride is close to that of soft tissue (8.2 and 7.4 respectively), and so both will have a similar absorption variation with photon energy. The small discs or sachets of powder may be placed around the fingers to assess the radiation dose received during manipulation of radioactive sources, or may be taped close to a crucial organ of a patient during radiotherapy (e.g. the eye) or even placed within a body cavity. After irradiation, the light emitted when the 'dosimeter' is heated is compared to that of a standard dosimeter to which a known radiation dose has been given, and the radiation dose calculated by direct proportion.

The great advantage of this method of radiation dose estimation is thus the ability to place the dosimeter in places and over tissues when it would be difficult or impossible to use the other methods. Also, the radiation doses at several different places may be estimated using the required number of lithium fluoride dosimeters (see also Fig. 33.2).

32.3.5 Photographic film

The photographic density produced by irradiation to X and γ-rays is not proportional to the absorbed dose within the emulsion (31.2.1). The calibration of the film density to absorbed dose is therefore necessary, and constitutes a major disadvantage of the method. Also, the film emulsion has significant photoelectric absorption at low energies and therefore the density-dose is dependent upon energy is this region.

Photographic film is useful (for example) in checking X-ray beam alignment with the optical axis of an X-ray unit, and for the estimation of the penumbra in therapy machines (3.4.1). Its major use, however, is as the detecting medium in the 'film badge' which is worn by 'classified' workers to verify that their radiation doses do not exceed their dose-equivalent limits (DEL-33.4.1). The film badge is described in more detail in the next chapter on radiation protection (33.5.2).

32.3.6 Semiconductor detectors

It was shown previously (19.1) that electrons raised to the conduction band of a semiconductor are able to take part in electrical conduction. The absorption of an X or γ-photon within the semiconductor produces an energetic electron (due to photoelectric or Compton interaction) which itself causes secondary electrons by ionisation, as in the case of the interaction of photons with air. A potential difference across the semiconductor 'sweeps' the electrons away from the site of their production, prevents recombination, and results in a pulse of electricity whose magnitude is proportional to the number of electrons produced and therefore to the absorbed dose within the semiconductor. The semiconductor detector is thus a solid-state 'ionisation chamber', and its great advantage over the air ionisation chamber is that about 10 times as many ion-pairs are produced in the semiconductor. This is because only about 3 eV is required to produce an ion-pair compared to about 33 eV for air. The electrical signal obtained from a semiconductor device is thus more precise, in that it has a smaller statistical uncertainty, and may be used to produce very accurate γ-ray spectra, for example.

There are many different types of semiconductor detector, some requiring to be used at liquid nitrogen temperatures for optimum performance. Germanium has a higher atomic number than silicon, and so has a greater variation of absorption with energy. Both types may be calibrated against a 'thimble' chamber, for example, for a given quality of radiation.

Semiconductor detectors are more suited to specialised detection and dosimetry applications than for general-purpose dosemeters. For example, a very small semiconductor detector may be made and used as a probe to measure dose rate within body cavities, e.g. as a rectal dosemeter.

Exercise 32.1

a.   Explain what is meant by the terms 'Exposure' and 'absorbed dose' as applied to a beam of ionising radiation. What are the units of each?

b.   In what way does the mass absorption coefficient of a medium determine the radiation dose absorbed in that medium? Illustrate your answer with reference to air, muscle and bone, and describe briefly the effect of varying the energy of X-rays.

c.   Define 'absorbed dose' and 'dose equivalent' and state the units in which each is measured. Why is the 'quality factor' of different types of ionising radiation different? Give examples.

d.   Write an account of the importance of 'dose equivalent' to the principles of radiation protection.

e.   Discuss the 'free-air' ionisation chamber and the 'thimble' chamber as methods for measuring Exposure and absorbed dose. State and explain any practical advantages of the latter for use in a hospital environment.

f.   Describe three methods of measuring Exposure or absorbed dose which might be used in a hospital environment. Discuss briefly the effect on each of these methods of the variation of the energy of X-ray beam.

SUMMARY

1.   Radiations capable of ionising the atoms of a medium through which they pass are called 'ionising' radiations. These include charged particle beams (electrons, protons, α-particles) as well as X and γ-radiation and neutrons.

2.   The Exposure is a measure of the ionisation produced by an X or γ-ray beam at a given point in air and is expressed as the total charge produced (primary and secondary electrons) per unit mass, i.e. coulomb per kilogram (C kg^{-1}).

3.   The 'absorbed dose' is the total energy absorbed in a small volume in the medium per unit mass and is expressed in gray, where 1 gray = 1 joule per kilogram. This unit applies to all types of ionising radiation and to any medium. (1 gray $\equiv$ 100 rad.)

4.   If the absorbed dose is known in a given medium, the absorbed dose which would have been present in another medium may be calculated by multiplying by the ratio of the two mass absorption coefficients. In practice, the absorbed dose in air is measured, and the absorbed dose in a biological material (e.g. bone) calculated.

5.   Different ionising radiations produce different densities of ionisations along their tracks in the medium. Those that produce dense ionisations (α-particles, protons, fast neutrons) do greater biological damage than those that produce less dense ionisation (electrons, X-rays).

6.   Each radiation has a 'Quality Factor' assigned to it which estimates its biological effect compared to X-rays. The 'dose equivalent' is obtained by multiplying the absorbed dose by the Quality Factor, and has the unit of 'sievert' (Sv), where 1 Sv = 1 joule per kg, as for the gray. This unit is very

useful for radiation protection purposes in assessing the doses received by personnel.

7.   Absolute methods of absorbed dose measurement include calorimetry and chemical methods, but the most sensitive and practicable is the 'free-air' ionisation chamber, as described in 32.2.2.

8.   Other methods of detecting ionising radiations include:

thimble chamber
Geiger–Muller counters
scintillation detectors
thermoluminescent dosimeters
photographic film
semiconductor detectors.

Each of these may be used to estimate radiation doses after calibration against a standard. Corrections for quality (i.e. energy of photons) is necessary if the average atomic number of the detector is different from that of the medium under consideration.

33. Radiation protection

33.1 THE PURPOSE AND SCOPE OF RADIATION PROTECTION

The purpose of radiation protection is to produce and maintain an environment, both at work and in the outside world, where the level of ionising radiation is 'safe' for human beings. 'Natural' ionising radiations have always existed in our environment in the form of cosmic rays, natural radioactivity in rocks etc. and radioactivity within our bodies, both ingested and inhaled. These natural sources of ionising radiation thus constitute a lower limit to the radiation doses received by the population at large, and radiation protection procedures can do little or nothing to reduce this limit. At the outset of any discussion on radiation protection, it is therefore apparent that our environment is, and always has been, *relatively* 'safe' from the effects of such radiations. It follows from this that one of the basic tasks of radiation protection is to establish the *levels of risk* to the population due to the natural, or 'background', radiation, and also to the 'man-made' sources of radiation such as nuclear 'fall-out' from atomic weapons testing, radiation leaks and discharges from nuclear power stations, and from the medical use of radionuclides and X-rays. Table 33.1 shows the relative amounts of natural and man-made sources of radiation.

Once the levels of such risks have been ascertained, appropriate maximum radiation doses (33.4) may be set whose associated risk is no greater (and

Table 33.1 Sources of ionising radiation

Source	Average annual whole-body dose-equivalent (mSv)	Percentage
Natural background	1	65%
Medical irradiation	0·5	33%
Radioactive fall-out (^{14}C, ^{90}Sr, ^{137}Cs)	0·01	0·7%
Occupational exposure	0·008	0·5%
Radioactive waste disposal	0·002	0·15%
Miscellaneous (^{226}Ra luminous watches, high altitude flying)	0·008	0·5%

frequently much less) than the risks experienced from other aspects of life, e.g. risk of accidents, contraction of fatal diseases etc. Such maximum permitted radiation dose levels help to prevent a repeat of the suffering and early deaths of the pioneering workers in radiology who were subject to gross over-exposure.

The study of radiation protection therefore embraces many other topics, including radiobiology, genetics, the fate of radioactivity released into the environment, the absorbing power of different materials to different radiations, the statistical analysis of risk, and the recommendation of various procedures to reduce the dose received by radiation workers and the population at large. Such a vast scope of study cannot be encompassed within one chapter, or even one book, and only a simplified treatment of some of these topics is considered in the following sections.

33.1.1 Ionising Radiations Regulations (1985)

The above comments indicate the tremendous scope of radiation protection and the need for multi-disciplinary collaboration in tackling some of its problems. Radiation protection is a developing subject where the acquisition of new knowledge is used in the formulation of safer procedures and lower doses. Prior to 1985, the main publications concerning the general aspects of radiation protection were:

a. *The Code of Practice of the Protection of Persons against Ionising Radiations arising from Medical and Dental Use* (published by HMSO).

b. *Recommendations of the International Commission on Radiological Protection* — ICRP publication 9 (published by Pergamon Press).

c. *Annals of the ICRP* — ICRP publication 26 (published by Pergamon Press).

d. *Official Journal of the European Communities*, Vol. 19, No. L 187. Available from HMSO.

e. *Ionising Radiations — Proposals for Provisions on Radiological Protection*. Health and Safety Commission. Available from HMSO.

Since joining the EEC, Britain has become subject to centralised policy decisions from Brussels. The 'Euratom Directive' (or 'EEC Directive') arises from a laudable attempt to standardise and modernise the radiation protection practice of all member states. This Directive in preliminary form is publication (d) above. However, since that document was prepared (1976), publication (c) was produced by the ICRP (1977) which contained some substantial changes of approach from the earlier ICRP publication shown in (b).

The original Euratom Directive has been influenced by the recommendations of ICRP 26 and other representations, and has resulted in the publication of the *Ionising Radiations Regulations 1985* (*IRR*). These regulations were laid before Parliament on 4th September 1985, and came into operation on January 1st 1986. They apply to work carried out with ionising radiations both in the private sector and within hospitals (i.e. Crown property). For the private sector, an inspector of the Health and Safety

Executive (HSE) is able to serve a notice to the employer in order to enforce compliance with the Regulations, and is also able to prosecute individuals within a court of law for offences against the IRR. On Crown property, however, although the HSE could serve a 'Crown Notice' in cases where the IRR was not being implemented in a satisfactory manner, the HSE would not take proceedings against an individual in circumstances where the employing health authority was responsible. Nevertheless, an individual who deliberately broke the law and thereby jeopardized the health or safety of others may be prosecuted.

The Ionising Radiations Regulations (IRR) is therefore a document which has a legal foundation, and so represents a considerable departure from the Code of Practice (reference a above), where radiation workers were expected to comply on a 'voluntary' basis. Even in this case, of course, considerable pressure could be exerted by the HSE when bad practice was encountered, and individuals who did not comply were liable to prosecution if an accident occurred as a result of their bad practice. Under the IRR, such an individual is liable to prosecution *before* an accident occurs. However, the full consequences of the IRR will not be worked out in detail for a number of years, owing to the range and complexity of work activities carried out with ionising radiations.

The Regulations contain the *fundamental requirements* needed to control the exposure to ionising radiation, both of radiation workers and members of the public. Details of acceptable methods of meeting those requirements are given in a supporting document: the *Approved Code of Practice (ACoP)** which was approved by the Health and Safety Commission on 3rd September 1985. The IRR contains a total of 41 Regulations divided into 9 parts, where the general principles of good radiation practice are laid down. In addition, there are 10 'Schedules' at the back of the publication which deal with specific points such as values of current dose limits, requirements for designation of controlled areas and information which the HSE requires from an employer before being able to start work with ionising radiation. The ACoP takes the Regulations in the IRR one at a time, and indicates acceptable ways in which they may be implemented. Some of the many recommendations in the ACoP are discussed later in this chapter. The reader is strongly advised to study both the Ionising Radiations Regulations and the Approved Code of Practice, as only a few essential Regulations may be considered here.

33.2 BIOLOGICAL EFFECTS OF IONISING RADIATION

It has been shown (25.5) that X and γ-rays are capable of ionising matter through which they pass — hence the term 'ionising' radiation. The ejection of electrons from the atoms and molecules of the material means that *atomic bonds are broken*. This is true even if an electron from the inner K shell is ejected (for example), since the resulting cascade of electrons falling down into lower orbits (25.5.3) produces an electron vacancy in the outer 'valence' shell

---

* all quotations from the IRR and ACoP are published with the permission of the Controller of Her Majesty's Stationery Office.

and so disrupts the 'valency' or bonding between the atoms (25.4).

If all the ions formed in tissue by the primary and secondary ionisation processes (32.1.1) were capable of recombining exactly as they were before, then no radiation damage whatsoever would occur in the tissue. Some such recombination takes place (in about 10^{-11} s), but the breaking of the chemical bonds produces 'free radicals', which are highly chemically reactive ions capable of forming new bonds to other ions. Thus, the absorption of energy from an X-ray beam (or internally administered radionuclide) produces *ionisation*, which produces *chemical changes*, which produces *biological damage*. The biological damage so caused may be categorised into two headings: 'stochastic' and 'non-stochastic'.

33.2.1 Stochastic effects

A stochastic effect is one which occurs as a result of the laws of chance, or probability. For radiation-induced effects, the probability of a stochastic effect occurring depends upon the radiation dose received, but there is no such thing as a 'safe' dose, i.e. no 'threshold' dose exists below which such an effect cannot occur.

The two important stochastic effects due to exposure to ionising radiation are the *induction of cancer* in its various forms, and the influence of the radiation on future generations, i.e. *genetic* effects. In both these cases, the lower the radiation dose received, the smaller is the chance of their occurrence, but this chance in always greater than zero.

Another important point concerning such stochastic effects is that the *severity of the effect is unrelated to the radiation dose*. Thus, as the radiation dose increases, the probability of cancer induction increases (for example), but the severity of the cancer does not depend upon the radiation dose which caused it.

Genetic effects

The cause of radiation-induced genetic effects is the damage to the genes and chromosomes of the germ cells (eggs in the ovaries and spermatozoa in the testes) caused by ionising radiation. Biological damage to the chromosomes is due to ionisation and subsequent faulty recombination of the molecules which make up the chromosomes. The biological 'code' contained by the genes on the chromosomes has thus been altered and constitutes an abnormality in structure which may be passed on to the chromosomes of the next (and succeeding) generations, if indeed successful reproduction is possible. Severe genetic effects (e.g. congenital malformations) tend to be eliminated from the population because of the increased likelihood of early deaths amongst those affected. However, less severe effects, involving slight physical or functional impairment, are more likely to become part of the common 'gene-pool' of the population by mating. Thus, future generations must be protected from an unacceptably high proportion of defective genes by the reduction of the radiation does received by the population. In practice, this means reducing the contribution of 'man-made' radiations to a minimum, by the use of the appropriate radiation protection procedures. The *gonad* dose in radiographic investigations must therefore be reduced as far as possible by the use of good equipment and technique (33.6).

Radiation-induced cancer

Cancers induced by radiation often develop many years after the radiation was received. This is known as the *latent period*, and may extend up to 30 years.

The risk of inducing a particular type of cancer is measured by the number of cancers produced in excess of those expected from the normal (i.e. unirradiated) population. The amount of risk is determined by the 'risk factor':

Definition

The *risk factor* is the estimated likelihood of the occurrence of a particular radiation-induced effect per unit dose-equivalent received by each member of the population considered.

As shown in the previous chapter (32.1.4), the unit of dose-equivalent is the sievert (Sv). The risk factor may be estimated for both stochastic and non-stochastic effects.

If the risk factor of a particular effect is r, then we may express r mathematically as:

$$r = \left(\frac{\text{no. of cases}}{\text{size of population}} \right) \Big/ \text{dose equivalent received} \qquad \text{Equation 33.1}$$

The units of r are 'fraction per sievert', i.e. Sv^{-1}.

Example

The risk factor for radiation-induced leukaemia is estimated to be about $2 \times 10^{-3} \ Sv^{-1}$. This means that, if the members of a population each receive 1 Sv, then the fraction of the population developing leukaemia is 2×10^{-3}. Hence, if the population consisted of a million individuals, then about $10^6 \times 2 \times 10^{-3} = 2000$ leukaemics will occur. The sievert is a very large unit of dose-equivalent (100 rem — see Appendix VI), so that the risk factor, although not zero, is very small.

Exercise 33.1

If 5 million people each receive 0·02 Sv, how many cases of radiation-induced leukaemia would you expect? (risk factor $= 2 \times 10^{-3} \ Sv^{-1}$).

The risk factors for other radiation-induced cancers (e.g. bone, lung, thyroid) are of a similar, or smaller value. Some tissues are more sensitive to radiation than others. For example, large-scale 'screening' of the breast by X-rays is not to be recommended, as the sensitivity of the breast to radiation may result in more induced cancers than are detected. Also the fetus is sensitive to radiation, particularly in the early stages of development. Hence women who may be pregnant should not, unless there is good reason, by X-rayed during this period (33.4.3).

As with radiation induced genetic changes, the incidence of radiation-induced cancers is reduced by minimising the radiation dose received (see 33.6).

33.2.2 Non-stochastic effects

A non-stochastic radiation effect is one whose severity increases with the radiation dose, and for which there may be a 'threshold' value below which the effect will not occur.

Conceptually, therefore, the difference between a stochastic and a non-stochastic effect is that, for a radiation dose above a given value, the non-stochastic effect *always* occurs while a stochastic effect *may* occur. Examples of non-stochastic effects include erythema (reddening of skin due to radiation), the formation of a cataract in the lens of an eye, radiation damage to the gut, and the production of temporary or permanent sterility in both males and females.

The radiation doses required to produce such effects are very large, and are likely to occur only in radiation accidents. For example, total absorbed doses of 20 Gy (2000 rad) are required to damage the skin, 15 Gy to produce a cataract, and about 7 Gy to produce permanent sterility in males by irradiation of the testes.

A whole-body dose of 50 Gy results in death within a few days as a result of damage to the bone marrow, gut, and central nervous system.

Insight

The classification of radiation-induced damage in terms of stochastic and non-stochastic effects is relatively recent. An alternative method of classification is *somatic* and *genetic*, where 'somatic' refers to damage to the individual, and 'genetic' to future generations. Thus, somatic damage includes both non-stochastic effects and radiation-induced cancer, the latter being a stochastic effect, as shown above.

33.3 RISK-BENEFIT, ALARA AND DETRIMENT

In view of all the possible effects of radiation on individuals and their future generations, no unnecessary radiation dose should be received by them. Thus, no radiological investigation should be embarked upon unless there are sound clinical reasons why the patient would be likely to benefit from such an investigation. The need to reduce the radiation doses received by patients and staff alike during these investigations has been stressed in previous chapters and is reiterated here. For example, the radiation dose received by the patient is reduced with use of proper beam filtration (Ch. 29) and the use of 'fast' screen/film combinations (27.5.1). Radiation doses received by staff are minimised by the use of good technique (33.6).

As described above, all exposure to ionising radiation is associated with certain risks in that there is a probability (albeit very small) of non-reversible damage to living tissues. However, it is not necessary to become alarmed or despondent about this, because the benefit received by a patient as a result of a radiograph may easily far outweigh any considerations of the potential hazards from the radiograph itself. For example, it is obviously better to take a radiograph of a patient who has a suspected skull fracture than to be over-concerned with the extremely small chance that he or she might thereby develop leukaemia in 20 years' time. This weighing of the possible risks against the likely benefits of a radiograph is called 'risk/benefit', and although many such clear-cut cases as the above exist, there is an area of uncertainty where the clinical judgement of the radiologist has to be made in the inevitable absence of reliable clinical information as to the patient's true condition or likely benefit.

Obviously, then, the risk of radiation-induced effects occurring is reduced when the radiation dose received is reduced. However, it is not practicable in modern society to reduce radiation doses to zero, particularly for *occu-pationally-exposed workers* (33.4.1), so that a balance must be achieved between the desired low doses and the cost or difficulty of achieving those low doses. This is the so-called ALARA Principle, introduced in ICRP 26, which is an acronym for '*As Low As Reasonably Achievable*'. The IRR has a very similar term for the same concept: '*As Low As Reasonably Practicable*'.

Radiation exposures due to a particular investigation (e.g. a radiophar-maceutical preparation or X-ray technique) are analysed in terms of the benefits likely to result and the cost and difficulty of reducing the detrimental effects of the radiation received to different levels. An appropriate practical solution is chosen where the expenditure of a lot more money and effort will have only a small effect on the radiation doses received. For example, the use of robotic arms for the dispensing of radiopharmaceuticals in a hospital laboratory would undoubtedly reduce the radiation dose received by the staff by a small amount, but at a very high cost in terms of financial outlay and at considerable inconvenience to the staff themselves. However, the use of lead shielding on benches is a much cheaper solution, and greatly reduces the radiation reaching the staff during these procedures. Further, the use of good technique, such as using long forceps and reducing the time taken for the radioactive dispensing by good work organisation, also has a significant role to play in minimising radiation doses. Thus, a high-cost high-technology solution is not always appropriate.

It would often be difficult to choose between various practicable solutions to working safely with radiation unless a *quantitative* assessment of the detrimen-tal effects of radiation were possible. The *detriment* due to radiation has a precise mathematical meaning, and is defined in ICRP 26 as:

'*The detriment is the expectation of harm incurred from an exposure to radiation, taking into account not only the probability of each type of deleterious effect, but also the severity of the effect.*'

The risk factors discussed above (33.2.1) are of value in assessing detriment.

33.3.1 Radiological examinations of women of reproductive capacity

The relative sensitivity of the fetus to ionising radiation (33.2.1) means that it is good radiographic practice to avoid all radiological investigations of the lower abdomen to women who may be pregnant unless there are overriding clinical considerations. Such considerations may include suspected fetal malformation or an essential investigation for the mother-to-be.

The ovum is particularly sensitive to radiation during the seven weeks prior to ovulation. Also, irradiations performed in the latter stages of pregnancy are not without hazard, albeit at a lower level of risk than the normal risks associated with any pregnancy. It is therefore important to attempt to ensure that the benefits of any radiological investigation of a pregnant woman, or one who *may be pregnant*, outweigh the risks involved, as outlined in the previous section.

The recommendation of the ICRP in 1970 was the women of reproductive capacity should only be X-rayed within 10 days of their last menstrual period (LMP), since pregnancy was then highly unlikely. This was known as the *Ten-Day Rule*. However, in 1984 the ICRP gave new guidelines as a result of a more accurate estimate of the risks and benefits associated with radiographs taken on such women before and after conception. The relevant paragraph reads as follows:

> *During the first ten days following the onset of a menstrual period, there can be no risk to any conceptus, since no conception will have occurred. The risk to a child who had previously been irradiated in utero during the remainder of a four week period following the onset of menstruation is likely to be so small that there need be no special limitation on exposures required within these four weeks.*

In addition, the National Radiological Protection Board (NRPB) added some recommendations in 1984, which are summarised below:

> a. *Any woman who has an overdue or missed period should be treated as though she were pregnant.*
> b. *If the woman cannot answer 'No' to the question 'Are you, or might you be, pregnant?', then she should be regarded as if she were pregnant.*
> c. *If the clinical indications are that an exposure must be made where the primary beam irradiates the fetus, then great care must be taken to minimise the number of views and the absorbed dose per view, but without jeopardizing the diagnostic value of the investigation.*
> d. *Provided good collimation is used, and properly shielded equipment, radiographs of areas remote from the fetus (e.g. chest, skull, hand) may be done safely at any time during pregnancy. (Reproduced by kind permission of the NRPB.)*

The demise of the Ten-Day Rule in favour of the new recommendations does not reduce the care which should be taken in reducing the potential radiation dose to the fetus. The change in emphasis of the recommendations is that special precautions need only be taken if the woman is, or may be, pregnant — where 'pregnant' is defined as beginning when a period is overdue. Other than this, there need be no special limitation on exposures during a cycle. Good technique should be used at all times, of course, to minimise doses for all investigations.

A *flowchart* showing the progress of a woman of reproductive capacity through a department of radiology is shown in the summary section of this chapter.

33.4 DOSE-EQUIVALENT LIMITS

The Ionising Radiations Regulations has followed the recommendations of ICRP 26 in using the term *Dose-Equivalent Limits* (DEL) in preference to *Maximum Permissible Dose* (MPD) as used in the 'old' Code of Practice. The author has attempted to use the newer terminology throughout this chapter.

The setting of dose limits to individuals and various groups of individuals is an extension of the risk/benefit principle outlined above (33.3). In the estimation of such limits, the effect of 'natural' background radiation and radiation from medical investigations is not included. This is because the former is largely beyond control so that no practical purpose is served in its inclusion, and the latter is because the individuals who are irradiated in the course of a medical investigation are assumed to benefit directly from such an irradiation. Thus, they fall outside the more general calculations of risk/benefit.

The limits discussed below should not be viewed as constituting boundary lines between safety and danger, should any particular limit be exceeded. Rather, they reflect levels of risks, either to the individual or to groups within the population, which are comparable to the risks from other activities within society which are already considered to possess an adequate degree of safety. There is therefore no abrupt increase in hazard if the radiation dose limit is exceeded; only an increasing (but still small) probability of a stochastic effect (33.2.1) occurring after some suitable latent period. If the limit is grossly exceeded, then various prompt non-stochastic effects (33.2.2) will occur.

Insight

The assessment of socially acceptable risk in various occupations and to the general public produces figures in the range of 10^{-6} to 10^{-5} per year, implying that there is a chance of between 1 in 100 000 and 1 in a million of an individual dying as a result of the hazards involved. If we take the figure of 10^{-5} and apply it to Equation 33.1, then the annual dose-equivalent limit is 1 mSv (see 33.4.2) if it is assumed that the total risk factor of all stochastic effects due to radiation is 10^{-2} Sv^{-1}. The use of stochastic effects to derive the dose-equivalent limits is chosen because such effects show no 'threshold' (33.2.1) and are therefore more significant than non-stochastic effects for the lower radiation doses. The dose-equivalent limits are thus chosen to prevent non-stochastic effects and to minimise the occurrence of stochastic effects to a socially acceptable level.

Effective Dose Equivalent

ICRP 26 introduced the concept of *effective dose equivalent* in order to take account of the fact that organs show different sensitivities to radiation. Thus a given dose delivered to an organ of high sensitivity carries greater risk than if the same dose was received by an organ of lower sensitivity. In the former case, a higher *effective* dose is said to have been received. Each organ is therefore given a 'weighting factor' which represents its sensitivity in relation to that of the whole body when the whole body receives the same dose. A more formal definition of a weighting factor is as follows:

Definition

The *weighting factor*, W_T, of a particular tissue or organ is the risk of stochastic effects being induced in the organ when singly irradiated compared to the total risk of inducing stochastic effects if the same radiation dose is received by the whole body.

The various weighting factors for different tissues are shown in Table 33.2. As shown, the gonads are the most sensitive tissues as they have the highest value of weighting factor. Notice that the sum of all the weighting factors is unity.

Table 33.2 Weighting factors for different tissues irradiated singly

Tissue	Weighting factor (W_T)
Gonads	0·25
Breast	0·15
Red bone marrow	0·12
Lung	0·12
Thyroid	0·03
Bone	0·03
Remaining 5 most sensitive tissues (5 × 0·06)	0·30

N.B. Sum of weighting factors = 1·0

The unit of the effective dose equivalent is just the same as that of dose equivalent, since the weighting factors are constants. Hence effective dose equivalents are expressed in sievert (Sv) or, more usually, millisievert (mSv) — see 32.1.4 for the definition of dose equivalent in sievert.

The *Ionising Radiations Regulations* has retained the use of effective dose equivalent for the determination of whole-body dose, but not in setting the dose equivalent limits for individual organs (these were obtained by ICRP 26 by dividing the annual whole-body dose equivalent limit by the weighting factor for each organ). See Table 33.3 for the relevant limits.

The following examples indicate how the weighting factors shown in Table 33.2 are used to determine the effective dose equivalent for two situations: when the whole body has been irradiated, and for a chest X-ray.

Example 1

Each tissue in the body receives a dose-equivalent of 2 mSv. What is the whole-body dose equivalent (i.e. the overall effect of these doses)?

The effect of the gonad dose is $2 \times 0\cdot25$; the breast $2 \times 0\cdot15$ etc., so that if all the factors are added together, we obtain:

$$\text{Effective dose equivalent} = 2 \times \text{sum of weighting factors}$$
$$= 2 \times 1 = 2 \text{ mSv}$$

which is the whole-body dose actually received.

Example 2

A chest X-ray produced the following doses: gonads $0\cdot01$ mSv; breast $0\cdot05$ mSv; red bone marrow $0\cdot005$ mSv; lung $0\cdot15$ mSv; thyroid $0\cdot02$ mSv; bone $0\cdot005$ mSv; stomach $0\cdot05$ mSv; small intestine $0\cdot01$ mSv; upper larger intestine $0\cdot002$ mSv; lower large intestine $0\cdot001$ mSv. What is the effective dose received by the patient?

Taking each value of dose-equivalent and multiplying by each weighting factor, we have:

$$\begin{aligned}
\text{Effective dose equivalent} = {} & 0\cdot01 \times 0\cdot25 + 0\cdot05 \times 0\cdot15 + 0\cdot005 \times \\
& 0\cdot12 + 0\cdot15 \times 0\cdot12 + 0\cdot02 \times 0\cdot03 + \\
& 0\cdot005 \times 0\cdot03 + 0\cdot05 \times 0\cdot06 + 0\cdot01 \times \\
& 0\cdot06 + 0\cdot002 \times 0\cdot06 + 0\cdot001 \times 0\cdot06 \\
= {} & 0\cdot033 \text{ mSv (3\cdot3 mrem)}
\end{aligned}$$

The chest X-ray is therefore equivalent to a whole-body dose of about $0\cdot03$ mSv, for radiation protection purposes.

Committed Dose

This section concerns the absorbed dose which a person receives as a result of the intake of radioactive material. In this case, the person will continue to receive a radiation dose for as long as any traces of radioactivity remain within the body. The factors which affect the activity which remain are the *physical* half-life (5.2.2) and the *biological* half-life of the radionuclide in question. The biological half-life is the time taken for half of the radionuclide to be removed from the body or an organ within the body, and depends upon the chemical form of the radioactive compound. In the event of an accidental intake of activity, it may be possible to reduce the biological half-life (i.e. increase the rate of its excretion from the body or organ) by the use of compounds which strongly chemically bind the radionuclide, but which are not themselves readily taken up by body tissues. It is not possible to reduce the physical half-life, of course, since this is a characteristic of the *nucleus* of an atom rather than the orbiting electrons (which give the atom its chemical properties).

The *effective* half-life is the combination of the physical and biological half-lives and is the time taken for the activity within the body (or organ under consideration) to reduce to one-half of its value.

Insight

The physical and biological decay of radioactivity may be combined in a simple mathematical formula by combining the individual decay constants λ_p, λ_b in the following manner (see Insight in 5.2.2):

The rate of physical decay $= \lambda_p$. N, where N is the number of atoms

The rate of biological decay $= \lambda_b$. N

The total ('effective') decay rate $=$ physical $+$ biological decay rates
$$= (\lambda_p + \lambda_b).\ N$$
$$= \lambda_e.\ N$$
where λ_e is the 'effective' (total) decay constant

Hence, we obtain the result:

$$\lambda_e = \lambda_p + \lambda_b$$
$$\text{or} \quad 1/T_e = 1/T_p + 1/T_b$$

since the decay constant and half-life are inversely related (5.2.2)

Thus, the effective half-life is obtained by adding the reciprocals of the physical and biological half-lives, and taking the reciprocal of the answer. Care must be taken to keep to the same units during the calculation.

The effective half-life is only one of a number of factors which determines the magnitude of the dose equivalent delivered to the body, however. The other factors are the *concentration* of the activity (e.g. in MBq per kg) in the organ, whether the concentration is uniform or localised in 'hot-spots' within the organ, the *decay-scheme* (Ch. 26) of the radionuclide, the Quality-Factors (32.1.4) of the radiations emitted (there may be more than one type), and the size and shape of the organ. The decay-scheme is particularly relevant because particulate radiation (alpha or beta emission) has such a short range in tissue that it can produce an intense localised doserate within the organ if the activity is sufficiently high, whereas gamma radiation, having an exponential absorption within matter (30.1.2), will be only partially absorbed within the organ. The higher the energy of gamma radiation the lower the attenuation, so that the absorbed dose becomes less. The sensitivity of the organs or tissues to radiation, as measured by the weighting factors in Table 33.2, must also be taken into account in order to assess the *effective* dose equivalent which the body has received as a result of the intake of radioactivity.

The *committed dose equivalent* is a quantitative assessment of the effect of a particular intake of radioactivity over the whole of a person's working life. It may be defined as follows:

Definition

The *committed dose equivalent* is the dose equivalent accruing over a period of 50 years following the intake of radioactive material.

The committed *effective* dose equivalent is obtained using the weighting factors in Table 33.2, and once this figure has been obtained for a dose intake occurring over a given period it is compared with equivalent limits laid down by the IRR for the same period (e.g. annual or 'calender-quarterly' limits) for the appropriate category of person (classified, member of public etc). The dose limits stipulated by the IRR are shown in Table 33.3.

Table 33.3a Dose limits specified by Ionising Radiations Regulations

Category of Person	Effective Dose Equivalent plus Committed Effective Dose Equivalent for WHOLE BODY		Dose Equivalent plus Committed Dose Equivalent for Individual Organs	for Lens of Eye
	Annual	Calender Quarter[a]	Annual	Annual
Employees aged 18 yrs or more	50 mSv	30mSv	500 mSv	150 mSv
Trainees aged less than 18 yrs	15 mSv	9 mSv	150 mSv	45 mSv
Any other person	5 mSv	3 mSv	50 mSv	15 mSv

Note a – Any of the inclusive periods January-March; April-June; July-September; October-December

Table 33.3b Dose equivalent limits to the abdomen for pregnant women and women of reproductive capacity

Category	Dose equivalent to abdomen
Woman of reproductive capacity at work	13 mSv in any consecutive 3 month interval
Pregnant woman at work	10 mSv during the declared term of pregnancy

Note: These limits do not take into account any committed dose equivalent to the fetus, so special care must be taken to restrict radioactive intake for a pregnant woman.

Table 33.3a shows the dose limits for two categories of person whose work may subject them to ionising radiation (adult employees and trainees) and for 'any other person' who is not involved in work with radiation and therefore has the same dose limits as a member of the general public. Note that, in all cases, the dose limits for trainees are 3/10 of those for adult employees, and the dose limits for 'any other person' are 1/10 of those for adult employees. The whole-body dose limits are expressed in *effective* dose equivalent units (including the contribution of the committed dose), whereas the dose limits to individual organs are in dose equivalent units. The use of weighting factors in the determination of effective dose equivalent is described above. These are required to calculate the effective whole-body dose whether the body has been irradiated uniformly or non-uniformly.

Table 33.3b concerns the dose limits specified by the IRR in order to protect the fetus. The dose equivalents shown refer to the maximum values that may be received from *external* radiation, i.e. the committed dose from the intake of radioactivity is not included. Hence there is a need to restrict the possible intake of radioactivity, especially in working environments where radioactivity is more easily dispersed into the air. Note that a woman who does not work with radioactive substances is already subject to the lower limit of 3 mSv in any calender quarter shown in Table 33.3a.

Insight
It is worth recalling at this point that the unit of dose-equivalent, the sievert, is the absorbed dose times the quality factor (32.1.4). Now, the absorbed dose in gray (Gy) is measured in joule/kg and so relates to *unit mass*. The total energy absorbed in a man weighing 70 kg who has received a whole-body dose of 3 Gy is therefore $3 \times 70 = 210$ joule. The same absorbed dose (in Gy) received by the lungs weighing, say, 0·15 kg results in an absorbed energy within the lungs of $3 \times 0.5 = 1.5$ joule.

Therefore, the same values of dose or dose-equivalent in different organs do not imply the same total absorption of energy, but the same energy per unit mass. The biological effects of the absorbed energy depend upon the sensitivity of the organ to radiation, as described above.

33.4.1 Designation of workers

If an employee is 'likely to receive a dose of ionising radiation which exceeds three-tenths of any relevant dose limit' (IRR-regulation 9) then that person must be designated as a *classified person*, provided that:

a.   the employee is aged 18 years or more
b.   the employee has been certified as fit to be designated as a classified person on medical grounds
c.   the employee is informed of being so designated.

For example, if an adult employee is likely to receive in excess of 15 mSv (i.e. 3/10 of 50 mSv — see Table 33.3a) in a year, then he or she must be classified, and informed of this fact.

The Approved Code of Practice, in paragraphs 64 to 66, discusses some of the practical ways of implementing the designation of employees as required by the IRR regulation 9, and these may be summarised as follows:

a.   It is not sufficient to rely on an individual's history of doses received if they are less than the 'three-tenths' limit. The potential doses which may be received in the set of circumstances related to that individual must be assessed.
b.   The reason for designation may be that the individual works in Controlled Areas (33.5.3), but this is not necessarily a sufficient reason for designation. This situation is more applicable to industrial rather than medical workers.
c.   Even if the Local Rules (33.5.1), when strictly obeyed, indicate that doses in excess of the 'three-tenths' limit will not occur, persons who work with sources of ionising radiation which are capable of producing an overdose in a few minutes will need to be classified. However, this has limited application in

the medical field, since it was intended to apply to personnel working with industrial rather than medical sources.

d. When considering classification of persons in relation to the intake of radionuclides, the factors which should be taken into account are: the potential of any intake to occur, the likely magnitude of any intake and the radiotoxicity of any intake (e.g. tritium is much less toxic than radium).

A person who has been classified must be subject to *medical surveillance*, with periodic reviews of health at least every 12 months, and the health records on such an individual must be kept on a suitable form for at least 50 years from the date of the last entry on it (IRR regulation 16). The employer must also arrange for the dose which the classified person receives to be measured by use of a suitable personal dosemeter (33.5.2), and measured by an 'approved dosimetry service' on the basis of accepted national standards. Again, the employer must keep records on all doses recorded on such individuals for at least 50 years (IRR regulation 13).

Note that this does not mean that persons who are not classified should not have dose records and medical records kept, but that there is no legal requirement to do so. However, the Radiation Protection Adviser (33.5.1) may use personnel and site dose records to monitor and to justify his designation (or lack of it) both for personnel and for working areas.

Any employee, whether classified or not, whose annual whole-body dose exceeds 3/10 of the limit for employees aged 18 years or more, shall be subject to an investigation to see if the working practices involved are in keeping with the ALARA principle (33.3), or whether improvements may be made which would lead to lower doses. Records of all such investigations must be kept for at least 2 years (IRR regulation 28).

In a medical environment, employees such as radiographers, medical laboratory scientific officers and medical physics technicians are involved in work with ionising radiations in the fields of therapeutic and diagnostic radiology (including dental and mobile radiography), nuclear medicine and pathology investigations using radionuclides. Each of these procedures has its own contributions to the doses received by the appropriate personnel, and these have to be analysed to determine whether a particular individual needs to become a classified person, to conform to the requirements of the IRR. For example, a diagnostic radiographer is subject to ionising radiation from scatter from the patient or from the walls of the room, while a therapy radiographer receives some radiation through the walls of the treatment room, and may receive an unexpected dose due to a therapy source sticking in the exposed position.

Persons involved in nuclear medicine will receive a dose to the hands due to the preparation of radiopharmaceuticals and the handling of 'flood sources' for gamma cameras, for example. They will also receive a whole-body dose due to being in proximity to patients who have received diagnostic or therapeutic quantities of radioactivity. Laboratory technicians who perform chemical tests using radioactivity will also receive a hand dose, and perhaps be more prone to producing spills and breathing in airborne contamination.

However, it is unlikely that any of these workers will need to be classified, although the radiological monitoring of their received doses and that of their environment is a precaution, and one which may be used to justify their non-classified status.

33.4.2 Dose limitation for overexposed employees

IRR regulations 29 and 30 lay down the procedures to adopt if it is known, or suspected, that an employee has been subject to an overexposure. This overexposure may be as a result of a single incident, or because the total dose received by that person during the period in question exceeds the relevant dose limit for that period. *Medical exposures* do not apply.

After an overexposure has been reported to the employer, he must notify the HSE and the appropriate medical doctor, and arrange for a detailed investigation into the circumstances of the overexposure to be carried out. The HSE, the appointed doctor and the employee must receive a copy of the report, and it must be kept for at least 50 years. The overexposed person may be allowed to continue to work with ionising radiation provided that the above notifications and investigations have been carried out, and under any conditions which the appointed doctor may specify.

The dose limit for the individual for the remainder of the calender year is given by the appropriate annual dose limit for that person multiplied by $m/12$, where m is the number of months remaining in the year.

33.5 PRACTICAL RADIATION PROTECTION

As described in the preceding sections of this chapter, radiation protection is based on three general principles:

a. every practice resulting in an exposure to ionising radiation should be justified by the advantages it produces

b. all exposures should be kept as low as reasonably achievable (ALARA)

c. the sum of doses and committed doses received should not exceed specified limits (shown in Table 33.3).

The first two principles show that it is not sufficient merely to observe the current dose limits, since the possible health detriment from a given exposure must be compared to the overall benefit of that exposure, and may result in some procedures involving ionising radiation being either discontinued, or not started on these grounds alone.

The Ionising Radiations Regulations (1985) indicates the legal and procedural framework in which these principles may be achieved in practice. Some of the requirements of the IRR are listed below:

a. the provision of suitable *environments* for all employees, such that those areas where they are likely to receive a significant dose are suitably restricted and controlled (33.5.3)

b.   the designation of employees into classified and non-classified groups on the basis of the doses which they are 'likely to receive'

c.   the establishing of a suitable personnel monitoring service to ensure that radiation doses received are measured and recorded on a regular basis (which of the non-classified employees are monitored depends upon the local circumstances)

d.   the keeping of records (health and doses) on classified workers for the statutory period (50 years) required by the IRR

e.   notification to HSE of unusual incidents and overexposures, and the writing of reports subsequent to investigations of these incidents

f.   the establishment of *environmental* monitoring to establish that the working conditions of employees and the doses received by the general public are in accordance with IRR

g.   the appointment of 'suitably qualified' persons (RPAs) to act in an advisory capacity to the employer and to monitor the day-to-day compliance with the protection procedures laid down for each department where work with ionising radiation takes place (RPSs)

h.   the writing of suitable *Local Rules* for the establishment of safe working practices for employees

i.   the drawing up of contingency plans (e.g. what to do in the event of a fire in a radiopharmacy or telecobalt treatment room).

The designation of workers, personnel record keeping and the notification of incidents of exposure have been discussed previously. The appointment of RPAs and RPSs, the formulation of local rules, personnel monitoring methods and the designation of working areas are considered in the following sections.

33.5.1 RPAs and RPSs

Regulation 10 of the IRR states that if any employee is subject to an instantaneous* dose rate which exceeds $7.5\ \mu Sv/hr$ ($0.75\ mr/h$) or where the employer has already designated a Controlled Area (33.5.3), then the employer must appoint one or more Radiation Protection Advisers (RPAs). Any RPA must be a 'suitably qualified and experienced' person, and is appointed for the purpose of advising the employer as to the observance of the IRR and on all other aspects of the safe use of ionising radiation. The Health and Safety Executive (HSE) must have been notified of the person's details, including qualifications and experience, at least 28 days before the appointment, or at shorter notice if this is unavoidable. In order that the RPA may perform his advisory role effectively, the employer must provide him or her with adequate information as to 'job description' (i.e. details of what areas of work the RPA is supposed to give advice upon), and the facilities (e.g. equipment) with which to perform the duties involved adequately.

The RPA will be expected to give advice on all aspects of dosimetry and monitoring, the designation and control of restricted areas; drawing up written

* instantaneous dose rate means a dose rate 'averaged over one minute' (IRR)

systems of work and local rules, investigation of radiation incidents, the training of staff, comment on the design of new or modified premises from a radiation protection aspect, and the drawing up of contingency plans.

The RPA is also usually involved in the selection of Radiation Protection Supervisors (RPSs), who are persons directly involved with work with ionising radiations on a day-to-day basis. In a medical environment, for example, each department working with ionising radiation would have an RPS to ensure compliance with safe working practices. For example, the RPS in a diagnostic X-ray or radiotherapy department may be the superintendent radiographer, the RPS in a pathology laboratory may be a senior medical laboratory scientific officer, and the RPS in a physics department may be one of the physicists. Each RPS must have sufficient knowledge and experience in order to carry out the continual monitoring process essential for successful radiation protection.

Local Rules

The employer has a legal responsibility to ensure that written local rules are produced in compliance with the requirements of the IRR, and must bring the appropriate local rules to the attention of the employees. In practice, the RPAs have the necessary knowledge and experience to formulate these rules, and it is the task of the RPSs to see that they are known and put into practice by colleagues in their own departments.

The local rules for a given department should be displayed in a prominent position or positions within the department concerned, and should contain the following information:

a. the name of the RPS for the department
b. a description of each restricted area (33.5.3)
c. details of any restrictions of access
d. written systems of work detailing the working procedures
e. details of any contingency plans.

33.5.2 Personnel monitoring

It is necessary to measure the radiation doses received by exposed workers during the course of their work in order to verify that the doses received by them are within the recommended limits (33.4). This is known as 'personnel monitoring' and is a check not only upon the actual doses received, but also on the various radiation protection procedures as formulated by the RPA. Also, there is no doubt that certain individuals are temperamentally more lackadaisical in their attitudes to radiation protection than others and are examples of 'familiarity breeding contempt'. Such individuals may be spotted during the course of routine monitoring by the higher doses they receive compared to other workers. They may thus be warned to mend their ways for the benefit of the patients and themselves before their neglectfulness reaches serious proportions.

The main method by which personnel monitoring has hitherto been carried out is by the use of film badges, as shown in Figure 33.1. The photographic film becomes progressively more optically dense as a result of exposure to ionising radiations (31.2.1) and hence may be used to measure the radiation dose received by the wearer. The use of the plastic, tin and aluminium filters enables the distinction to be made whether the dose was as a result of beta particles or high or low energy X and γ-rays. Such films may either be processed within a department or sent routinely to a centre specialising in such a service, i.e. the National Radiation Protection Board (NRPB) at Harwell. Records of all doses so measured on a classified worker must be kept and a copy sent to any future employer where ionising radiations are used. The main disadvantage of the use of film badges is that any untoward dose received is measured *retrospectively* and may therefore be difficult to relate to the event which caused it. Secondly, photographic film is expensive, cannot be reused

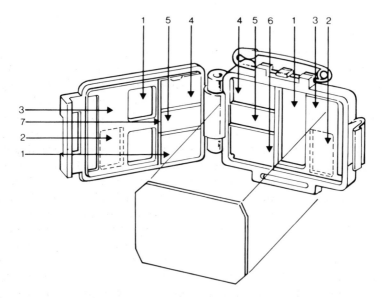

Fig. 33.1 A 'film-badge holder' and film as issued by the National Radiological Protection Board (NRPB), Harwell. The optically sealed film has a 'fast' emulsion on one side (facing the front of the badge) and a 'slow' emulsion on the other. If a high exposure to radiation has occurred, the fast emulsion may be removed and an estimate of the dose made from measurements on the slow emulsion. Various filters are used so as to separate the effects of different types and energies of radiation. These filters are numbered in the above diagram as follows: 1 — open window; 2 — thin plastic (0·020"); 3 — thick plastic (0·110"); 4 —0·040" of dural (an alloy of aluminium); 5 — 0·028" tin + 0·012" lead; 6 — 0·028" cadmium + 0·012" lead. 7 is a 0·012" strip of lead which shields filters 5 and 6, so avoiding any 'cross-over' effects between them. Beta particles are absorbed in filters 3 onwards. Only high-energy X- and γ-rays are able to penetrate the tin–lead filter (5) significantly so that an estimate may be made of the relative amounts of low- and high-energy X- and γ-rays by comparing the photographic densities beneath filters 4 and 5. The cadmium–lead filter (6) is used to estimate the exposure to thermal neutrons (for workers in the nuclear industry), because neutron-capture by the cadmium nuclei results in gamma emission which exposes the film. (*This illustration is reproduced by kind permission of the National Radiological Protection Board, Harwell.*)

and suitable emulsions may become increasingly difficult to obtain because of the withdrawal of Kodak from the market.

The use of *thermoluminiscent dosimeters* (27.4) obviates many of the disadvantages of the film badge. The dosimeters, in powdered form or as discs, are reusable and may be measured as frequently as desired on relatively inexpensive equipment. Further, the materials which make up the dosimeter (lithium fluoride) are not in short supply and there are several manufacturers who supply suitable designs. The small size of many specialised dosimeters enables them to be worn comfortably on the fingers, for example, so that a good estimate of the finger dose received in various procedures may be obtained. Thus, thermoluminescent dosimetry (TLD) is a flexible and efficient way of monitoring personnel, and it has the additional advantage of being suitable for computerisation, even in small departments, so that much of the time-consuming clerical involvement may be reduced. TLD is expected to gradually take over the functions of personnel and site monitoring from the film badge. However, it still suffers to some extent by being a retrospective test, as is the film badge. An example of a TLD 'badge' for personnel monitoring is shown in Figure 33.2.

Specialised devices which measure the radiation dose received by personnel and indicate any unusually high dose rates *at the time of exposure* have become available over the past few years. These are worn in the pockets of laboratory coats and are hence known as *pocket dosemeters*. There are a wide variety of different makes and models of such devices, which usually contain a very small Geiger tube to detect the radiation, and some battery-powered micro-electronics. When the dose rate exceeds some pre-set value, a warning noise is emitted and the wearer is able to take appropriate action. The more expensive pocket dosemeters also record the dose received and display it in digital form (rather like a digital watch). The choice of which occupationally exposed workers need to wear such a device is governed by an assessment of the likelihood of their receiving an unexpected high dose, as determined by the RPA (33.5.1). This is a more serious problem in radiotherapy departments than radiodiagnostic departments due to the potentially more serious consequences of an accident involving beams of radiation of very high intensity. Thus, it is quite common for radiotherapy radiographers to wear pocket dosemeters (in case, for example, a teletherapy source is stuck and the alarm in the treatment room also fails to work), but it is more usual for people in a diagnostic department to wear such devices when involved in special procedures, such as the holding of a restless patient.

33.5.3 Designation of working areas

In order to protect employees and members of the public from unnecessary amounts of radiation when on an employer's property, the Ionising Radiations Regulations 1985 (IRR-Regulation 8 and Schedule 6) makes a distinction between two types of area: *supervised* and *controlled*. The differences between these areas are summarised in Table 33.4. The employer, once having designated an area under his control as a controlled area, must demarcate or

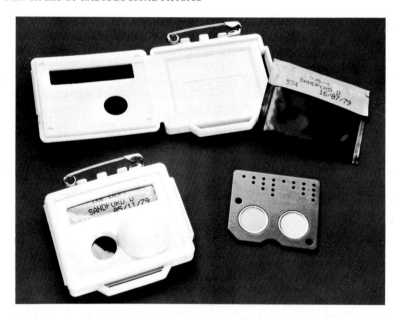

Fig. 33.2 The 'Thermoluminescent Dosimetry Badge' as supplied by the National Radiological Protection Board (NRPB), Harwell. The photograph shows the component parts of the NRPB body thermoluminescent dosemeter — the holder (*top left*) and the insert cover (*top right*) below which is shown the insert itself, with its two lithium fluoride/PTFE disks. Each insert is coded by holes punched in it, so enabling computerised record-keeping by the NRPB after automatic measuring of the doses received, under computer control. The holder has an open window over its 'thin' TLD disk (40 mg cm^{-2}) which is used to estimate the dose received by the skin (i.e. from electrons and low-energy X- or γ-radiation). The other 'thick' disk (90 mg cm^{-2}) is held under a 700 mg cm^{-2} thick dome of plastic and is used to estimate the whole-body dose (i.e. that due to X- or γ-radiation of higher energies). (*This photograph is published by kind permission of the National Radiological Protection Board, Harwell.*)

Note: The true thickness of a material (in centimetres, say) is obtained by dividing the value of the 'thickness' expressed in mg cm^{-2} by the density of the material in mg cm^{-3}.

otherwise delineate the area by some suitable means, and must restrict access to it. The area may be described with respect to existing walls, if this is convenient, but this is not possible if the source of radiation is mobile as in the case, for example, of a mobile X-ray unit. Access is best restricted by use of physical barriers rather than continuous supervision of the area unless the work concerned is of a short duration.

The only conditions under which a person may enter a controlled area are:

a.   the person is designated as classified (33.4.1)

b.   entry under a written scheme of work designed to ensure that, for an adult employee, 3/10 of any relevant annual dose limit is not exceeded. For any other person, the annual dose received must not exceed any relevant dose limit

c.   if the person is a patient undergoing diagnostic or therapeutic procedures.

Table 33.4 Description of designated areas

Name of Designated Area	Requirements for Designation	Permitted Access
Controlled Area	a. Area where instantaneous* dose rate exceeds 7·5 μSv/hr b. Area where adult employee is likely to receive more than 3/10 of any relevant dose limit (e.g. 15 mSv whole-body dose per annum)	a. Classified person b. Any other person under a written scheme or work c. Patient undergoing therapy or diagnostic procedures
Supervised Area	Area where any person would be likely to receive in excess of 1/3rd of the value required for designation of a controlled area (e.g. 5 mSv whole-body dose per annum)	Those whose presence is necessary

* dose rate averaged over 1 minute

Although the full implications of the requirements to designate supervised and controlled areas have not yet fully been worked out, it seems probable that, for diagnostic radiology, all X-ray rooms will become controlled areas, with no place for supervised areas. Obviously rooms used for therapy with external beams will also need to be designated as controlled areas, and areas may need to be demarcated outside these rooms if the instantaneous dose rate exceeds 7.5 μSv/hr. The designation of supervised and controlled areas around radioactive sources used for therapy depends upon the local situation, and it will be the task of the RPA to give advice on individual practices.

Each mobile and dental X-ray unit will have a controlled area associated with it during exposures whose extent may be approximated by 1 metre from the X-ray tube or the patient when operating up to 70 kVp, or 1·5 metre if operating above this value. No supervised area is necessary outside this area.

33.6 GOOD RADIOGRAPHIC PRACTICE

The importance of minimising the radiation doses received by patients and staff has been stressed in this and previous chapters. Methods by which this is accomplished are given in Table 33.5 (for patients) and Table 33.6 (for staff). It may be noted that some of the items listed are within the control of the radiographer (e.g. field size, screen/film combination etc.) and some are not (e.g. tube and wall shielding). By careful attention to detail the radiographer is able to produce excellent radiographs with the lowest practicable dose to the patient.

Fluoroscopy results in higher doses than conventional radiography, and it is here that good technique is essential to reduce these to a minimum. The use of image intensification has undoubtedly played a major role in this. Modern techniques of image intensification reduce the doses even further by, for

Table 33.5 Minimisation of radiation dose to patients

Factors not within radiographer's control:
Filtration of beam (Ch. 29)
Rectification (Ch. 20)
Tube shielding

Factors within radiographer's control:
Limitation of field size
Use of fast screen/film (consistent with required unsharpness)
Reduction of number of repeat exposures by careful alignment and selection of kV_p and mAs
Optimum film processing
Highest practicable kV_p
Use of autotimers to control exposure time
Use of gonad shields as appropriate
Selection of appropriate grid
Compression on obese patients

In fluoroscopy:
Adequate dark adaptation
Image intensification (with properly adjusted settings)
Radiation not to be continuous
Use of modern 'store and replay' systems (see text)

Table 33.6 Minimisation of radiation dose to staff

Only those whose presence is essential should be within the room
All staff should stand behind the protective barrier during the exposure.
X-ray units must have adequate shielding*
Use of immobilisation devices for restless patients, or patient held by member of family if possible

When required in front of barrier:
Staff must wear properly fastened lead–rubber aprons and gloves
Field size must be less than screen size
Staff should stand outside path of primary beam and as far away as practicable, because of scatter
Scatter reduced by use of lead–rubber flaps on image intensifier apparatus

* $2 \cdot 58 \times 10^{-6}$ C kg^{-1} in 1 hour ($\equiv$ 10 mR in 1 hour)

example, storing an image and replaying it to the TV monitor 'mixed' with the signal from the intensifier tube. The picture on the monitor is therefore composed partly of the pictures that went before and partly of the picture being produced in the intensifier, so that a much lower X-ray intensity is needed to maintain a picture of sufficient brightness on the monitor. Dose reductions by a factor of 10 are possible with this technique, and it is expected that such apparatus will gradually become increasingly common.

33.7 ROOM DESIGN

The purpose of an X-ray room is to provide an enclosure for the X-ray unit(s) in order to limit access to the radiation area (33.5.3) and to provide adequate shielding of the X-rays to the rest of the environment. In addition, provision is made for a 'barrier' inside the room behind which staff may be protected from radiation as they operate the units. If there is more than one unit within the room, then visual indication as to which tube is selected must be present and safety interlocks must ensure that it is possible to expose only one unit at a given time.. Also, protective barriers are necessary in order to protect one patient from the scattered radiation from another patient.

The thickness of absorbing barriers and walls is usually expressed in terms of their 'lead equivalent':

Definition

The *lead equivalent* of an absorbing material is the thickness of lead which would absorb the same amount of radiation as the given material when exposed to the same radiation.

The lead equivalent thus forms a basis of comparing one absorber to another at a given energy of beam.

At 'diagnostic' energies (up to about 150 kV_p), the photoelectric absorption within lead is significant, owing to the high atomic number of lead (30.4), so that protective barriers of a few millimetres of lead (laminated with wood) are adequate for the protection of staff within the room. 'Lead glass' windows are fitted into such barriers, enabling visual contact between the patient and radiographer to be maintained. The protection afforded by the window must be of at least the same amount as the protective barrier itself and there must be no gaps where radiation is able to penetrate. The siting of a barrier should be such that radiation must be scattered at least twice before reaching the opening of the barrier, thus greatly reducing its intensity.

Wall thickness must be such that any transmitted radiation will not produce a radiation dose exceeding 0·1 mSv in one week (i.e. 5 mSv per annum — the dose limit to the general public — 33.4.2). This figure is calculated from the measured transmission of X-rays through doors, walls, ceilings, floors and windows and applying a *use* factor. The use factor is the fraction of the time which the beam will be pointing towards a given area. As a result of this factor, the maximum weekly dose likely to be received by one person is estimated, and must be less than 0·1 mSv (10 mrem), as stated above.*

The materials used in the construction of the walls, floors and ceiling of a particular diagnostic X-ray room may contain thin lead sheeting, or be of sufficient thickness of other materials such as concrete to provide adequate absorption of the primary and scattered radiation produced within the room.

---

* The use of the so-called Occupancy Factor (the fraction of time for which a particular area will be occupied by people) has been discontinued, because it is often the case that the same person is involved in radiation work at different sites, particularly in industrial environments.

There is in addition a small component due to 'leakage' radiation through the shield of the unit. The lead equivalent of concrete walls 15 cm thick is approximately 1·5 mm within the diagnostic energy range, reflecting the superior absorption of lead to concrete. The use of 'barium sulphate plaster' as a coating on such walls shows increased absorption owing to the relatively high atomic number of barium (56) — the same reason why barium is used in 'barium meals'.

As the energy of the beam increases, the advantage of lead over concrete (say) diminishes because of the strong dependence of the photoelectric absorption on energy (30.4), so that the lead equivalent will increase with energy, i.e. a correspondingly thicker piece of lead will be required to produce the same absorption as the concrete. In the region of 1 MeV, where the Compton process predominates, there is no real advantage in using lead because all materials show very similar mass attenuation coefficients (30.1.3). This example is relevant to radiotherapy rather than radiography, but does serve to show that the lead equivalent of a material varies with energy of the X-ray beam.

In conclusion, the design of the room, its wall thicknesses and barriers must be such that the radiation dose received by staff and members of the general public is reduced to a minimum, in accordance with the main aims of radiation protection as discussed previously in this chapter.

Exercise 33.2
    a.   What is the purpose of radiation protection?
    b.   Outline briefly what is meant by the following terms:

    (i) stochastic effects
  (ii) non-stochastic effects
 (iii) somatic effects
 (iv) genetic effects

as applied to the biological effects of ionising radiation.
    c.   What factors determine the frequency of occurrence and the severity of the effects listed in the previous question?
    d.   What is meant by the term 'risk/benefit' when applied to the medical uses of ionising radiations? Give some examples of situations involving:

    (i) little risk with high benefit
  (ii) great risk with low benefit.

    e.   What is meant by the term dose equivalent limit (DEL)? What are the annual and quarterly values of the 'whole body' DEL for

    (i) occupationally exposed workers ('classified')
  (ii) occupationally exposed workers (16–18 years)
 (iii) members of the general public

Why are the doses received from 'natural radiations and medical investigation not included?
    f.   Explain why and how the '10-day rule' has been superseded.

g. Describe the organisational chain of command and responsibility which is set up in your hospital to ensure good radiation protection procedures (your answer should include reference to the employer, RPA, RPS, local rules and safety committees).

h. Discuss the relative advantages and disadvantages of personnel monitoring using film badges, thermoluminescent dosimeters and pocket dosemeters.

i. Define the 'lead equivalent' of a material. Explain why this may vary with energy of X-ray beam.

j. What factors must be taken into account in the design of an X-ray room in order to achieve adequate radiation protection to patients, staff and members of the general public?

SUMMARY

1. The purpose of radiation protection procedures is to reduce the radiation doses to a value which is 'As Low as Reasonably Achievable' (ALARA), consistent with achieving the maximum benefit which the use of ionising radiations can produce.

2. Stochastic effects of radiation are those whose likelihood increase with the dose received, but not the severity (e.g. genetic effects and cancer). There is no known threshold below which such effects will not occur.

3. Non-stochastic effects are those which exhibit a threshold and whose severity increases with the dose. Examples include cataracts and induced sterility.

4. The Ionising Radiations Regulations 1985 (IRR) and the associated Approved Code of Practice (ACoP) provide the legal and procedural framework for all aspects of radiation protection in the UK using ionising radiations, and has developed from the Euratom Directive of 1976.

5. The IRR lays down dose equivalent limits for various categories of persons which must not be exceeded (see Table 33.3).

6. Those employees who are likely to receive a dose of greater than 3/10 of the relevant dose equivalent limit (e.g. 15 mSv whole-body dose in one year) must be designated as classified.

7. Those areas in which employees are likely to receive greater than 3/10 of the relevant dose equivalent limit must be designated as controlled areas, the area demarcated, and access limited to either classified persons or persons who may enter under a written scheme of work.

8. Those areas in which employees are likely to receive a dose of greater than 1/3rd of that required to designate a controlled area are to be designated as supervised areas.

9. Radiation Protection Advisers (RPAs) are appointed to advise on all aspects of the safe use of ionising radiation, to help the employer draw up Local Rules for each department and to advise on the design of rooms and equipment from a radiation protection aspect.

10. Radiaton Protection Supervisors are appointed to ensure compliance with the Local Rules on a day-to-day basis.

11. Personnel and site monitoring are used to ensure adequate radiation protection techniques and procedures. Classified workers must be monitored, and records kept for at least 50 years.

12. All radiological investigations should minimise the radiation dose received by patients and staff (see Tables 33.4 and 33.5) but without jeopardizing the diagnostic value of the procedure.

13. The design of X-ray rooms should ensure that the staff are adequately protected by the use of protective barriers, and that the general public is protected by adequate shielding on walls, floors and ceilings and the appropriate levels of 'Use Factor'. The thickness of protective materials is normally expressed in 'lead equivalent', which will vary with energy if the material used is not lead (e.g. concrete).

14. The 'Ten Day Rule' for the diagnostic X-ray examination of women of reproductive capacity has been discontinued as a result of a more detailed examination of risk to the fetus. The flowchart summarises one procedure to adopt when a woman presents herself to be X-rayed. (Individual departments may have slightly differing procedures which still comply with ASP8.)

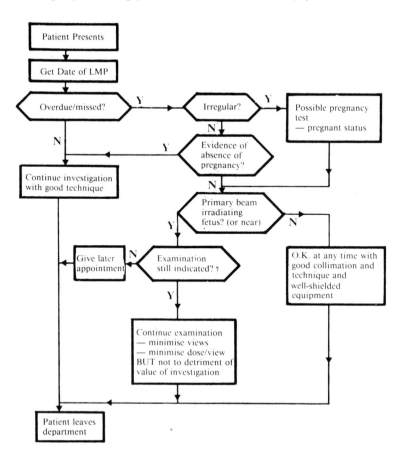

Part G
RADIOTHERAPY

34. Basics of radiotherapy

It is impossible to cover adequately in one chapter all aspects of the techniques of radiotherapy in the treatment of cancer. Only the general principles of this use of ionising radiation are discussed therefore, with reference to some of the material contained in earlier chapters.

The biological principles common to all forms of radiotherapy are discussed first, and then the three techniques of teletherapy, brachytherapy and radionuclide therapy are considered.

34.1 BIOLOGICAL PRINCIPLES

Cancer is second only to cardiovascular disease as the main cause of death in Western countries today. This situation has arisen partly as a result of the successes of modern medicine in the control of other diseases and the subsequent increased longevity of the general population.

The finding of a 'cure' for cancer is presently beset by many problems, not the least of which is lack of detailed knowledge of what a cancer cell actually is, or how it became that way. Even the behaviour of normal cells in a living organism is by no means completely understood, so that the behaviour of cancerous cells is a formidable problem.

For the purposes of this chapter, we may take the very simplified view that a cancer cell is one which has lost its ability to perform its specialised functions (e.g. as a liver or brain cell) and will therefore not respond correctly to the chemical 'messages' it receives from the adjacent normal cells and bodily fluids. It has therefore developed some form of internal control which cannot be overridden or regulated effectively by the organism as a whole. Such cells are often characterised by a higher metabolic rate than normal cells, and may reproduce quickly, so that a fast-growing ('malignant') tumour develops. Such cancer cells are described as being 'well' or 'poorly' *differentiated*, depending upon the degree to which they are like or unlike the normal cells from which they have grown.

The treatment of cancer lies in attempting to use a form of therapy which is able to turn the aberrant characteristics of the cancerous cells against them. Thus, the success of the therapy used depends upon the degree to which it affects the cancerous cells to a greater extent than the normal cells.

The three main forms of cancer therapy are surgery, chemotherapy and radiotherapy. These may be used in isolation or together to produce an optimum treatment regime for a given form of cancer in a given patient. The success of a particular treatment is measured in terms of the resulting *survival rate*, where the percentage of patients surviving beyond a given time is quoted, e.g. the 3-year survival rate for cancer of the bladder treated by radiotherapy is about 65%.

The reason for the relative success of radiotherapy in the management of cancer lies in the fact that cancerous cells are more sensitive to ionising radiation than normal cells within the same organ. Thus, it is possible to deliver a lethal dose of radiation to a tumour while normal tissues will be able to recover from the effects of receiving the same radiation dose. Some cancerous cells are much more *radiosensitive* than others, however. For example, an absorbed dose of 35 Gy (3500 rad) in 3 weeks is sufficient to destroy seminoma cells (a cancer of the testis), while 50 Gy (5000 rad) is required to destroy a meningioma (a cancer of the brain). Seminomas are therefore more radiosensitive than meningiomas, and hence more likely to respond successfully to treatment by radiotherapy. In general, the faster-growing tumours respond better to radiation than the slower-growing types, and this is due to the increased sensitivity of cells during mitosis (reproduction). Cell damage caused by radiotherapy treatment may be sufficient to prevent mitosis of the next generation, or subsequent generations, of cancer cells.

The radiotherapist decides from the details of a given patient whether the radiotherapy treatment is to be *radical* or *palliative*; the former being an all-out effort to achieve a cure, and the latter being used to relieve pain and other distressing symptoms present in the final stages of the disease.

34.1.1 Fractionation

Small volumes of the body are able to withstand the large doses required to destroy particular tumours. For example, cancer of the lip may be treated with a single dose of about 20 Gy (2000 rad). However, the treatment of larger volumes, particularly within the abdomen, requires the total treatment dose to be delivered over a number of treatments, rather than just a single treatment. This technique is known as *fractionation*, and has the great advantage of allowing the tissues to recover somewhat between treatments. Typically, 15 to 30 fractions may be given over a period of 3 to 6 weeks. The cancerous cells also recover to some extent between the fractions, so that the overall radiation dose must be increased slightly as the number of fractions increases in order to produce the same effect. A given patient may not be able to tolerate the normal number of fractions given to other patients with the same condition, so his treatment may be modified as a result of the effect of the first few fractions.

34.2 TELETHERAPY

Ionising radiation may be used in the treatment of patients in two ways: by the use of external beams impinging on the patient, or by sources of radiation being placed in contact with or within the patient's body. The first of these alternatives requires a source of ionising radiation to be at a distance from the patient, and is therefore known as *teletherapy* ('tele' — 'at a distance'), and is considered in this section. The second alternative is considered in the following section (34.3).

Many different types of ionising radiation have been used in radiotherapy, from X and γ-rays to electrons, protons, neutrons and negative pi-mesons (25.1). However, the vast majority of clinical radiotherapy departments have access only to therapy machines employing the relatively well-understood therapeutic properties of electromagnetic radiation, i.e. X and γ-rays, which are therefore the only types of radiation considered further in this chapter.

Historically, teletherapy using X-rays has been a story of ever-increasing beam energies. This is because the greater the (average) beam energy, the greater the penetration of the beam into the tissues, since the linear attenuation coefficient decreases with energy for both the photoelectric and Compton effects (30.4 and 30.5), and the contribution due to pair production (30.6) is very small in biological tissues of low atomic number. Thus, the beams of lower energy are suitable for the treatment of superficial lesions only, while the high-energy beams may be used to treat the more deep-seated lesions.

It was shown previously (28.2) that the energy of radiation generated by an X-ray unit is dependent upon the potential difference applied across the tube, and it is for this reason that X-ray beams used for therapy are broadly categorised in the following manner:

(i) *superficial* therapy beams (60–150kV$_p$)
(ii) *kilovoltage* or *orthovoltage* beams (200–300 kV$_p$)
(iii) *megavoltage* therapy beams (2–20 MeV).

All of these beams show a continuous spectrum of X-ray energies with an 'end-point' (28.2), and are heavily filtered (29.1) to remove the damaging 'soft' X-rays. Such continuous spectra are in contrast to the 'line' spectra obtained from the γ-ray emissions of radioactive sources (26.2), which may also be used to provide a beam of ionising radiation for the treatment of cancer patients. Such sources are known as *telecurie* sources and are well shielded with lead or depleted uranium (for example) owing to their very high radioactivity, e.g. 300 TBq (8100Ci). A consequence of the differences in the spectral shapes between the X-rays and γ-rays is that, in order to be equally penetrating in tissue, the X-ray beam must have an end-point which is of higher energy than the energy of the gamma ray(s) emitted by the radioactive source. For example, a 4 MV linear accelerator produces X-rays with an end-point energy of 4 MeV, and this is about as penetrating as the 1·17 and 1·33 MeV gamma rays emitted from a telecurie source of cobalt-60 (the decay scheme of ^{60}Co is shown in Figure 26.5 (26.3)). However, telecurie radiation beams have disadvantages compared to megavoltage beams, notably in their large penumbra (3.4.1), lower dose rates, need for periodic source renewal and their inability to be switched off. This latter point is important when the radioactive source may have stuck in the exposed position as a result of mechanical failure, such as the breaking of a spring. The patient is therefore overdosed on that treatment, and there is an obvious hazard to staff who have to enter the treatment room to move the source to the 'safe' position by other methods.

34.2.1 Beam characteristics

The absorption of a therapy beam within the patient's tissues results in a complicated pattern of absorbed dose within those tissues. In order to predict this, the pattern of absorbed dose within water is measured, usually by means of a small ionisation chamber (32.3.1) or semiconductor detector (32.3.6), since water corresponds well to the behaviour of the soft tissues of the body. The presentation of the absorbed doses so measured may be given in various forms. For example, Figure 34.1 shows the graphical representation of the absorbed doses measured along, and at right-angles to, the central axis of two different X-ray beams: 250 kV$_p$ and 4 MV. The graphs of dose at right-angles to the beam axis are often termed 'beam profiles'. As expected, the effect of increasing the energy of the beam is to make it more penetrating, as evidenced by the reduced fall-off of the dose with depth in tissue (left-hand figures). The maximum dose for the 4MV beam is below the surface of the tissue (point P in the figure) unlike the beams of lower energy. This is due to the greater range of the electrons produced in the Compton scattering process (30.5) in the first few millimetres beneath the surface. Such energetic electrons travel mainly in the

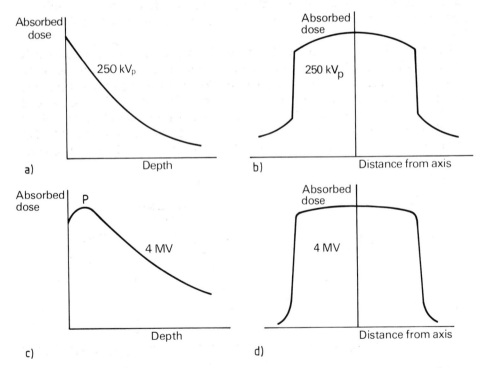

Fig. 34.1 Central axis and 'profile' absorbed doses due to a 250 kV$_p$ and a 4 MV beam of X-rays. Central axis doses are shown in (a) and (c), while profiles are shown in (b) and (d). The measurements are made in water.

same direction as the beam, and deposit energy in the tissue as they are slowed down by collisions. They thus come to rest at a significant distance from the site of the original Compton interaction, unlike those produced by the lower-energy X-ray beams in the figure (see discussion on kerma and absorbed dose in 32.1.2). This effect is known as *skin sparing* because the radiation dose received by the skin is less than that just below its surface — an important consideration in treating deep-seated lesions with a high dose, owing to the relatively high radiosensitivity of the basal layers of the skin.

The dose profiles, as illustrated by the right-hand figures of Figure 34.1, are characterised by small penumbra (a few millimetres) owing to the small effective size of the source of radiation, i.e. the 'focal spot' on the anode (3.4.1). The central portion of the beams is thus relatively fat, but reduces in value very sharply over the penumbral region. The 'tails' on the profiles beyond the penumbra are due to the scattering of the X-rays out of the primary beam. This scattering effect reduces as the energy of beam increases, as shown by the reduced size of the 'tails' on the 4 MV beam compared to the 250 kV$_p$ beam.

The low-energy X-ray beams deliver a higher absorbed dose to the bones than to soft tissue because of the significant contribution of photoelectric absorption to the overall absorption processes at these low energies. The megavoltage beams, on the other hand, are subject to relatively small amounts of photoelectric absorption compared to Compton events $\tau \propto \rho Z^3 / E^3$; $\sigma \propto \rho x$ electron density$/E$ — see 30.7), so that the absorbed dose in bone is similar to that of soft tissue, owing to the similar values of the electron densities of the two substances.

The axial dose variation and beam profile for a ^{60}Co telecurie source is shown in Figure 34.2, where 'skin sparing' is illustrated, as in the case of the 4 MV X-ray beam of the previous figure. The point of maximum dose (the 'build-up' point) is situated 5 mm below the skin surface. The penumbral width shown on the beam profile for ^{60}Co is significantly wider than that of the X-ray beam owing to the larger size of the radioactive source compared to that of the X-ray focus — typically 1 cm to 2·5 cm compared to 3 mm to 10 mm.

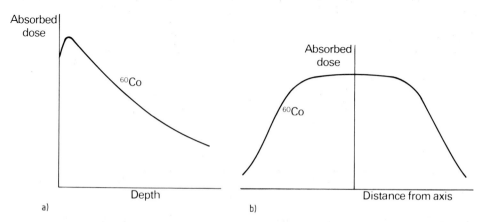

Fig. 34.2 (a) Central axis and (b) profile absorbed doses due to a beam of ^{60}Co gamma radiation in water.

Exercise 34.1

Estimate the size of the geometric penumbra at a distance of 100 cm from the source if the radioactive source has a diameter of 1·5 cm and the source-to-diaphragm-distance (SDD) is 30 cm. (Hint: see 3.4.1.)

The absorbed dose at a point within the beam has two components: the absorbed dose due to the unscattered ('primary') beam reaching the point, and the absorbed dose due to photons scattered within the whole beam reaching the point. The intensity of such scattered radiation depends in a somewhat complicated manner on the energy of the radiation, since the energy dictates the likelihood of scatter occurring, together with the attenuation and angular distribution of the scattered photons. (See also 31.1.3 for a more complete description of scatter and beam energy.)

The intensity of scattered radiation reaching a point within the beam always increases as the size of the beam (the 'field size' — 3.2) increases because of the additional scatter produced within the large beam compared to the smaller beam. Thus, large beams are said to be *more penetrating* than small beams of the same radiation since they produce a greater absorbed dose at the same depth, reflecting the greater absorbed dose due to the increased scatter. (The absorbed dose due to the primary beam does not depend upon the field size, of course.) Also, the *relative* amount of scatter compared to the primary beam also increases with depth in tissue. This relative increase in scatter is fairly rapid immediately below the surface, but then increases more slowly as the depth increases. This effect is due to the extra attenuation experienced by those photons scattered near the surface of the medium as they travel towards the deeper levels. Below a given depth, the magnitude of which increases with beam energy, the ratio of scattered radiation to primary radiation increases very slowly, and may be considered to be a constant. This reflects the almost complete attenuation of those photons scattered from points remote from these deeper levels.

As an illustration of the above points, consider first the gamma rays emitted from ^{60}Co, which form a 'line spectrum' with an average energy of 1·25 MeV (26.3). The passage of the gamma ray beam through tissue produces attenuation and absorption (30.2) of the beam due mainly to Compton scatter, where photons of lower energy are produced subsequent to the interaction process. The energy of the primary beam is unaltered in the attenuation events, although its intensity is reduced, of course. The relative amounts of scattered radiation compared to the primary beam increases with depth in tissue, as described in the previous paragraph, so that the overall spectrum of gamma rays has become 'softer', i.e. the average energy of primary plus scattered beam is less than the 1·25 MeV of the primary alone.

The spectra emitted by X-ray machines are continuous (28.2) and the primary beams are therefore subject to modification as they pass through tissue, unlike the case of ^{60}Co discussed above. The spectral modification is due to the preferential absorption of the 'soft' X-rays at the lower end of the energy spectra. (The effect of the resultant 'beam hardening' or the primary is taken into account in modern CT scanners Appendix IV.) Again, the relative importance of scattered photons increases with field size and depth for X-ray beams so that the absorbed dose at a point is significantly increased by the effect of such scatter.

A very useful way of presenting the information contained in the previous figures is obtained by plotting the pattern of absorbed dose in terms of lines of equal dose — the *isodose lines*. Examples of isodose lines forming isodose *charts* are shown in Figure 34.3, where the previous comments concerning penetration of beam with energy, skin sparing and size of penumbra are evident.

34.2.2 Wedges and compensators

A particular clinical condition may not be able to be treated adequately by teletherapy when using any combination of fields such as shown in Figure 34.3. This is because these 'open' fields may give rise to an unacceptably large variation in absorbed dose across the tumour volume ('unacceptable' normally means greater than 10%). However, it is possible to modify the isodose charts of these fields by the use of shaped absorbers called *wedges* placed in the path of the beams. Wedges modify the isodose charts by absorbing one side of the beam to a greater extent than the other, so that asymmetrical isodose lines are produced, as illustrated in Figure 34.4. The wedge symbol shown in the figure is drawn on the chart so that the thick end corresponds to the side of reduced penetration of the beam. The *wedge angle* is the angle at which the 50% isodose line cuts the central axis — as shown in the figure. An example of the use of wedges is shown in the next section.

The surface of the body is not flat, of course, so that the isodose charts obtained from measurements using a flat water surface will be modified by the presence of slope or curvature of the surface of the patient. This effect must be

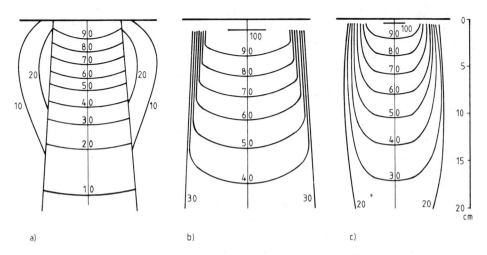

Fig. 34.3 Isodose charts for (a) 250 kV$_\mathrm{p}$ X-rays, (b) 4 MV X-rays, (c) ^{60}Co gamma rays. See text for the similarities and differences between these charts.

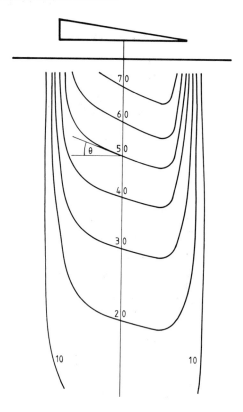

Fig. 34.4 A 'wedged' isodose chart. A wedge placed in the path of the beam absorbs one side of the beam more than the other, so producing 'sloped' isodose lines. The 'wedge angle' is given by the value of θ.

taken into account to achieve accurate treatments. It may be found that the isodose lines are not sufficiently symmetrical to produce a uniform dose distribution within the treated volume. This may be corrected by the use of another type of beam modification produced by *compensators*, which are individually designed absorbers placed in the path of the beam. The principle of the use of a compensator is shown in Figure 34.5, where it is seen that the presence of the compensator supplies the required amount of attenuation of the beam to correct for the 'missing' tissue. This has the effect of making the isodose lines similar to those of the corresponding 'open' fields (Fig. 34.3). Note that both wedges and compensators retain the 'skin sparing' effect of the high-energy beams, although this may be lost if the compensator is placed close to, or in contact with, the patient's skin. Compensators may be made of any suitable absorbing material, e.g. shaped wax or lead foil of different thicknesses.

34.2.3 Principles of beam summation

Even the most penetrating beams of electromagnetic radiation available to the

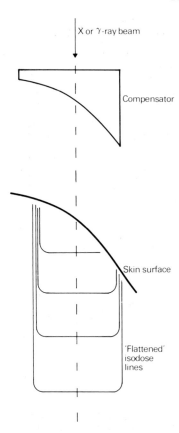

X or γ-ray beam

Compensator

Skin surface

'Flattened'
isodose
lines

Fig. 34.5 The action of a 'compensator' in flattening the isodose lines. In the absence of the compensator, the isodose lines would appear very like those shown in the previous figure.

clinician for the treatment of cancer will produce a smaller absorbed dose to a deeply seated treatment volume than to structures at shallower depths. Moreover, the dosage delivered by a single beam (or 'field') will vary significantly across the treatment volume so that some parts of the tumour will receive greater doses than others. The ideal situation is where an accurately known and constant dose is delivered to the whole of the specified treatment volume and no dose is given to the surrounding healthy tissue. This is impossible to achieve in practice, of course, but with careful placing of two or more beams it is possible to maximise the dose received by the tumour compared to normal tissue and to ensure that it receives a reasonably constant dose across it. The calculation of the overall effect of several fields is known as *beam summation*, and may be accomplished in two main ways: 'hand-planning' and by computer.

In the case of hand-planning, isodose charts such as shown in Figures 34.3 and 34.4 are placed on a cross-sectional view of the patient. The charts are then positioned at particular orientations (determined from experience), and the overlapping parts of the fields area added together and joined by coloured pencil to form the isodose distribution of the completed plan. These isodoses the represent the treatment which the patient will actually receive in practice. Some of the factors which are in the control of the hand-planner are:

a. number of fields
b. field sizes
c. distance of source from skin (SSD)
d. directions of fields
e. wedge types (if any) and their orientations
f. compensators (if any)
g. 'weighting factors' of each field, i.e. the amount by which the isodose values of a given field must be multiplied to achieve the desired result on the final plan.

The main disadvantages of the hand-planning method are its inherent inaccuracy and the slowness of the calculations. It is therefore possible to try only restricted number of plans, and the one chosen may not be the best that can be used. In addition, it is difficult to correct the isodose values satisfactorily for the effect of skin curvature and for tissue inhomogeneity (e.g. the effect of the presence of lung tissue).

The use of a computer to perform the task of beam summation is much faster than hand-planning and potentially more accurate. This is possible because of the high-speed computing power of modern computers, which enables the rapid automatic calculation of the doses received at a large number of points within the cross-sectional area. Skin curvature and tissue inhomogeneity may be automatically corrected for, and the resulting plan may be quickly inspected on a television monitor prior to being drawn on paper under computer control. The computer program is able to correct for the effect of different SSD's on the isodose charts, and may even be able to optimise the final plan by altering the field sizes, weighting factors, wedge types etc.

The increasing use of CT scanners (Appendix IV) has made it possible for the computer to receive the detailed information of the patient's internal structure to use to correct the isodose plan for the effect of tissue inhomogeneity in a much more accurate manner than hitherto; something which is far beyond the capability of hand-planning techniques. However, it is true to say that any plan is only as good as the data used to produce it, and (perhaps more importantly) only as good as the accuracy of the setting-up procedure of the therapy machines for a given treatment. The achievement of the best possible treatment to the patient is therefore more than a matter of performing accurate calculations, but such calculations set a goal to which the more practical aspects of radiotherapy must aspire.

Examples of computer-produced isodose plans are shown in Figure 34.6.

34.2.4 Simulators and CT scanners

In order to achieve a satisfactory dose distribution to the treatment volume and to give as little dose as possible to normal tissue, it is necessary to choose the smallest practicable field sizes and to align them accurately with respect to the patient's anatomy. It is possible to take 'check films' using the therapy machines set up in the treatment position and thereby check the accuracy of the alignment of the fields. However, the quality of the radiographs so obtained is poor owing to the lack of subject contrast (31.1.4), reflecting the dominance of Compton scatter at these high energies. It would therefore be difficult to be sure from the radiographs obtained that the treatment beams were the correct size, or even passed through the treatment volume at all.

This problem of poor contrast is overcome by the use of radiotherapy treatment *simulators*, which are able, by definition, to simulate (i.e. copy) the

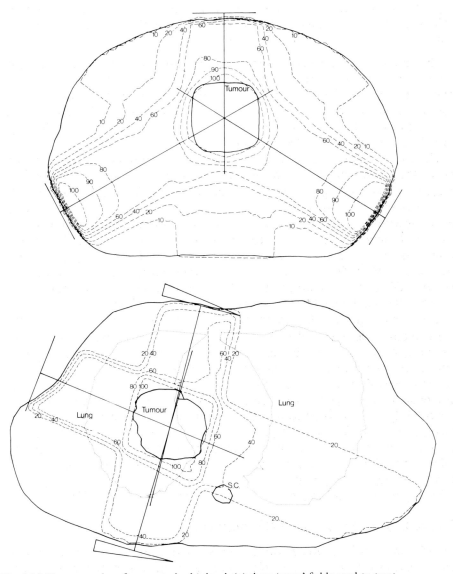

Fig. 34.6 Two examples of computerised 'plans': (a) three 'open' fields used to treat carcinoma of the bladder, (b) one 'open' and two 'wedged' fields used to treat carcinoma of the lung.

behaviour of the therapy machines in all respects other than the giving of the actual treatment. A conventional X-ray tube is used as the source of radiation in order to produce pictures of the same standard as the usual 'diagnostic' images, such pictures being produced either on a radiograph or on television monitors connected to an image intensifier. As in diagnostic radiology, contrast media may be used to delineate the treatment volume more accurately.

The use of a simulator enables the type of radiotherapy plan to be decided in some detail, including the sizes of fields and their angles of entry into the patient. In addition, if parts of the patient must be shielded from a beam, then it is possible to verify that the lead (or 'heavy alloy') absorbing blocks to be used on the treatment machine are of the correct shapes and sizes and positioned accurately before treatment actually begins. The progress of the patient's treatment may also be followed if desired, e.g. to estimate the amount of tumour regression and any corresponding changes in the treatment which may be required.

One main problem encountered when attempting to achieve accurate and reproducible treatments on a given patient is that the positioning of the patient may change slightly from treatment to treatment, or even during the same treatment. This is a practical problem which, if not solved, can make a nonsense of very careful and detailed beam summation calculations, to the detriment of the potential benefits received by the patient. Radiation fields to the head and neck are often of the smaller sizes, and it is in these cases particularly that the patient needs to keep still. This is accomplished using a *shell*, which is made of thin plastic moulded to the shape of the individual patient. Such a shell is fitted to the patient prior to each treatment, and firmly attached to the treatment couch to minimise any movement. Verification of field sizes and angles of entry may be performed using the simulator (see above) with the patient wearing the shell in the same way that it would be fitted for the therapy session itself. An example of a shell is shown in Figure 34.7.

Computerised Tomography (CT) has revolutionised many aspects of diagnostic radiology, and will doubtless have a profound effect on radiotherapy. The anatomical detail in the cross-sectional CT image enables the extent and location of a cancerous growth to be estimated to a high degree of accuracy, and is therefore of obvious advantage in planning the patient's treatment. It may well influence the decision as to the best way to proceed with the treatment (i.e. which combination of surgery, chemotherapy and radiotherapy) and whether the treatment should be radical or palliative. Also, as mentioned above, the 'CT numbers' on the image may be used to produce an idodose plan which is corrected for the difference in tissue composition (i.e. inhomogeneity).

The most modern simulators are able to perform all the usual functions of a conventional simulator and, in addition, to produce cross-sectional CT images. It is a logical extension of this to use the same computer which calculates the CT images to calculate the beam summations as well, so that future development in this field may involve much more computer control and automation of the simulator/planning system. This might include the

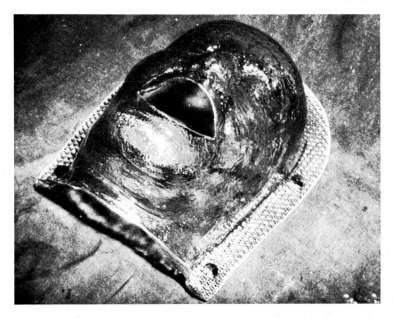

Fig. 34.7 An example of part of a 'shell' used in the immobilisation of a patient during radiotherapy treatment. (My thanks are due to Mr S. White, who made the shell and supplied me with this photograph.)

automatic estimation of size and position of the tumour and the production of an optimised plan before the patient has even left the simulator couch!

A relatively recent advance in the use of computers (or microprocessors) in radiotherapy is the automatic checking of therapy machine settings in an attempt to achieve consistently high accuracy and to reduce the chances of operator error.

34.3 BRACHYTHERAPY

External beam therapy (teletherapy) described above is not necessarily the best form of treatment using ionising radiation for all types and locations of cancers. Those localised lesions situated close to the surface of the body, or within a body cavity, may often best be treated by the use of sealed radioactive sources. This technique is known as 'brachytherapy', and consists of choosing a distribution of sources such that the treatment volume receives a uniform absorbed dose of sufficient magnitude to destroy all the cancerous cells while keeping the dose received by normal cells as low as possible in order to avoid non-reversible damage. In this way, the chances of either a recurrence of the tumour of the necrosis of healthy tissue are minimised.

The great advantage of brachytherapy over teletherapy lies in the rapid fall-off of dose rate with distance from the sources, owing to the effect of the Inverse Square Law (Ch. 4). It is thus possible to deliver a high dose to one area, and a much lower dose to another, fairly adjacent, area.

There are three types of brachytherapy; *surface, interstitial* and *intracavitary*, which are discussed briefly in turn. Surface 'applicators' or 'moulds' are arrangements of sealed radioactive sources which are applied to the surface of the body but kept at a small distance (usually 0·5 to 1 cm) from it. This technique is therefore suitable only for superficial conditions, such as skin and lip cancers, and is beneficial also in the treatment of cancerous conditions of the eye.

In interstitial therapy, the radioactive sources are introduced into the patient's tissues, and hence are often termed 'implants'. The sources may be inserted into the tissues directly, such as is the case for radium needles, or into narrow plastic tubing which has previously been positioned in or through the treatment volume (see 34.3.1 on afterloaders). The characteristics of some of the sources used are shown in Table 34.1.

The implant may be removable, as in the case of radium, or permanent in the case of gold-198 'grains'. This is because the half-life (5.2.2) of radium is very long (1620 years), but is only 2·7 days for ^{198}Au. Example of implants include treatments to the tongue by radium needles, gold grain implants into the pituitary gland, and various gynaecological treatments. 'Afterloaders' using radioactive wire for interstitial therapy are described below.

Intracavitary therapy is, as its name implies, the insertion of radioactive sources within the body cavities in order to treat the cancerous conditions found within them. These mainly involve cancer of the cervix, uterus and vagina. Radium or caesium-137 sources within plastic or nylon balls ('ovoids') and rods are introduced into the vagina and cervix. These sources are arranged to give as uniform a dose to the cancerous tissue as possible, but without overdosing adjacent radiosensitive areas such as the urethra and rectum.

34.3.1 Afterloaders

In recent years, the use of radium for radiotherapy has gradually declined in favour of other radioactive sources which produce similar clinical results, but which do not present as much of a potential hazard to the patient nor as much of a problem in radiation protection (Ch. 33). The latter is due to the very penetrating gamma rays emitted from a radium source (see Table 34.1), and the potential hazard to the patient is due to the high radioactive and chemical toxicity of radium which is taken up into the paitent's bones if the needle or tube should leak. Also, the long half-life of radium (1620 years) ensures that any leakage will be in the environment for a long time, and the radioactive radon gas emitted in the decay of radium and the emission of alpha particles from the other daughter products of radium (Table 34.1) are an additional hazard.

The use of other sources with less energetic gamma emissions such as ^{137}Cs and ^{60}Co present fewer problems with leakage or the protection of medical personnel during the insertion of the sources or with the subsequent nursing procedures during the treatment time. The radiotherapist inevitably receives the greatest dose, particularly to the fingers. This problem of high doses received by personnel is one reason why teletherapy has become a more generally preferred method of treatment compared to brachytherapy.

Table 34.1 Characteristics of sources used in brachytherapy

Source	Half-life	Decay	Main gamma emissions	Other Emissions*	Decay products	Applications
$^{192}_{77}$Ir	74·4 days	$\beta-\gamma$	0·296 to 0·605 MeV	β^-	$^{192}_{78}$Pt (stable)	Radioactive wire for interstitial therapy
$^{182}_{73}$Ta	115 days	$\beta-\gamma$	0·068 to 1·23 MeV	β^-	$^{182}_{74}$W (stable)	Radioactive wire for interstitial therapy
$^{137}_{55}$Cs	30 years	$\beta-\gamma$ (delayed)	0·662 MeV	β^-	$^{137}_{56}$Ba$^{m} \longrightarrow\, ^{137}_{56}$Ba $+ \gamma$ (0·662)	Teletherapy sources and intracavitary sources
$^{60}_{27}$Co	5·27 years	$\beta-\gamma$	1·17 and 1·33 MeV	β^-	$^{60}_{28}$Ni (stable)	Teletherapy sources and intracavitary sources
$^{226}_{88}$Ra	1620 years	α	0·188 MeV from $^{226}_{88}$Ra; 0·61 to 2·43 MeV from $^{214}_{83}$Bi (radium C)	α and β^-	See note †	Needles and tubes for interstitial therapy and gynaecological inserts

* Absorbed by outer sheath of platinum
† Simplified decay scheme:

$$^{226}_{88}\text{Ra} \xrightarrow[\substack{(1620\ \text{y})}]{\alpha} {}^{222}_{86}\text{Rn} \xrightarrow[\substack{(3\cdot8\ \text{d})}]{\alpha} {}^{218}_{84}\text{Po} \xrightarrow[\substack{(3\ \text{m})}]{\alpha} {}^{214}_{82}\text{Pb} \xrightarrow[\substack{(27\ \text{m})}]{\beta} {}^{214}_{83}\text{Bi} \xrightarrow[\substack{(20\ \text{m})}]{\beta} {}^{214}_{84}\text{Po} \xrightarrow[\substack{(0\cdot0002\ \text{s})}]{\alpha}$$

$$^{210}_{82}\text{Pb} \xrightarrow[\substack{(21\ \text{y})}]{\beta} {}^{210}_{83}\text{Bi} \xrightarrow[\substack{(5\ \text{d})}]{\beta} {}^{210}_{84}\text{Po} \xrightarrow[\substack{(138\ \text{d})}]{\alpha} {}^{206}_{82}\text{Pb (stable)}$$

However, much of the radiation doses received by doctors, nurses and technicians can be very substantially reduced by the use of an *afterloader*. An afterloading method may be used in superficial, interstitial and intracavitary therapy. Its use ensures that the geometrical arrangement of sources is correct before loading the sources into position.

In an interstitial treatment of the tongue with an afterloading technique, for example, inactive 'guide' needles may be inserted into the tongue and their positioning checked by the use of fluoroscopy and/or a radiograph. Once the radiotherapist is satisfied that the positions are satisfactory, radioactive wires of the correct shape and size (supplied by the manufacturer) are inserted into the guides. The guides are then removed so that the sources are left in the tongue. On completion of the required treatment time, the sources may be easily removed. The time-consuming operation of ensuring adequate source 'geometry' is thus performed with inactive materials, and hence constitutes no hazard to the staff, while the loading of the radioactive wires is comparatively quick so that the doses received by staff are minimised. Reductions of doses to radiotherapists by a factor of 100 are possible with this afterloading technique.

The use of iridium wire (^{192}Ir) in afterloaders for interstitial therapy is becoming more popular owing to its mechanical flexibility and relatively low energy gamma emissions (see Table 34.1) which allow the use of lighter and thinner absorbing barriers for radiation protection purposes. Thin (0·3mm diameter) iridium wire may be bent to a wide variety of shapes and hence put to uses which are impossible for rigid sources such as radium needles. Further, the wire may be cut to length for a given treatment with no danger of subsequent source leakage and contamination.

The use of afterloaders in the intracavitary treatment of gynaecological cancer has had a major effect on the reduction of radiation doses to radio-therapists and nursing staff. It may also allow a greater number of patients treated in a given working day. As in the case of afterloading in interstitial therapy described above, the first stage is the insertion of the inactive source holders: the intrauterine tubes (placed through the dilated cervical opening) and the ovoids (placed in the fornices to treat the vaginal vault). When these have been located properly (verifiable by 'check' films), flexible plastic tubes are connected from a machine which is capable of automatically sending selected sources from a lead safe within the machine to the intrauterine tubes and ovoids along the plastic tubes. Air pressure is used to force the sources along the flexible tubes, and a partial vacuum brings them back again at the end of the treatment time, or when a door to the treatment room is opened. The patient may thus be isolated in a treatment room for the duration of the therapy (although visual and voice contact is maintained) so that the medical personnel receive almost no radiation dose. The use of very active sources can reduce treatment times to about 30 minutes, if desired. Alternatively, nursing staff may approach the patients in their rooms with no hazards to themselves, because the sources are returned to the 'safe' position whenever the door of the patient's room is opened. Treatment continues automatically after the door is closed, when the nursing staff operate a remote switch.

Both ^{60}Co and ^{137}Cs sources have been used in such afterloading devices, the

^{137}Cs being easier to shield against because of its lower-energy gamma emissions (see Table 34.1).

34.3.2 Dosage calculations

As mentioned previously, the purpose of the use of sealed sources in brachytherapy is that the cancerous cells should receive a high uniform absorbed dose and that normal tissue should be 'spared' as much as possible. The combination of the activities of the sources used and the prescribed treatment time determines the magnitude of the radiation dose received by the tumour, while the distribution of sources determines the degree of uniformity of the dose received. Obviously, the shapes and sizes of tumours vary greatly, so that an optimum configuration of sources for a particular treatment is a complicated three-dimensional problem. In addition, there are practical constraints to be taken into consideration, such as the number and types of sources available to the radiotherapists, and which of the possible source configurations is able to be reproduced accurately in the therapy situation.

Before the advent of small, powerful computers, various tried and tested 'rules of thumb' (such as the 'Manchester System') were derived so that a practical source distribution could be quickly chosen from a fairly limited number of options. The lengths, separations, activities and positions of the sources are clearly defined in such rules, and an acceptably uniform dose obtained (usually within about 10%). However, if a 'check film' shows that a source has been incorrectly placed, or has moved, it is a difficult and time-consuming procedure to investigate the effect on the overall dose distribution and what, if any, corrective action to apply.

An adequate description of the dose distribution around a particular arrangement of sealed sources may be achieved only by the use of a computer. The dose distribution in any plane may be calculated and displayed as a series of isodose lines (34.2.1). Such computer calculations show the variation in dose in much greater detail than is possible with manual calculation methods, and may reveal the presence of local areas subject to under-dosage or over-dosage in an otherwise normal-looking arrangement. The high calculating speed of the modern computer makes it possible to display the dose distribution in a large number of selected planes and to include other factors in the calculations, such as attenuation and scatter of the gamma rays in the tissues. (Manual methods of calculation assume that the effects of attenuation and scatter cancel each other, so that the dose may be determined simply by the Inverse Square Law.)

The positions of the sources may be determined from two 'check films' taken at right-angles to each other. This information is fed into the computer, which then calculates the absorbed dose at any required point or in any plane. The effect of the addition of any required 'top-up' sources in regions of under-dosage may be investigated on the computer prior to their use.

As the price of computer hardware continues to fall, an increasing number of radiotherapy departments will be able to take advantage of the accurate dose distribution calculations they can provide, and thereby improve the service to the patient both in teletherapy and brachytherapy treatment planning.

34.4 RADIONUCLIDE THERAPY

Radionuclides in various chemical forms may be used to treat some abnormal clinical conditions, as outlined briefly below.

Iodine is taken up by the thyroid gland (see Appendix II) and organified to produce various hormones. If the thyroid becomes overactive ('hyperthyroid' or 'thyrotoxic') it shows a higher uptake of iodine than normal. Hence, doses of 185 to 370 MBq (5 to 10 mCi) of ^{131}I in the chemical form of sodium iodide (NaI) may be given orally to the patient to treat this condition. The thyroid takes up some of the radioactive iodine (most of the rest is excreted in the urine), and consequently receives a sufficiently high radiation absorbed dose due to the beta emission of ^{131}I (Table 26.3) to reduce its metabolic functions towards the normal range, with the resulting reduction of clinical symptoms. Overdosage may result in the later onset of the reverse condition, i.e. hypothyroidism, necessitating a diet which includes some thyroid hormone.

Thyroid cancer requires a more complicated treatment involving much higher activities of radioactive iodine. Those tumours which show a good uptake of iodine may be successfully treated in this way. The thyroid is first removed by surgery, or 'ablated' with a high dose of ^{131}I (e.g. 296 MBq, or 80 mCi), or a combination of both. When a radionuclide 'scan' (Appendix II) shows poor uptake by the thyroid, or what is left of it, a very high dose of ^{131}I (up to about 5·55 TBq, or 150 mCi) is given in an attempt to destroy any 'secondary' deposits which may be present throughout the body. Further scans and large doses of ^{131}I are used in a long period of follow-up to ensure management of the disease.

Phosphorus-32 (^{32}P) in the form of sodium phosphate (Na$_2$PO$_4$) is used to treat the blood condition 'polycythaemia rubra vera', which is characterised by the patient having very viscous blood containing a high percentage of red cells. The heart and blood vessels are put to great strain by this disease, which is caused by an overactive bone marrow. Injections of sterile radioactive sodium phosphate produce a radiation dose to the bone marrow, because it metabolises phosphorus. The beta emission of ^{32}P delivers the necessary absorbed dose and reduces the rate of production of red blood cells. This treatment usually gives the patient many extra years of life.

Colloidal solutions of gold-198 (^{198}Au) or yttrium-90 (^{90}Y) have been used for a variety of purposes, from the treatment of malignant growths in peritoneal cavities to the treatment of osteoarthritis in knee joints. The colloidal form of the solutions is composed of particles of sufficient size to ensure that the injected material stays in whatever bodily space it is injected.

Exercise 34.2

a. What is meant by the terms 'teletherapy' and 'telecurie therapy'? Describe the similarities and differences in the patterns of absorbed dose in tissue between beams of X-radiation of energies of about 250 kV$_p$ and 4 MV, by reference to the appropriate isodose charts.

b. Sketch the effect on an isodose chart of using a *wedge*, stating the energy of beam considered. What is meant by the term 'wedge angle'?

c. Show how two wedged fields as described in the previous question may be used to produce a uniform absorbed dose over a treatment volume.

d. What is the purpose of a radiotherapy simulator? Describe three uses for such a machine, two of which employ the use of radiographic contrast media.

e. Describe the impact of computerised tomography on both diagnostic radiology and radiotherapy.

f. Discuss the role of a computer in a modern radiotherapy department. (*Note:* Include more than just scientific calculations, e.g. medical records, teaching aids etc.)

g. Show how the use of 'afterloading' techniques in radiotherapy is able to reduce the radiation dose received by medical personnel.

h. Describe briefly:

(i) the advantages and disadvantages of flexible radioactive wire (e.g. ^{192}Ir) compared to rigid sources for interstitial radiotherapy
(ii) the uses of radiochemicals in the management of hyperthyroidism (thyrotoxicosis).

SUMMARY

1. Radiotherapy is the treatment of cancer by the use of ionising radiations, of which X and γ-radiations are the most common.

2. The aim of all radiotherapeutic regimes is to deliver a sufficiently high and uniform dose to the tumour so that it is destroyed, while sparing the normal tissue as much as possible. The magnitude of the dose required depends upon the type of tumour, i.e. its *radiosensitivity.*

3. The dose required to kill a tumour cannot normally be given in one treatment, apart from very small areas of treatment, owing to the intolerance shown by the patient. Dose *fractions* are therefore used to enable the tissues to recover somewhat between successive treatments.

4. Teletherapy employs external radiation beams impinging on the patient which are arranged in such a way as to satisfy 2 above. Megavoltage X-ray beams produce large depth doses (i.e. good beam penetration), high dose rates, narrow penumbra and very little preferential absorption in bone compared to soft tissue. For characteristics of other beams, see text.

5. Wedges and compensators may be used to modify the shape of the beam, as measured by the *isodose chart.*

6. Simulators and CT scanners may be used to increase significantly the accuracy of radiotherapy planning procedures, as does the fitting of 'shells' for patient immobilisation.

7. Computers are able to produce rapid calculations of beam summation, and a suitably optimised plan selected. Computers are also useful in brachytherapy calculations (see below).

8. Brachytherapy is the arrangement of radioactive sources on ('moulds'), in ('interstitial') or within ('intracavitary') the body for the treatment of cancer.

The rapid fall-off in dose rate from these sources due to the Inverse Square Law is an advantage in sparing normal tissue adjacent to the treatment volume. The hazard to medical staff is greater than for teletherapy, but may be reduced by the use of afterloading techniques.

9.   The ingestion or injection of radionuclides in suitable chemical forms is used in the control of various disorders, mainly thyrotoxicosis and thyroid cancer (^{131}I) and polycythaemia rubra vera (^{32}P).

APPENDICES

Appendix I

FLEMING'S LEFT AND RIGHT-HAND RULES

Fleming's Left (LH) and Right-Hand (RH) Rules are used to determine the direction of force on a current-carrying conductor in a magnetic field (the Motor Principle), and the direction of induced current when a conductor is moved in a magnetic field (the Generator Effect). The particular Hand Rule used depends upon whether electron flow or 'conventional' flow is considered. We shall consider only electron flow in this section, in which case the RH Rule is used for the Motor Principle and the LH Rule is used for the Generator Effect, as shown in the figure.

In each case it is necessary to know the directions of *two* of the variables in order to determine the direction of the third. In the case of the RH Rule, the forefinger and middle finger are aligned with the direction of the magnetic field and the electron current respectively, as shown in Figure I.1(a). The direction of the thumb then gives the direction of the force on the current-carrying conductor.

For the LH Rule it is the forefinger and thumb which are aligned with the directions of the magnetic field and movement of the conductor. The middle finger then gives the direction of the induced current.

These Hand Rules may be applied to the examples in Chapters 13 and 14, where an alternative method of determining the directions of force in the Motor Principle, and induced current in the Generator Effect is described.

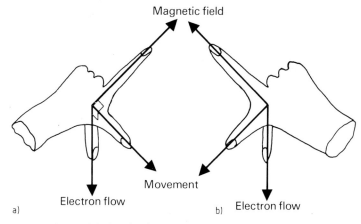

Fig. I.1 Fleming's left and right-hand rules.

Appendix II

SCINTILLATION COUNTERS

A scintillation counter may be used to detect minute amounts of X or γ-radiation, usually emitted in radioactive decay. There are two main types of scintillation counter: one where the detector is a crystalline solid (e.g. NaI(Tl)) and the other having a liquid scintillation material as a detector. The former is suitable for the detection of individual quanta of X and γ-radiation, and the latter may be used for either X and γ-radiation or β-particles (for which it is particularly suitable).

II.1 NaI(Tl) crystals and photomultipliers

A crystal of sodium iodide into which thallium has been introduced as an impurity is one of the most efficient scintillators developed. The thallium impurities act as 'luminescent centres' (27.2) and about 10–15% of the energy deposited in the crystal is transformed into light energy with a maximum emission at about 420 nm (i.e. blue light). Sodium iodide crystals are mounted in sealed containers ('cans') to prevent them absorbing moisture from the atmosphere and becoming cloudy. One face of the crystal is cemented to a transparent glass 'window' and all other surfaces are in contact with a reflecting powder (magnesium oxide) in order that as much light as possible escapes through the window.

A sodium iodide crystal in optical contact with a photomultiplier is shown in Figure II.1. A gamma ray is absorbed in the crystal at point P (say), and results in the emission of light in all directions. Some of this light reaches the 'photocathode' of the photomultiplier which is a thin coating of alkaline compounds deposited on the inside face of the photomultiplier. About 10–25% of the light photons reaching the photocathode eject electrons from it by the photoelectric effect (25.5.1), and these electrons are accelerated to a succession of positively charged plates ('dynodes') which are coated with a 'secondary emitting' layer. Each dynode produces about six times as many electrons as fall on it and so the number of electrons produced from the last dynode may be very considerable. One photoelectron released from the photocathode may well result in the collection of over one million electrons by the collecting plate (the 'anode') of the photomultiplier. The collection of this charge by the anode occurs over a very small time (less than 10^{-6} s) and so produces a 'pulse' of electricity, the magnitude of which is proportional to the

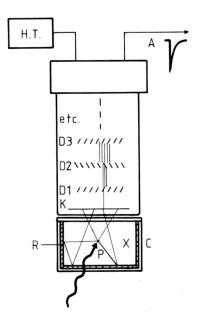

Fig. II.I A scintillation detector using sodium iodide. Key: X — NaI(Tl) crystal;
R — powdered reflector; C — crystal can: K — photocathode; D1, D2, etc. — dynodes.

energy of the absorbed gamma ray. For example, if there are n dynodes each of
which releases 6 electrons for each incident electron, then the *electron gain* of
the photomultiplier is just 6^n. Thus, the release of one electron from the
photocathode of a 10-dynode tube produces a total number of electrons of 6^{10}
at the anode. This is just over 60 million electrons, and represents a charge of
about 10 picocoulomb.

A spectrum of these pulses does not show the discrete gamma energies
emitted by a radioactive source (26.2), however, because of the statistical
nature of the light production in the crystal and the electron multiplication
within the photomultiplier. This is shown in Figure II.2 where the number of
pulses of a given height produced at point A in Figure II.1 are plotted. The
ideal spectrum would be a line placed at the centre of the 'photopeak', i.e.
the peak corresponding to the total absorption of the gamma rays by the
photoelectric effect (25.5.1). In addition, some gamma rays undergo Compton
scatter (30.5) within the crystal and then escape from the crystal with no
further interactions. Such events result in an energy being deposited in the
crystal of less than the full energy of the gamma ray, so that smaller pulses are
produced from the photomultiplier. These pulses produce a 'Compton peak' as
shown in Figure II.2.

Some very small pulses are produced by the release of single electrons from
the photocathode of the photomultiplier by the process of thermionic
emission. (Ch. 18). Also, some positively charged ions strike the photocathode
and release electrons. These 'noise' pulses are shown in Figure II.2.

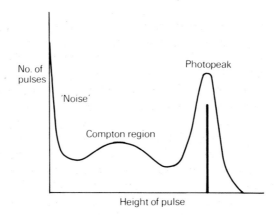

Fig. II.2 A typical gamma-ray spectrum using sodium iodide.

II.2 Scintillation counters in medicine

It is the usual practice to count only the pulses which occur in the photopeak of the spectrum, particularly when investigating the amount and/or distribution of a radioactive 'tracer' within a patient's body. This is accomplished by means of a 'pulse-height analyser' (PHA) which only produces an electrical output signal if the input pulses lie within a certain range: the range being adjusted to cover the photopeak. Pulses from the PHA are accumulated on a 'scalar' for a time determined by a timer, as shown in Figure II.3. The number of counts obtained is related directly to the activity being measured and may be compared to a previously determined normal range of counts.

For example, the uptake of radioactive iodine (as sodium iodide) is illustrated in Figure II.3. Here, the γ-rays, emitted from the thyroid are detected in the lead-shielded sodium iodide crystal, and the absorbed gamma rays whose energies lie within the photopeak are counted, as described above.

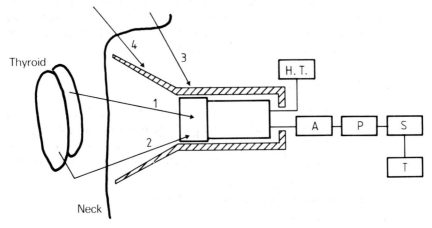

Fig. II.3 A scintillation detector used to measure activity within a thyroid gland. Key: A — amplifier; P — pulse height analyser (PHA); S — scalar; T — timer.

The collimator and lead shield serve to reduce the effect of activity which is not within the thyroid (rays 3 and 4 in the figure), and the selection of photopeak events by the PHA rejects events which are Compton scattered within the patient (ray 2 in the figure). The uptake figure is obtained by expressing the counts obtained from the patient's thyroid as a fraction of the counts which would have been obtained if the whole of the activity administered to the patient had been taken up by the thyroid. Typical values of a '24-hour uptake' lie between 10% and 25%. An overactive thyroid has a higher figure than this, and an underactive thyroid has a lower figure.

A scintillation counter may also be used to measure the amount of activity present in an organ with time. For example, the ability of the kidneys to take up a radioactive tracer (e.g. 'hippuran') and to excrete it to the bladder may be shown by taking the outputs to two scintillation counters to a chart-recorder. Similarly, blood-flow to the brain may be recorded from a number of such scintillation counters arranged around the skull. The injection of a suitable tracer (e.g. radioactive xenon) produces a sequence of responses from each detector, from which it may be ascertained if an abnormal cerebral blood flow is present.

II.3 The gamma camera

The gamma camera (first developed by H. O. Anger in 1958) is a special type of scintillation counter where the *position* of the scintillations within a large-diameter thin NaI(Tl) crystal is obtained by an electronic combination of the signals from many photomultipliers. It may therefore produce a *picture* of the distribution of radioactivity within the patient, and follow the progress of activity through the heart (for example).

A picture of a 'positive' brain scan is shown in Figure II.4, where the area shown marked corresponds to the increased radioactive uptake due to the presence of a brain tumour.

The ability of the gamma camera to measure the *physiological status* of the bodily organs together with its 'dynamic' (i.e time-varying) measurement capabilities make it a very powerful diagnostic instrument in the detection of many different types of abnormal conditions.

II.4 Liquid scintillation counting

Radioactive nuclides which decay solely by beta decay (26.3) are not suitable for detection by NaI(Tl) crystals because of the low efficiency of detection. Many electrons are absorbed by the 'can' around the crystal, and others are scattered out of the crystal. A *liquid* scintillation solution is composed of:

    a. a solvent (e.g benzene, toluene)
    b. a scintillation solute (the 'primary' solute)
    c. a 'secondary' solute.

The sample containing the beta-emitting radionuclide is dissolved in a solution containing (a), (b) and (c) above. The beta particles from the

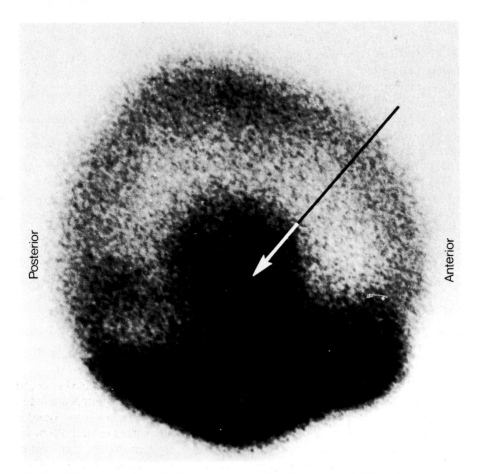

Posterior

Anterior

Fig. II.4 A brain scan obtained using a gamma camera. The area marked is an increased uptake due to a brain tumour.

radioactive sample travel through the liquid and produce ionisation and excitation (25.5) in the molecules of the solvent. The excitation energy is transferred quickly (in less than 10^{-9} s) to the primary solute, which fluoresces (i.e. produces a photon of electromagnetic radiation) when the excited electrons 'drop' to the original lower-energy state. The secondary solute is introduced into the solution as a 'wavelength shifter', i.e. it absorbs the photons emitted by the primary solute and re-emits them at a longer wavelength, since the wavelengths emitted by the primary solute are generally too short for efficient detection by the photocathodes of photomultiplier tubes. A typical efficiency of the liquid scintillation process is 3%, i.e. 3% of the energy of the electrons are converted to photons.

A typical arrangement for the counting of radioactive samples by liquid scintillation is shown in Figure II.5. Two photomultipliers A and B view a plastic or glass bottle into which has been introduced the liquid scintillator (usually 10 ml or less) and contains the dissolved radioactive sample. A scintillation

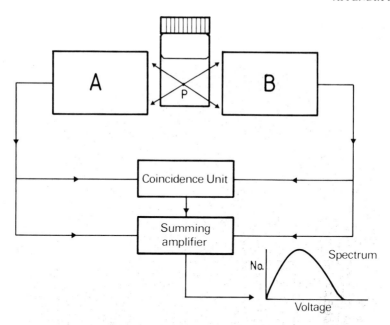

Fig. II.5 A basic liquid scintillation counter.

event at P within the liquid produces light photons which are shared between photomultipliers A and B. The outputs of these two photomultipliers are fed to a summing amplifier which is only switched on when the pulses from A and B occur at the same time (i.e. in 'coincidence'). In this way, the random noise pulses (see II.2) from each tube are almost entirely eliminated. The output pulses from the summing amplifier are then a measure of the original continuous beta spectrum (26.3) of the radioactive sample and may be counted with a scalar and timer (II.2).

Liquid scintillation counting is a very sensitive method of measuring the activity of a beta-emitting sample because of the intimate contact between the sample and the scintillator. This means that all but the very lowest energies of the emitted beta particles are detected. The familiar very sensitive 'carbon-dating' method of dating naturally occurring objects uses liquid scintillation counting to detect the tiny activities of carbon-14 present in such samples.

Appendix III

MODULATION TRANSFER FUNCTION (MTF)

The MTF is a mathematical method of assessing the performance of an imaging system, whether it be optical, radiographic or radioactive (e.g. gamma camera — II.3). The use of the MTF for this purpose was pioneered in the field of optics when it was discovered that a lens which was excellent at imaging the structure of very fine objects was not necessarily as good as another lens of lower resolving power when imaging coarser (i.e. larger) objects.

III.1 Spatial frequencies and modulation

The concept of spatial frequencies is inherent in any description of the MTF and will therefore be considered first before the MTF is defined in III.2.

An object with a spatial frequency of v cycles per cm (say) is shown in Figure III.1. The object has an amptitude which is sinusoidal (15.1) with a wavelength of λ. The spatial frequency is the number of cycles per unit length, and is there-fore given by $1/\lambda$. The *modulation* of the object, m_0, is defined as

$$m_0 = \frac{a - b}{a + b} \qquad \text{Equation III.1}$$

where a and b are the height of the peaks and the troughs of the waveform respectively.

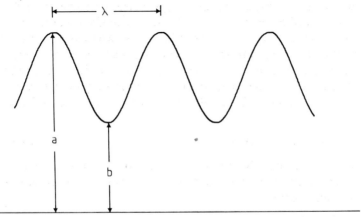

Fig. III.1 The definition of modulation (see text).

The amplitude of the sine-wave is the intensity of light for lenses, the activity for gamma cameras and the X-ray intensity in radiography. If it is supposed that an absorber is placed in the path of an X-ray beam such that it would produce a sinusoidal variation of intensity of the transmitted beam, then a perfect imaging system would produce a sine-wave of photographic exposure on the film of the *same* modulation. The *image modulation* would then be the same as the *object modulation*. However, in practice, the relative amplitude of the image modulation is reduced by the finite size of the focal spot and the characteristics of the film/screen combination, which tend to spread the image onto a larger area than theoretically desirable. Thus, the 'peaks' of the sinusoidal exposure tend to contribute to the 'troughs', so that an overall reduction in amplitude (and therefore modulation) is experienced.

This effect of a reduction in image modulation is small when the sinusoidal object has a long wavelength (low spatial frequency), but is of increasing importance as the wavelength is reduced to about 1 mm or less (spatial frequencies of 10 per cm or more). The image modulation therefore depends upon the spatial frequency of the object, and this forms the basis of the MTF described below.

III.2 MTF and spatial frequency

the Modulation Transfer Function is defined as:

$$\text{MTF} = \frac{\text{image modulation}}{\text{object modulation}} \qquad \text{Equation III.2}$$

In a perfect imaging system, the image is an exact copy of the object and so has the same modulation at all spatial frequencies. The MTF is therefore always unity for such a system. However, we have seen that the image modulation is reduced as the spatial frequency increases (III.1) and so a graph of the MTF plotted against spatial frequency has a general appearance as shown in Figure III.2. Three cases are considered: an 'ideal' imaging system, where the MTF is 1·0 and is independent of the spatial frequency, a curve where the MTF is reduced at the higher frequencies due to geometric unsharpness (3.4) only, and a curve obtained when using screens. It is to be expected that the imaging of fine detail (high spatial frequencies) would be worse when using screens because of the spreading of the light from the fluorescent screens (27.5) over the film. The MTF is particularly useful in separating the individual causes of image degradation. MTF's due to each cause may be measured separately (MTF_1, MTF_2, ... etc.) and may be combined to produce the overall MTF of the system:

$$\text{MTF} = \text{MTF}_1 \times \text{MTF}_2 \ldots \qquad \text{Equation III.3}$$

It thus becomes possible to predict the response of the overall system with various combinations of focal spot size, film/screen combinations etc. if the MTF of each is known.

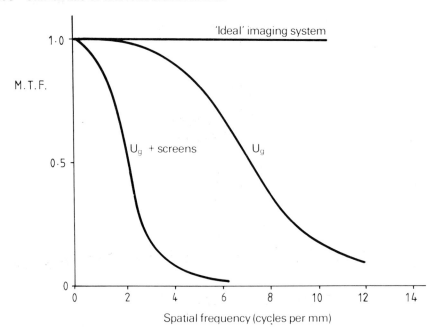

Fig. III.2 The variation of the modulation transfer function (MTF) with spatial frequency for an ideal system, that due to geometric unsharpness (U_g), and that due to geometric unsharpness and screens (U_g + screens).

III.3 Objects as spatial frequencies

A 'sinusoidal' object does not bear much similarity to the objects which are normally radiographed. However, it may be shown that the shape of any object may be obtained from the summation of sine and cosine waves of different amplitudes and frequencies (Fourier's Theorem). Thus, if the MTF of the X-ray unit is known at each frequency, the overall response to the object may be determined.

As an example of the summation of amplitudes of different frequencies forming a shape, consider the flat-topped object shown by the dotted lines in Figure III.3(a). The height of the object may be considered to represent the degree of absorption of the X-rays by the object, and the width is the physical size of the object. It may be shown that such a shape may be obtained by adding an infinite series of cosine waves (which are just sine waves displaced by 90°) of increasing frequency (f), where the amplitudes (g) are given by

$$g = \frac{\sin(\pi f d)}{2\pi f} \qquad \text{Equation III.4}$$

The sum of the first 500 terms of such amplitudes is shown in Figure III.3(a). The effect of including 2500 terms (i.e. containing higher frequencies) is shown in Figure III.3(b), where a closer approximation to the square shape is obtained. The agreement is exact when an infinite number of terms is

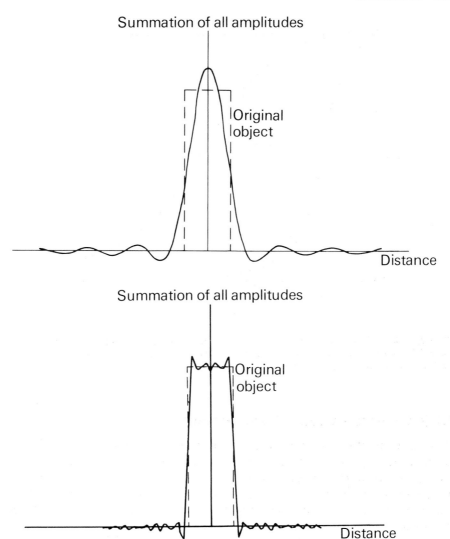

Fig. III.3 The representation of a 'square' object (dotted lines) by the summation of frequencies of different amplitudes: (a) 500 terms, (b) 2500 terms. An infinite number of terms reproduces the object exactly.

included. However, the higher spatial frequencies present in the object are poorly reproduced in the image, because the MTF is low at high frequencies. Since the high frequencies are responsible for the 'squareness' of the corners for objects such as shown in Figure III.3, sharp objects will be shown as being slightly blurred or 'out of focus'. This is in accordance with the concept of *unsharpness* as discussed earlier (3.4), and the two approaches are just two ways of looking at the same thing. The MTF is more mathematically rigorous as a complete description of the imaging properties of the X-ray unit, but even this does not consider other problems such as statistical 'noise' within the image, known as 'quantum mottle'.

III.4 Measurement of MTF

It would be difficult in practice to manufacture sinusoidal objects in the
numbers and the small wavelengths required. It would also be time-consuming
to measure the object and image modulation for each conceivable combination of frequency, position of absorber and screen/film combination. Fortunately, there is no need to do this, since the MTF may be calculated from the
Line Spread Function (LSF). This calculation is best accomplished using a
computer program and is beyond the scope of this book. The LSF is the profile
of the intensity curve obtained by shining the X-ray beam through a very
narrow slit (Fig. III.4).

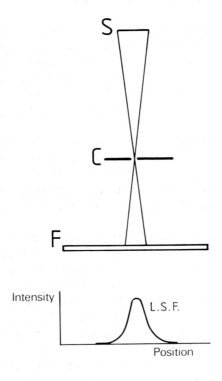

Fig. III.4 The line spread function.

Appendix IV

COMPUTERISED TOMOGRAPHY (CT)

The principles of linear tomography are outlined in section 3.6. This technique enables the imaging of selected depths within a patient's body by the choice of the appropriate geometrical settings. However, adjacent areas above and below the selected depth form an 'out-of-focus' or blurred background image which is superimposed upon the focused image. The effect of this is to blur detail to some extent and may raise difficulties of interpretation of the radiograph.

The very successful technique of computerised tomography (CT), first developed by EMI Ltd, forms a picture of the cross-section of a patient's anatomy without the contribution of areas on either side of the chosen cross-sectional 'slice'. The method requires both sophisticated equipment and very specialised computer programs to obtain images of the quality presently achievable.

The intensity of radiation which is transmitted through a patient's body when it is irradiated by a thin parallel beam of X-rays gives some information about the average attenuation of that beam, but very little about the details of the internal structures within the body. In order to determine this, much more information is needed, and this is obtained by subjecting the body to a very large number (approx. 30 000) of such thin beams at different angles, and measuring how much is transmitted in each case. Each beam gives a small amount of information as to what lies along its path; a large number of beams gives a lot of information which a computer is able to subsequently unravel and present in the form of a picture whose brightness increases with the attenuation of its internal structures. Examples of such pictures are shown below.

The earliest type of CT scanner consisted of a single scintillation detector placed directly opposite the X-ray tube on either side of the patient. The tube and detector were then scanned across the patient, rotated around the patient by a few degrees and then scanned again. The signal from the detector was, of course, fed into the computer along with other information such as the angle of scanning. The simplicity of such an arrangement was somewhat offset by the problems of mechanical reliability which were encountered, particularly with the early models. A natural extension to this arrangement was the inclusion of more scintillation detectors in the plane of the 'slice' for greater sensitivity.

More modern machines have superseded the sideways scanning movements

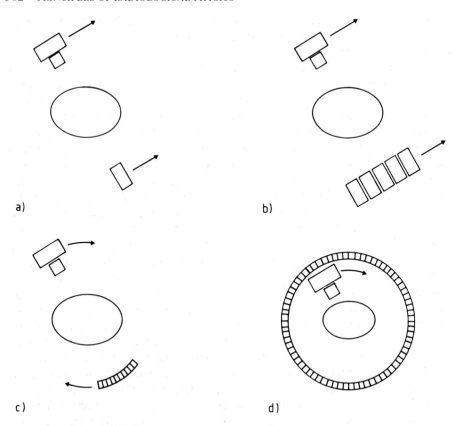

Fig. IV.1 Different configurations of CT scanner: (a) single detector, (b) multiple detectors, (c) rotating source and multiple detectors, (d) rotating source and stationary multiple detectors.

by the rotational movement of the X-ray tube around the patient, and have a large number of detectors on an arc opposite the tube or on a complete circle (see Fig. IV.1). In the former case the detectors need to move with the X-ray tube, but may be stationary in the latter. The advantages of either of these two systems is that of reduced mechanical complexity and *speed*, where a complete rotation may take five seconds or less, compared to a time of about four minutes to complete all the scanning movements of the early machines. The reduced time required to obtain a complete section scan results in fewer artifacts due to movement of the patient.

The types of scintillation detector used include sodium iodide (Appendix II), bismuth germanate (BGO), and calcium fluoride. Gas proportional counters employing xenon under pressure are frequently used on the rotational machines owing to the ease with which they may be closely packed together and their relative inexpensiveness.

Further practical considerations include the need for the reduction of the effects of scatter by an appropriate collimator system between the detectors (e.g. tungsten sheets) and the generation of an X-ray beam of constant quality (Ch. 29). This is achieved by the use of three-phase rectification circuits

(20.4.3) and adequate filtration, the latter being to reduce the effect of the 'hardening' of the beam as it passes through the tissues because of the preferential absorption of the 'softer' X-rays.

The mathematical methods (i.e. the 'software') by which the computer is able to 'reconstruct' the structures within the body by operating upon all the information it has received from the detector(s) are somewhat too complicated to describe in any detail in this book. Perhaps the easiest method to visualise is the 'back-projection' method, a version of which (the 'filtered back-projection' method) is used in many commercial machines. Consider two small structures A and B (Fig. IV.2(a)) which have been scanned in the 'X' and 'Y' direction to produce two attenuation profiles as shown. If these profiles are projected back onto the object, then the two projections overlap at A′ and B′ as shown in (b). However, there is also an unwanted component making up the final image due to the parts of the back-projection which do not overlap. In this way 'ghost' images and other artifacts occur in such a simple reconstruction method, and it is the purpose of the 'filtered back-projection' method to modify the shapes of all profiles so that, when back-projected, no significant artifacts occur.

When used alone or in conjunction with other procedures such as nuclear medicine and ultrasonics, 'head' and 'body' CT scanners constitute a powerful diagnostic tool. Differences in values of the linear attenuation coefficients (30.1.2) of about 0·5% are visualised on the display, which in turn reflect small changes in the values of electron density and average atomic number (30.7) of different tissues. Thus it is possible to visualise (for example) abscesses, blood clots and tumours which are often difficult to detect by other methods (see Fig. IV.3). However, the CT scanner measures anatomy rather than physiology, so that 'dynamic' studies with a gamma camera yielding information on the physiological status of an organ (e.g. cardiac and renal studies) still have an important part to play.

One very interesting development from CT scanning is its use in the accurate planning of dose distributions in radiotherapy, where the effects of

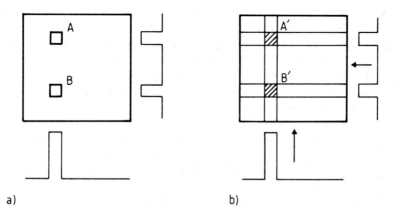

a)   b)

Fig. IV.2 Principle of CT reconstruction. The profiles obtained in (a) are 'back-projected' in (b) to form image (see text).

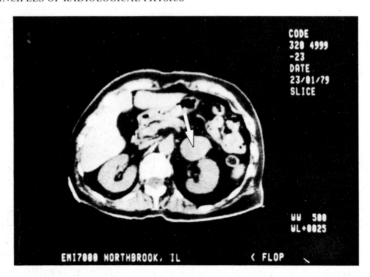

Fig. IV.3 A CT scan of the trunk showing a soft-tissue mass, which arises from the lower pole of the left adrenal gland (as shown marked). This 5 mm 'slice' was taken on an EMI 7070 scanner in a time of 3 seconds, and is published by kind permission of Thorn-EMI Medical Limited.

the inhomogeneity of the tissues (as measured quantitatively on the CT scan) are corrected for by a suitable computer program.

The future is certain to produce CT images of increasing quality obtained in shorter times, and it will be interesting to see the full potential of this technique realised both diagnostically and for therapy planning.

Appendix V

COUNTING STATISTICS

V.1 Poisson statistics and the standard deviation

Whenever a radioactive sample is 'counted' by detecting the radiations it emits in a suitable counter (see Appendix II), the number of counts so obtained is subject to statistical fluctuation. For example, a series of readings taken over consecutive 10-second intervals might produce 1243, 1402 and 1196 counts respectively. The reason for this lies in the decay of a radionuclide being subject to the laws of probability, so that it is not possible to tell when a particular nucleus will decay. Hence, the 'law of radioactive decay' and the exponential radioactive decay discussed in Chapter 5 are expressions of the *average* decay rate of the radionuclide, and any particular measurement of the decay rate may deviate somewhat from this average figure.

Radioactive decay is governed by 'Poisson statistics', which is a result of the fact that the probability of decay of any nucleus of a particular radionuclide over a *very short* time is constant.

If the probability of a nucleus decaying over a very short time τ is p, then the probability that it does not decay over the time τ is $(1 - p)$ and the probability, q, that it does not decay over a time t is $(1 - p)^{t/\tau}$. If $p = \lambda\tau$, where λ is a constant depending upon the particular radionuclide, then

$$q = (1 - \lambda\tau)^{t/\tau}$$
$$= [(1 - \lambda\tau)^{-1/\lambda\tau}]^{-\lambda t}$$

$$\left(\text{since } \frac{1}{\lambda\tau} \cdot \lambda t = \frac{t}{\tau}\right)$$

Substituting n for $-1/\lambda\tau$, we obtain

$$q = \left[\left(1 + \frac{1}{n}\right)^{n}\right]^{-\lambda t}$$

As the time τ is reduced to zero, the magnitude of n increases, and the limiting value of $[1 + (1/n)]^n$ is just e (i.e. $2 \cdot 7183 \ldots$). Also, the value q is equivalent to the fraction of the number of atoms left undecayed after time t, i.e. N_t/N_0, so we obtain finally

---

$$N_t = N_0 e^{-\lambda t}$$

Equation V.1

---

thus deriving the formula introduced in Chapter 5.

Further mathematics may be used to show that the probability, p_N, of measuring a count N if the average count is μ is given by the relationship:

$$p_N = \frac{\mu^N e^{-\mu}}{N!} \qquad\qquad \text{Equation V.2}$$

An example of the shape of the curves given by this equation is shown in Figure V.1 for different values of the average count, μ. Notice that the width of the curves increases as the average count, μ, increases, and the curves become more symmetrical about the peak (they become so-called 'Normal Distribu-

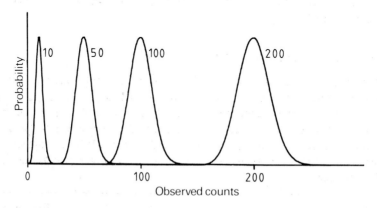

Fig. V.1 The probability of observing a particular number of counts when the average number of counts is as shown by the peaks.

tions'). The widths of the peaks are described by the 'standard deviation', σ, where 68·3% of all the counts exist between $(\mu + \sigma)$ and $(\mu - \sigma)$. A narrow peak will thus have a small value of σ and a wide peak will have a large value of σ. It might be thought from these considerations that it is more accurate to collect a few counts rather than a large number of counts because the standard deviation would be less. However, this is not the case, since the quantity which is of importance is the 'relative standard deviation' (6.6.1). It may be shown that, for a Poisson distribution:

$$\sigma = \sqrt{\mu}$$

so that
$$\frac{\sigma}{\mu} = \frac{1}{\sqrt{\mu}} \qquad\qquad \text{Equation V.3}$$

For example, if we obtain an average count of 10 000, then the standard deviation (SD) is $\sqrt{10\,000} = 100$ and the relative SD is $\dfrac{100}{\sqrt{10\,000}} = \dfrac{1}{100}$, or 1% (sometimes called the 'coefficient of variation'). The practical result of these considerations is that if we require to estimate the activity of a sample to within about 1%, then we need to detect at least 10 000 counts.

Exercise V.1
   a.   What are the standard deviations of a set of counting measurements if the average values are

   (i) 100
   (ii) 900
   (iii) 6400
   (iv) 10 000
   (v) 90 000?

   b.   What are the relative standard deviations in each of the above cases?
   c.   How many counts need to be collected if a relative standard deviation of 0·5% is required?

V.2 Effect of background counts

The standard deviation as discussed in the previous section does not take into account the effect of counts from other, unwanted, sources. One of these sources is 'background' due to cosmic rays and small amounts of radioactivity in the environment. The effect of background is to increase the statistical uncertainty of the counts obtained using a scintillation counter, Geiger counter etc., but the overall uncertainty may be estimated from the following useful relationship:

$$\sigma^2 = \sigma_b^2 + \sigma_s^2 \hspace{4cm} \text{Equation V.4}$$

Here, σ is the overall standard deviation obtained when counting in the presence of a background, and σ_b, σ_s are the standard deviations due to the background counts and the sample respectively. The square of the standard deviations is known as the *variance*, so that equation V.4 shows that the overall variance is just the sum of the individual variances.

If a separate counting experiment establishes that the background counts obtained in the same time as the measurement of the sample (N_s) is N_b, then we know from equation V.3 that $\sigma_b = \sqrt{N_b}$ and $\sigma_s = \sqrt{N_s}$.

The variance of the net counts ($N_s - N_b$) is the same as that of the total counts ($N_s + N_b$) since the errors are always assumed to add to each other rather than to subtract. Thus, the variances of the net counts, σ^2, are given by:

$$\sigma^2 = N_s + N_b \hspace{4cm} \text{from V.4}$$

so that $\sigma = \sqrt{(N_s + N_b)}$

and the relative standard deviation is $\dfrac{\sqrt{(N_s + N_b)}}{N_s + N_b}$

If N_b is so small as to be negligible, then this last expression simplifies to

$$\frac{\sqrt{N_s}}{N_s} = \frac{1}{\sqrt{N_s}}$$

as before (equation V.3).

The *optimum* distribution of counting times shared between background and sample which reduces the errors obtained to a minimum may be shown to be in inverse proportion to the square root of their count rates, i.e.

$$\frac{t_s}{t_b} = \sqrt{\frac{n_b}{n_s}}$$

Equation V.5

If the two count rates are known approximately, the overall counting time available may be split up as shown by this equation to achieve the best final statistical accuracy of the count rate due to the sample.

V.3 Dead time

There is an upper limit to the count rate at which any electrical counting circuit is able to cope. This is because if two consecutive pulses arrive within a very short time of each other, the circuit has not recovered sufficiently from the first pulse to be able to count the second. This time is known as the 'dead' time since the circuit is effectively dead, or non-operative, during this short period. Figure V.2 illustrates the situation when there is an average value of the

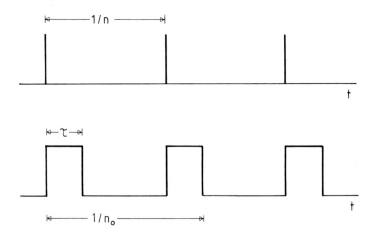

Fig. V.2 The average time separation of pulses for no dead-time (upper trace) and a dead-time of τ (lower trace).

observed count rate n_0, and a true rate of n. On average, each incoming pulse is separated by a time of $1/n$ (e.g. if there is a count rate of 100 per second, the pulses are separated by 1/100th of a second). However, the circuit is 'dead' for a time τ as shown in the figure — the 'dead time'. Thus the overall observed time between pulses is $1/n + \tau$, and this is just $1/n_0$.

$$\therefore \quad \frac{1}{n} = \frac{1}{n_0} - \tau = \frac{1 - n_0\tau}{n_0}$$

i.e. $\quad n = n_0/(1 - n_0\tau)$

Equation V.6

Note that if $\tau = 0$ (i.e. the electronic pulse counting circuit is perfect) $n = n_0$, i.e. there are no 'lost' pulses and the observed count rate is equal to the true count rate. A typical value of the dead time is $5\mu s$ (5×10^{-6} s), and the differences between the observed count rates are negligible except at high count rates. At an average observed count rate of 1000 per second, for example, the true rate is 1005 with such a dead time. However, at an observed count rate of 100 000 per second, the true rate is 200 000!

The use of longer dead times (which may be approximately 300 μs in a Geiger counter — see 32.3.2) makes the corrections important even at relatively low count rates.

Exercise V.2
Using equation V.6, draw a graph of observed count rate against true count rate for a dead time of 10 μs and hence find the true rate at which there is a 10% loss in the observed rate.

Appendix VI

THE ROENTGEN, RAD AND REM

The SI units of Exposure, absorbed dose and dose-equivalent are defined and discussed in Chapter 32. The previous units, which will probably be used concurrently with the SI units for some time, are the roentgen, rad and rem respectively. These are defined below.

An Exposure due to one roentgen (R) of X-ray or γ-radiation produces a total charge of one sign of $2 \cdot 58 \times 10^{-4}$ coulomb/kg in air by ionisation.

(The SI system does not have a special name of unit to represent the Exposure; it is just expressed directly in coulomb per kilogram.)

An absorbed dose of one *rad* exists when an energy of $1/100$ joule/kg is deposited in a medium.

(The SI unit of absorbed dose is the gray, where 1 gray = 1 joule/kg (32.1.2). Thus 1 gray $\equiv$ 100 rad. Both the rad and the gray apply to any beam of ionising radiation absorbed in any medium whereas the roentgen applies only to ionisation in air.)

The *rem* is a unit of dose-equivalent, and is used for radiation protection purposes. It is obtained by multiplying the absorbed dose in rads by the 'quality factor' (32.1.4) for the radiation under consideration.

(The sievert is the SI unit for dose-equivalent, and is equal to 100 rem (32.1.4).)

Tables of conversion factors between these units are given at the end of this book in Table C.

Appendix VII

DEFINITIONS OF SI BASE UNITS

The *metre* is the length equal to 1650 763·73 wavelengths in vacuum of the radiation corresponding to the transition between the levels $2p_{10}$ and $5d_5$ of the krypton-86 atom.

The *kilogram* is the unit of mass; it is equal to the mass of the international prototype of the kilogram.

The *second* is the duration of 9 192 631 770 periods of the radiation corresponding to the transition between the two hyperfine levels of the ground state of the caesium-133 atom.

The *ampere* is that constant current which, if maintained in two straight parallel conductors of infinite length, of negligible circular cross-section, and placed 1 metre apart in vacuum, would produce between these conductors a force equal to 2×10^{-7} newton per metre of length.

The *kelvin*, unit of thermodynamic temperature, is the fraction 1/273·16 of the thermodynamic temperature of the triple point of water.

The *mole* is the amount of substance of a system which contains as many elementary entities as there are atoms in 0·012 kilogram of carbon 12.

Appendix VIII

ELECTRON ORBITS AND QUANTUM MECHANICS

The electron configuration of the elements is explained by quantum mechanics by the use of four 'quantum numbers' (n, l, m, s) and the Pauli Exclusion Principle.* n is the principal quantum number, l is a number denoting the angular momentum, m is the number describing the orientation of an orbit to a magnetic field and s is the intrinsic spin of the electron itself. Each of these numbers is 'quantised', i.e. can take only certain discrete values, thus producing a limited number of combinations of possible electron orbits. It may be shown that for each value of n, l may take the values 0 to $(n - 1)$. Also, for each value of l, m may take the values $-l$ to $+l$. s is always $+\frac{1}{2}$ or $-\frac{1}{2}$.

To take an example, suppose $n = 3$ (i.e. the M shell), then l may have the values 0, 1, 2. For the value $l = 0$, m has only one value, i.e. 0, and s always has 2 possibilities (i.e. $+\frac{1}{2}$ or $-\frac{1}{2}$), so that the total number of electron orbits for $n = 3$, $l = 0$ is just 2. For $l = 1$, however, m may have the values $-1, 0, 1$ each of which may be combined with $s = \pm \frac{1}{2}$, so that there are **6** possibilities. For $l = 2$, m may have the values $-2, -1, 0, 1, 2$ each combining with $s = \pm \frac{1}{2}$, giving **10** possibilities. There are therefore a maximum of **18** electrons in the M shell, with subsets consisting of 2 and 8 electrons.

---

* The Pauli Exculsion Principle states that no two electrons may have the same values of n, l, m and s, so that each new added electron takes up a separate orbit. If this were not so, a shell would be able to have an indefinite number of electrons.

TABLES

Table A Powers of 10

Prefix	Symbol	Factor
exa	E	10^{18}
peta	P	10^{15}
tera	T	10^{12}
giga	G	10^{9}
mega	M	10^{6}
kilo	k	10^{3}
milli	m	10^{-3}
micro	μ	10^{-6}
nano	n	10^{-9}
pico	p	10^{-12}
femto	f	10^{-15}
atto	a	10^{-18}

Table B Becquerel to Curie conversion

The following table is based on the relationship: $1\ \text{Ci} = 3\cdot7 \times 10^{10}\ \text{Bq}$

Curie to Becquerel		Becquerel to Curie	
1 μCi	37 kBq	1 Bq	27 pCi
2 μCi	74 kBq	10 Bq	270 pCi
5 μCi	185 kBq	100 Bq	2·7 nCi
10 μCi	370 kBq	1 kBq	27 nCi
20 μCi	740 kBq	10 kBq	270 nCi
50 μCi	1·85 MBq	100 kBq	2·7 μCi
100 μCi	3·7 MBq	1 MBq	27 μCi
200 μCi	7·4 MBq	2 MBq	54 μCi
500 μCi	18·5 MBq	5 MBq	135 μCi
1 mCi	37 MBq	10 MBq	270 μCi
2 mCi	74 MBq	20 MBq	540 μCi
5 mCi	185 MBq	50 MBq	1·35 mCi
10 mCi	370 MBq	100 MBq	2·7 mCi
20 mCi	740 MBq	200 MBq	5·4 mCi
50 mCi	1·85 GBq	500 MBq	13·5 mCi
100 mCi	3·7 GBq	1 GBq	27 mCi
200 mCi	7·4 GBq	10 GBq	270 mCi
500 mCi	18·5 GBq	100 GBq	2·7 Ci
1 Ci	37 GBq	1 TBq	27 Ci
10 Ci	370 GBq	10 TBq	270 Ci
100 Ci	3·7 TBq	100 TBq	2·7 kCi

Table C Exposure conversion

This table is based on the relationship: $1 \text{ R} = 2{\cdot}58 \times 10^{-4} \text{ C kg}^{-1}$

Exposure		Exposure rate	
10^{-6} C kg^{-1}	3·876 mR	10^{-10}C kg^{-1}s^{-1}	1·395 mR h^{-1}
10^{-5} ,,	38·76 mR	10^{-9} ,,	13·95 mR h^{-1}
10^{-4} ,,	387·6 mR	10^{-8} ,,	139·5 mR h^{-1}
10^{-3} ,,	3·876 R	10^{-7} ,,	1·395 R h^{-1}
10^{-2} ,,	38·76 R	10^{-6} ,,	13·95 R h^{-1}
10^{-1} ,,	387·6 R	10^{-5} ,,	139·5 R h^{-1}
1 ,,	3876 R	10^{-4} ,,	1395 R h^{-1}

In addition, 1 gray (Gy) = 100 rad, where 1 Gy = 1 J kg^{-1} and 1 sievert (Sv) = 100 rem, where Sv = Gy × quality factor

Table D Physical constants

Quantity	Value
Avogadro's Number, N_A	*6·02 × 10^{23} mole^{-1}
Velocity of light in a vacuum, c	3·00 × 10^8 m s^{-1}
Permittivity of vacuum, ε_0	8·8 × 10^{-12} F m^{-1}
Permeability of vacuum, μ_0	1·26 × 10^{-6} H m^{-1}
Electron rest mass, m_e	9·11 × 10^{-31} kg
Proton rest mass, m_p	1·672 × 10^{-27} kg
Neutron rest mass, m_n	1·675 × 10^{-27} kg
Planck's constant, h	6·63 × 10^{-34} J s
Electronic charge, e	−1·60 × 10^{-19} C

* Or 6·02 × 10^{26} (kg-mole)$^{-1}$

Table E Important conversion factors

1 atomic mass unit (amu)	= 1·66 × 10^{-27} kg
1 electron volt (eV)	= 1·60 × 10^{-19} J
1 joule (J)	= 6·24 × 10^{18} eV
Electron mass	= 0·511 MeV
Proton mass	= 938 MeV
Neutron mass	= 940 MeV
1 angstrom (Å)	= 0·1 nm

Table F Greek symbols and their common usage

Name	Symbol capital	lowercase	Usage
Alpha	A	α	α-particle (He nucleus)
Beta	B	β	β-particle (electron or positron)
Gamma	Γ	γ	γ-ray; slope of photographic density curve
Delta	Δ	δ	Δx or δx used to indicate change in x
Epsilon	E	ε	
Zeta	Z	ζ	
Eta	H	η	
Theta	Θ	θ	Used to represent an angle
Iota	I	ι	
Kappa	K	κ	
Lambda	Λ	λ	Wavelength; decay constant
Mu	M	μ	Attenuation coefficient
Nu	N	ν	Frequency of electromagnetic radiation
Xi	Ξ	ξ	
Omicron	O	o	
Pi	Π	π	Circumference/diameter of circle; Pair production
Rho	P	ρ	Density of matter
Sigma	Σ	σ	Standard deviation (σ); Summation of terms (Σ)
Tau	T	τ	
Upsilon	Y	υ	
Phi	Φ	φ	Used to represent an angle
Chi	X	χ	
Psi	Ψ	ψ	
Omega	Ω	ω	Symbol for resistance in ohm (Ω)

ANSWERS TO EXERCISES

Exercise 1.1 (a) $1/12$ (b) $1\frac{4}{9}$ (c) 10 (d) $1\frac{1}{60}$
(e) $19/99$ (f) $12 \cdot 5\%$

Exercise 1.2 (a) 4 (b) -6 (c) -36 (d) 39 (e) -28

Exercise 1.3 (a) $-1\frac{1}{7}$ (b) $-11/21$ (c) $4/243$

Exercise 1.4 (a) $3a + 8$ (b) $6x - 6y + 18$ (c) $9a - 26$

Exercise 1.5 (a) $x = 6$ (b) $y = 18$ (c) $q = -18/35$ (d) $I = 5\frac{1}{2}$

Exercise 1.6 (a) $50\,\text{mA}$ (b) $125\,\text{kV}_\text{p}$ (c) $65\,\mu\text{F}$ (d) $0 \cdot 00000055\,\text{m}$

Exercise 1.8 (a) $\sin C = c/b$; $\cos C = a/b$; $\tan C = c/a$
(b) 1 (by Pythagoras)

Exercise 3.2 (b) $0 \cdot 78$ mm (c) 2 mm
(d) (i) field size of $12 \cdot 5$ cm $\times$ 15 cm at 50 cm from focus
(ii) field size of 8 cm $\times$ $9 \cdot 6$ cm at 32 cm from focus
(e) magnification factor of $1 \cdot 2$, giving true object size of 10 cm
(f) (i) $0 \cdot 1$ mm (ii) $0 \cdot 0625$ mm

Exercise 4.1 (a) $21 \cdot 6$ mAs (d) 405 mAs (e) 360 mAs (*Note*: kV_p^2, not kV_p^4)

Exercise 5.1 (b) 4 MBq ($108\,\mu\text{Ci}$) (c) $\lambda = 0 \cdot 5\,\text{s}^{-1}$ decays faster

Exercise 5.3 (c) $8 \times 10^{-7}\,\text{C kg}^{-1}$ (d) (i) 7 (ii) 10 (iii) 13

Exercise 6.1 (a) $0 \cdot 1$ (10%) (b) 6%
(c) 10% error in kV_p means approximately 21% intensity change
(d) 100%, 50%, 10%, 2%, 1%
(e) (i) $36 ; 36$ (ii) $9 ; 10$ (iii) $47 \cdot 7 ; 47$
(f) mean $= 70 \cdot 07$; S.D. $= 0 \cdot 111$; S.E. $= 0 \cdot 035$
2 S.D. limits are $69 \cdot 85$ to $70 \cdot 29$

Exercise 8.1   The body with the smaller specific heat capacity

Exercise 8.2   (a) a good conductor has a high value of k
(b) watt $m^{-1} K^{-1}$

Exercise 9.1   (b) 207·5 volt

Exercise 9.2   (b) 0·05 coulomb in both cases (or 50 mC)
(c) (i) in parallel
     (ii) in series
(d) 20 μF
(f) (i) nil   (ii) nil   (iii) no capacity possible
     (iv) charges on plates 'shorted' together
(g) (i) 480 mC   (ii) 448 mC   (iii) 56 kV
     (iv) 56 kV

Exercise 10.1   (b) 2 metres

Exercise 10.2   (a) (i) nil   (ii) nil   (iii) resistance increased
(b) (i) 70 Ω (ii) $5\frac{5}{7}\Omega$
(c) $I = 0·25$ A; $i_1 = 0·20$ A; $i_2 = 0·05$ A
    $V_1 = 2$ volts; $V_2 = 4$ volts

Exercise 13.1   (a) Into the paper   (b) Out of the paper

Exercise 13.2   (a) mutual repulsion   (b) mutual attraction

Exercise 13.3   (b) (i)   an arc away from the first path
     (ii) deflection in an arc in the opposite sense to the
           electron beam

Exercise 14.1   (a) (i) at 90° to lines of flux, i.e. in or out of the paper
     (ii) at 0° to lines of flux, i.e. to the left or right
(b) (i) clockwise, looking from above
     (ii) anti-clockwise, looking from above

Exercise 15.1   (c) (i) 0·1 A   (ii) 0·1414 A   (iii) zero   (iv) 1 watt
(d) 0·1 A (same as rms value)

Exercise 16.1   (b) 55kV (77·8 kV_p)
(b) 0·2 A (0·19 A, if perfect transformer)

Exercise 16.2   (e) zero (AC required)

Exercise 17.1   (c) (i) 0·5 Ω   (ii) 0·22 Ω   (iii) 0·01 Ω   (iv) 0·001 Ω

Exercise 17.2   (a) 95 kΩ   (b) 80 mV   (c) 2 Ω; 0·67 Ω; 2 kΩ

Exercise 17.3   (a) no deflection of pointer
(b) pointer does not stop on scale
(c) steel is magnetic, and would align itself along the lines of flux

Exercise 17.4   (e)   (i) 0·02 Ω shunt resistor
(ii) 10 kΩ series resistor
(iii) rectification and 0·028Ω shunt resistor (to give f.s.d. for 100mA RMS)

Exercise 21.1   If no PD across tube, no mA will flow even though a filament current is possible

Exercise 23.2   (d) $1·50 \times 10^{-10}$ joule (or 938 MeV)
(e) $1·989 \times 10^{-15}$ joule

Exercise 24.1   (d) (i) 0·124 nm   (ii) 0·025 nm   (iii) $6·2 \times 10^{14}$ m
(e) 0·0124 nm

Exercise 26.2   A '$\beta - \gamma$' decay, where the γ produces internal conversion

Exercise 26.3 Z decreases by 2, and A by 4

Exercise 27.1   (b) 4   (c) 4 mAs

Exercise 33.1   200 cases

Exercise 34.1   3·5 cm

Appendix V   (a) (i) 10   (ii) 30   (iii) 80   (iv) 100   (v) 300
(b) 10%; 3·3%; 1·25%; 1%; 0·3%
(c) 40 000

Index